Food & Your Health

Selected Articles from Consumers' Research Magazine

Beatrice Trum Hunter

Food Editor, *Consumers' Research Magazine*

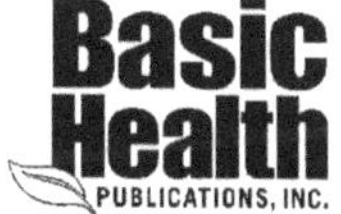

The information contained in this book is based upon the research and personal and professional experiences of the author. It is not intended as a substitute for consulting with your physician or other healthcare provider. Any attempt to diagnose and treat an illness should be done under the direction of a healthcare professional.

The publisher does not advocate the use of any particular healthcare protocol but believes the information in this book should be available to the public. The publisher and author are not responsible for any adverse effects or consequences resulting from the use of the suggestions, preparations, or procedures discussed in this book. Should the reader have any questions concerning the appropriateness of any procedures or preparations mentioned, the author and the publisher strongly suggest consulting a professional healthcare advisor.

Basic Health Publications, Inc.
An imprint of Turner Publishing Company
Nashville, Tennessee | www.turnerbookstore.com

Editor: Cheryl Hirsch • Typesetter: Gary A. Rosenberg
Series Cover Designer: Mike Stromberg

Library of Congress Cataloging-in-Publication Data

Hunter, Beatrice Trum.
Food and your health / Beatrice Trum Hunter.
p. cm.
Includes bibliographical references and index.
ISBN 978-1-59120-032-1 (Pbk.)
ISBN 978-1-68162-720-5 (Hardcover)

1. Nutrition. 2. Health. 3. Food. I. Title.

RA784.H795 2003 2003007766
613.2—dc21

CONTENTS

Preface, v

1. Diet and Health: Making Wise Food Choices, 1
2. Special Food and Health Concerns throughout Life, 31
3. Form and Function: The Body Knows Best, 95
4. Basic Foods and Beverages with "New and Improved" Uses, 134
5. Sugar: Desired but Undesirable, 170
6. Fats and Oils: What You Should Know, 191
7. Dispelling Some Popular Health Myths, 213
8. Food Additives and Your Health, 261
9. Avoiding Foodborne Illnesses, 312
10. Contaminants in Our Food, 361
11. Agricultural Practices That Affect Our Food and Health, 388

Index, 428

About the Author, 439

Dedicated to the memory of
Nathan and An Keats,
and F.J. Schlink

PREFACE

Since the inception of *Consumers' Research Magazine* in 1928, its readers have been given reliable and useful information regarding the subjects of food and nutrition, and their relationship to health. These important topics are discussed in each issue, along with other topics affecting consumers.

Characteristically, much of the food and nutrition information has been given far in advance of official concern or public awareness. For example, the problems of the food-borne illness inflicted by *E. coli* 0157:H7 were discussed in May 1991—several years prior to the publicized incident in a fast food restaurant that affected many children. Information on the now-banned pesticide, Alar, was printed as early as November 1985, and the value of homocysteine as a biomarker for health problems, as early as May 1996. Readers had been warned about the dangers of pesticide residues in foods decades before the publication of *Silent Spring*, and had been alerted to the problems of heavy metal poisonings from lead, cadmium, and mercury, many years prior to official acknowledgments that these substances were public health problems. *Consumers' Research Magazine* was in the forefront in exposures of blatant advertisements and nutritional shortcomings of many highly sugared breakfast cereals, long before congressional hearings were called on this subject.

In selecting articles for the present series, it was apparent that some of the topics are still in advance of official policy or public understanding. For example, "The Downside of Soy" offers information contrary to mainstream claims. In the future, however, the minority view expressed will be validated and acknowledged by health professionals and understood by the general public.

From the beginning, Consumers' Research has attempted to make consumers aware of the importance of making wise choices, on the basis of sound information. Also, the organization has pointed out the problems, pitfalls, and need for appropriate actions by official agencies making public policy:

> ". . . let your voice be heard loudly and often, in protest against the indifference, ignorance, and avarice responsible for the uncontrolled adulteration and misrepresentation of foods, drugs, and cosmetics. In this adulteration and misrepresentation lurks a menace to your health that ought no longer be tolerated."

Lest the reader think that this advice came out of the burgeoning consumer movement of the 1960s, and 1970s, be assured that it was written far earlier. It appeared in 1933, in *100,000,000 Guinea Pigs* (Vanguard Press), co-authored by F.J. [Frederick John] Schlink, founder and president of Consumers' Research, Inc. and publisher of *Consumers' Research Magazine.* This best-selling book exposed the dangers in everyday foods, drugs, and cosmetics. The book was based on information from the extensive files of the organization. The work shocked many individuals into an awareness of many hazards in consumer goods, and was an important influence leading to congressional hearings and strengthening of federal and state regulations for food, drug, and cosmetic safety.

The files of Consumers' Research continued to be utilized for programs of public enlightenment, with the issuance of both periodicals and books. In 1934, *Skin Deep* (Vanguard Press) exposed dangerous substances used in cosmetics. The book was written by a staff member, M.C. Phillips (Mary Catherine Phillips, wife of F.J. Schlink). *Eat, Drink, and Be Wary* (Covici, Friede, Inc.), by F.J. Schlink, published in 1935, was another hard-hitting exposé of what was happening to the food supply.

Consumers' Research, Inc. is a unique organization. It has been in the forefront of the consumer movement. Its sole purpose remains to serve the ultimate consumer. Its various activities center around the needs of its subscribers, to whom it dedicates its facilities, special knowledge, and skills. The organization accepts no commercial advertisements, nor contributions from industry, manufacturers, and dealers. Nor does it receive any funding from governmental sources. It is a non-profit organization.

Consumers' Research offered to its readership in 1971 a philosophy of lasting value:

> "The right choice of specific foods and types of foods, makes, for millions of persons, the difference between health and vigor on the one hand, and a lack of energy and resistance to disease on the other. A good diet is not merely a matter of having money to spend. Deficient nutrition is common among people who can buy whatever foods they choose, but make the wrong choices, for lack of knowledge. Like millions of teenagers, these people tend to 'follow the crowd' to hot dogs, French fries, cakes, candy, soft drinks, and ice cream, unaware of what they are missing.
>
> "The path to good eating and good health is not an easy or simple one . . . Partly, this is because of the

abundance of choices available under modern industry's efficiency in manufacture and distribution. Partly, it is because tradition no longer plays an important part in choices of basic foods for the table."

Chapter 1

Diet and Health: Making Wise Food Choices

AMERICANS' EATING HABITS: POOR, AND GETTING POORER

"In America, today, poor diets are typically too high in calories and fats, and too low in fruits and vegetables—problems associated with certain chronic diseases and obesity."

These words, in the introductory remarks of a report issued by the U.S. Department of Agriculture's (USDA) Economic Research Service (ERS), depict (long-term) changes in American eating habits, and the consequences resulting from the changes. The report is one in a series of several critical reports issued by ERS on the status of the current American diet, and the implications. Other reports focus on the growing trend of eating away from home, and its impact on the decline of quality in the American diet; the current diet of American children; and an assessment of actual food consumption by Americans, compared with official recommendations.

These reports, examined in toto, confirm and give added weight to concerns already expressed by many nutritionists, dietitians, health practitioners, and public health officials. All groups have reported findings, based on clinical studies, that current American eating habits are poor, and apt to get poorer, due to changes in eating patterns.

The reports serve as a wake-up call. They deserve study and discussion. These are some of the highlights:

"More Americans than ever are overweight, fiber consumption is low, and snack foods are as popular as ever. . . . Americans are eating more and exercising less. . . . Consumers eat three meals a day, quench their thirst with carbonated beverages, and constantly nibble on snacks. Is it any wonder that by the end of the day few of us know how many calories we have ingested, let alone our fat intake? . . . Clearly, counting grams of fat is more difficult for food purchased from the local hamburger joint, a sidewalk vendor, or a supermarket deli [than from home-prepared foods] . . ."

Eating Away from Home. The frequency of eating away from home rose by more than two-thirds over two decades, from 16 percent of all meals and snacks in 1977–78 to 27 percent by 1995 (the latest year examined in the report). It is anticipated that the trend will continue. Regarding the health consequences of this trend, ERS found that foods prepared and eaten at home generally contain less fat and less saturated fat, but more fiber, calcium, and iron, than foods eaten away from home. The report notes that, in recent years, the nutritional content of foods eaten at home had improved more than those eaten away from home.

"American consumers are inching ever closer to a dining watershed," the report notes. "The continued growing popularity of eating away from home has brought Americans to the verge of spending as much on food away from home as they do on food prepared at home." In 1970, 34 percent of the food dollars was spent on food away from home; today, it has risen to 46 percent. If a baseline had been chosen for a time period prior to 1970, the percentage would have been extremely low.

The consequences of this trend are especially important with American children. A USDA survey found that 88 percent of children aged six to eighteen have poor diets. An ERS report raised questions about nutrient intake by children eating more and more of their meals away from home. This trend indicates a lessening of control over what children eat, how the food is prepared, and the nutrient quality of the diet. For example, broccoli and kale are not likely to be on menus where children choose to eat. The potatoes are likely to be deep-fried, not baked. White potatoes will be available, but sweet potatoes are not apt to be on the menu. The limited food offerings probably will be high in fat, low in essential nutrients such as calcium and iron and contain added sugars and salt.

Recommended vs. Actual Food Consumption. Perhaps the most discouraging news of all is contained in ERS's report: *A Dietary Assessment of the U.S. Food Supply*. The study compares actual food consumption with official recommendations. Many shortcomings in the American diet are apparent. The two that are the most discouraging concern the underconsumption of vegetables and fruits, and the overconsumption of added sugars.

The official recommendation for vegetable intake is to eat nearly four servings of dark-green leafy and deep-yellow vegetables, starchy ones including beans, and other vegetables daily. In reality, an average of only a half serving of one vegetable is actually eaten. (A half serving is equivalent to about one-quarter cup of cooked vegetables, one-quarter of a baked potato, or about five French fried potatoes—a very scant amount.) Only five vegetables, out of a choice of some eighty that are available in food stores, account for half of all the vegetables chosen. Of those, poor choices are made. Nutrient-low head lettuce is popular, not the dark-green, nutrient-rich greens. The starchy vegetables are weighted heavily with white potatoes, especially in frozen, fried, and chipped forms, rather than baked or boiled. Intake of beans, as well as other vegetables, is far below the official recommendation. Also, the popularity of only five vegetables suggests that Americans are not having sufficient variety in their daily intake of vegetables. Yet variety is one of the basic concepts of good nutrition, and helps to contribute many nutrients from different sources.

Fruit consumption, too, falls far short of recommendations. The average American consumes less than half of the modest minimum recommendation, and consumes only 1.3 servings daily of fruits in various forms.

The shortfalls of vegetable and fruit consumption by many Americans are particularly worrisome. A wealth of scientific studies affirm that the consumption of many vegetables and fruits lowers the risks of various chronic diseases, including some types of cancers.

Added Sugars. The official recommendation is to use added sugars sparingly or moderately. A suggested upper limit for daily consumption of added sugars is twelve teaspoons. In reality, the food supply provides an average of thirty-two teaspoons of caloric sweeteners (dry weight)—nearly three times the recommended level. According to the ERS report, this amount is equivalent to the amount found in about three and one-half bottles of twelve-ounce regular soft drinks per person daily.

Sweeteners are added to processed products such as baked goods, pre-sweetened cereals, soft drinks, and candies, as well as to numerous other food products in which one does not expect to find added sugar. According to the USDA, "in a sense, sugar is the number one food additive. It turns up in some unlikely places, such as pizza, bread, hot dogs, boxed mixed rice, soup, crackers, spaghetti sauce, lunch meat, canned vegetables, fruit drinks, flavored yogurt, ketchup, salad dressing, mayonnaise, and some peanut butter."

In another USDA publication, *Sugar and Sweetener: Situation and Outlook Yearbook* (May 1999) the most recent figure for the average American's annual consumption of sugar is a whopping 156.4 pounds. The yearly consumption of added sugars translates to two-fifths of a pound daily (fifty-three teaspoons)—far more than is advised. The USDA's Food Guide Pyramid suggests that people who consume a daily diet of 1,600 calories restrict added sugar intake to six teaspoons daily; 2,000 calories, ten teaspoons; 2,200 calories, twelve teaspoons; and 2,800 calories, eighteen teaspoons.

Some people need to limit sugar intake due to health problems (for example, diabetes), and others choose to restrict sugar intake due to nutritional concerns. Therefore, there must be some people who consume more sugar annually than the average 156.4 pounds.

Each year, the amount of sugar consumed keeps increasing. The steep rise in sugar consumption since the mid 1980s coincides with the large increased consumption of carbonated soft drinks—from twenty-eight gallons per person annually in 1986 to forty-one gallons in 1997. More than one-fifth of all added sugars in the present American diet are in carbonated soft drinks. The USDA's Continuing Survey of Food Intake by individuals found that nearly 25 percent of children aged five years or younger drink carbonated soda on a regular basis.

The human body may not distinguish between naturally occurring sugars present in foods (such as fruits) and sugars added to food and beverage products. But the naturally occurring sugars are accompanied by nutrients that help metabolize them; the added sugars supply calories, but few nutrients, if any.

Official dietary guidelines recommend limiting foods and beverages with high levels of added sugars. Frequently, such foods and beverages replace nutrient-rich foods, such as vegetables, fruits, and whole grains.

The ERS report notes that consumers have difficulty in moderating their intake of added sugars. Although they can restrict the amounts they choose to add to foods and beverages, they cannot control the amounts added by others in food and beverage manufacture. Although the current food labels require manufacturers to disclose total sugar contents of foods and beverages, the label does not distinguish between total sugar content and added sugar content. This lack of information makes it difficult for consumers to know how much added sugar they are consuming, and whether the total amount is within the suggested limit for added sugar.

More Food, More Calories, Larger Portions. All food supply measurements suggest that Americans are consuming more food, and several hundred more calories per person daily, than Americans did a half-century ago. In addition, portion sizes are larger. These trends relate to increased obesity and its associated health problems. These are some findings by the USDA.

The aggregate food supply in 1994—the latest year for which nutrient data from the USDA's Center for Nutrition Policy and Promotion are available—provided 3,800 calories per person daily. This amount is 500 calories more than the 1983 level, and 800 calories more than the record low in the mid-1950s. Some calories are lost to spoilage, plate waste, cooking, and other factors, so the ERS's estimates of the current caloric intake probably is somewhat lower than the 3,800 calories—just below 2,700 calories, However, even with this adjustment, ERS data suggest that the average daily caloric intake increased 14.7 percent between 1984 and the present.

Larger portion size is one aspect in the dietary dilemma. In the mid-1950s, the typical hamburger offered by a fast-food outlet consisted of a little more than one ounce of cooked meat. Currently, it consists of up to six ounces. This is the age of the forty-ounce restaurant served steak, the fast-food "supersized" meal, the "Big Foot," one-foot-by-two-foot slab of pizza, "all you can eat" fish fries, and limitless repeats at buffets. In the mid-1950s, the soda serving was eight ounces; currently, it is thirty-two to sixty-four ounces. A muffin was less than one- and one-half ounces; currently, five to eight ounces. Similarly, serving sizes have increased exponentially for portions of items such as ice cream, coffee, and beer. The larger servings seem to be associated with the "Good Life." Yet, the current concept by many Americans of serving sizes far exceeds those that are recommended by the USDA's Food Guide Pyramid.

In a recent study, Brian Wansink, Ph.D. and associates at the University of Illinois found that food products packaged in large containers appear to be consumed at greater rates than those in small packages. Formerly, a theater serving of popcorn was a three cup measure. Now, a sixteen cup measure is contained in the "medium" size container. Wansink and his colleagues found that moviegoers, given extra-large containers of popcorn, ate 44 percent more than people who were handed popcorn in slightly smaller containers. The extra-large size added about 120 extra calories to the intake. Wansink concluded: "If you have it, you'll eat it." Wansink found that consumers use more from larger packages because the product is perceived as cheaper. In addition to the findings with popcorn, Wansink had similar results with spaghetti, bottled water, and cooking oils. "People use more from larger sizes—typically between 9 and 36 percent more because they perceive the per-unit cost is cheaper in the larger size."

The largest American manufacturer of restaurant dinnerware, Homer Laughlin China Company, reports that the demand for big plates and bowls has increased greatly. The best sellers are big, deep bowls for pasta. Some are so large that they hold up to forty ounces for one serving of pasta (two and one-half pounds of cooked food).

Restaurant surveys confirm this trend. According to Alan Ripp, who conducted a restaurant survey for Zagat's restaurant guide: "In the eighties there were mini-portions. Now there are eye-splitting mega-portions."

Packaged foods now list serving sizes, but the sizes do not necessarily match those recommended in the Food Guide Pyramid. A typical serving of pasta is two cups, which comes to about four servings in the pyramid. A New York-style bagel typically is about four ounces, or about four servings in the pyramid. And a two-ounce hamburger bun is two servings.

As caloric intake levels have risen, along with more food intake, physical activity levels have appeared to decline for the majority of Americans. According to the Centers for Disease Control and Prevention (CDC), more than 60 percent of American adults are not physically active on a regular basis; and 25 percent of American adults are not active at all. Increasing physical activity is a "formidable public health challenge in a technologically advanced society," according to the CDC. "Few occupations today require significant physical activity, and most people use motorized transportation to get to work and to perform routine errands and tasks. Even leisure is increasingly filled with sedentary behaviors, such as watching television, 'surfing' the Internet, and playing video games."

The benefits of good nutrition are not observed immediately, or they are elusive. Some people may forestall practicing good nutrition. In the short run, they may prefer convenience foods over more healthful alternatives.

A variety of factors has led to changes in our food consumption patterns in the past half century. Among them are changes in relative prices and increases in real disposable income. Additional contributing factors include the development and expansion of food advertisement and new food product innovations (especially more convenient ones) that shift consumption to growth in the away-from-home food markets.

Sociodemographic trends, too, influence changes in food choices, according to the USDA. These include smaller households, more two-earner households, more single-parent households, an aging population, and increased ethnic diversity.

Being aware of the problems of too much food, too many calories, and too large portions is the first step in addressing the dietary dilemma. Wise food selections, smaller portions, and physical activity need to be learned and practiced at all ages.

Effects of Eating Habits. *America's Eating Habits* notes that, often, the benefits of good nutrition are not observed immediately, or they are elusive. Some people may forestall practicing good nutrition. In the short run, they may prefer convenience foods over more healthful alternatives. In the long run, taste considerations may prevail. For many, healthy eating is not worth what some people might perceive as an effort and a sacrifice. Obviously, convincing people about long-range benefits of good nutrition is made more difficult if immediate gratification is given high priority.

The official dietary recommendations, based on time-honored basic concepts as well as solid scientific evidence, face overwhelming obstacles for implementation. The ERS report notes: "With a bewildering array of food items to select from, research indicates that the average consumer takes only twelve seconds to make a brand selection. Of course, Madison Avenue spends $11 billion [annually] in advertising to help us here. Not surprisingly, most of these advertising dollars promote prepared and convenience foods, snacks, and alcoholic beverages. By contrast, the federal government spends a mere $350 million annually to promote healthy eating."

USDA Reports

For readers who are interested to obtain further details of the critical findings about various aspects of the current American diet, these are important reports:

- *America's Eating Habits, Changes & Consequences,* edited by Elizabeth Frazao. USDA, ERS, Agriculture Information Bulletin Number 750, issued 1999.
- *Away-From-Home Foods Increasingly Important to Quality of American Diet.* BiingHwan Lin, Joanne Guthrie, and Elizabeth Frazao. USDA, ERS, Agriculture Information Bulletin Number 749, issued January 1999.
- *A Dietary Assessment of the U.S. Food Supply: Comparing Per Capita Food Consumption With Food Guide Pyramid Serving Recommendations.* Linda Scott Kantor USDA, ERS, Agricultural Economic Report Number 772, issued December 1998.
- *The Diets of America's Children: Influences of Dining Out, Household Characteristics, and Nutrition Knowledge.* Biing-

MODERN FOOD PROCESSING: NUTRITIONAL SHORTCHANGES

"Today, Western man has revolutionized the production, storage and distribution of his food. He superheats it, freezes it, cans it, processes it, extracts it and divides it . . . He also refines it . . . His diet is unbalanced," warned Henry A. Schroeder, M.D., a world authority on trace minerals. How has our present diet become imbalanced to the point that it has been termed a "national disaster" by a prominent researcher?

Growing and Harvesting. Present practices in food pro-

Hwan Lin, Joanne Guthrie, and James R. Blaylock. USDA, ERS, Agricultural Economic Report Number 748, issued December 1996.

- *U.S. Trends in Eating Away From Home, 1982–1989: A Survey of Eating Occasions, Type of Foodservice Establishment, and Kind of Food.* Jesus C. Dumagan and John W. Hackett. USDA, ERS, Statistical Bulletin Number 926, issued December 1995.
- "Annual Spotlight on the U.S. Food System, 1999," *Food Review,* ERS, USDA September/December 1999.

For information about these reports, contact USDA, Economic Research Service, 1800 M Street NW, Washington, D.C. 20036-5831, or go to *www.econ.ag.gov.* To order the reports, call (800) 999-6779.

For additional information about ERS publications, databases, and other products, both paper and electronic, the ERS Home page on the Internet is at *www.econ.ag.gov.*

duction have drastically altered nutritional values in our food supply. For example, animals are routinely fed, not with natural feedstuffs, but with special types of feedstuffs known as "concentrates." Such feeding results in meat that contains smaller amounts of the desirable unsaturated fatty acids; in some instances, it adds antagonistic fatty acids that increase our dietary need for the essential polyunsaturated ones.

A nutritionist comments: "In his eagerness to produce more kernels per row, more rows per ear, and more ears per stalk, the plant breeder has sacrificed nutrient content. In his desire to produce lovelier apples, sweeter oranges, blander vegetables, ship resistant foods, he has often produced varieties which are less nutritious." An analysis of common food crops grown in the United States compared to similar ones grown in Mexico and Central America showed that the Latin American varieties usually had higher contents of nutrients. Another study showed that the average amount of ascorbic acid (vitamin C) per 100 grams (g) of orange juice was 61 milligrams (mg) from California Navels; 49 mg for California Valencias; and 37 mg from Florida Valencias. In several thousand samples of oranges, the ascorbic acid content ranged from 20 mg per g of juice to more than 80 mg, a fourfold difference.

The mineral content in common vegetables may vary over a wide range. The late Dr. Firman E. Bear of Rutgers University analyzed crops and found that some contained nearly seventy times more of a particular mineral than others; with trace minerals, he found as great a variation as two thousand to one.

Soil may be a factor in nutrient content. In certain regions, the soil may be deficient in nutrients. Animals raised for food production on such soils, or crops grown on such soils, may reflect such deficiency.

Present practices in harvesting, shipping, and storing crops can lessen their content of nutrients. A few examples will illustrate the point. Some crops, picked prematurely and shipped unripe, never develop their full potential in nutrients or in flavor. It was found that postponing the date of harvest for early grown carrots could develop greater nutritive value. Because falling temperature favors the formation of the protein and unsaturated fatty acids in soybeans, late harvesting of this crop can increase its nutritional content. Tomatoes grown in greenhouses during the wintertime may have only half the amount of ascorbic acid of tomatoes that are vine-ripened and grown outdoors in sunlight.

Storing. Prolonged storage, especially under conditions of high temperature and humidity, results in a progressive deterioration of the protein value of foods. Canned vegetables, stored at 65°F, lost 15 percent of thiamine (vitamin B_1) within a year; with storage at a higher temperature, the loss was more severe. The thiamine in canned meat was reduced by 30 percent when the meat was stored for six months at 70°F. Pyridoxine (vitamin B_6) was lost in appreciable amounts from Army C Rations stored at 100°F for twenty months. Commercial chilled orange juice lost 57 percent of the ascorbic acid that was present in the fresh orange juice. Vitamin E deteriorated in stored food, even when the food was frozen.

Refining. Drastic nutritional losses result when food is refined, overprocessed, or modified. About 80 percent or more of our calories presently come from flour and cereal products, sugar, potatoes, and fats, but most of the vitamins and minerals also present in them are removed or destroyed when these foods undergo typical modern processing. It has long been recognized that a large percentage of vitamins, minerals, and trace minerals are lost in the milling of flour and the polishing of rice.

Fortifying. The "enrichment" program was launched as an attempt to restore some of the lost nutrients. However, the shortcomings of this program become apparent upon close analysis. Although a number of vital nutrients are removed in the milling, only relatively few are restored in enrichment. It is well established that changing the level of one nutrient affects the levels of other nutrients intimately associated with it. Unless a proper balance is maintained, serious deficiencies and excesses can result. For example, cadmium competes with and displaces zinc in human metabolic processes. Any appreciable content of cadmium is hazardous to human health. In whole wheat, the ratio between cadmium and zinc is 1:120, with the presence of zinc opposing or buffering the potentially harmful effects of cadmium. In refined flour, much of the zinc, an essential trace element, is lost. The altered ratio between cadmium and zinc becomes 1:20. The buffering action of the zinc is decreased and the threat of excessive cadmium intake is increased sixfold.

Drastic nutritional losses occur when food is refined, overprocessed, or modified. About 80 percent or more of our calories presently come from flour and cereal products, sugar, potatoes, and fats, but most of the vitamins and minerals also present in them are removed or destroyed when these foods undergo typical modern processing.

Food processing frequently alters such subtle balances. This is demonstrated again, in the enrichment program. Although iron is restored to the flour and cereal, copper is not restored. Yet copper is needed for utilization of the iron. The choice of an iron preparation used by the baking industry may be made because of some desirable baking or storing feature, rather than nutritional suitability. There is no assurance that the form of iron chosen is one that will be well assimilated by the body.

Infant feeding formulas made with partially skimmed cow's milk need to be supplemented with tocopherol (vitamin E) in order to balance the ratio of tocopherol with polyunsaturated fatty acids, to approximate the ratio found in breast milk.

Packaging. Mineral balances found in raw produce undergo extreme alterations in canning. As an illustration, examine sodium and potassium, two "competing" minerals. The processing of canned peas lowers the potassium found in raw peas by 66 percent; at the same time, sodium is increased by 1,400 percent. Other canned produce undergoes similar alterations. Potassium decreases in typical canned foods: 47 percent in spinach; 51 percent in tomatoes; 60 percent in green beans; and 65 percent in carrots. At the same time, sodium increases in canned foods in an extraordinary way: over 350 percent in spinach; 370 percent in carrots; 450 percent in tomatoes; and over 45,000 percent in green beans.

This sodium load, already heavy, is further increased by the food processors, who find that the use of salt is helpful for their purposes. It can mask the unpleasant flavor of odorous foods. It inhibits the growth of molds and bacteria. It can bleach and prevent discoloration, and thus "improves" food color. It is an aid for peeling, sorting, and floating, in food processing, and it is useful in the drying and freezing of foods. Still more sodium is added to processed foods in the use of many chemical food additives that are sodium-containing compounds (*sodium* nitrite, mono*sodium* glutamate, *sodium* propionate, *sodium* bisulfite, *sodium* phosphate, etc.).

Certain practices in processing of foods rob foods of essential metals, while other practices may contaminate foods with undesirable ones. Our iron intake is reduced by improved food packaging that reduces contamination by the iron in "dust." Food processors may remove iron particles magnetically or use chemical agents to bind the iron and so inactivate it. Canners, who try to reduce the pitting and "detinning" of cans or who attempt to preserve the integrity of the enamel coating, seek techniques to avoid even slight iron contamination of foods. On the other hand, undesirable amounts of certain other metals may contaminate foods from modern processing methods. These hazards may result from metals present in the tinplate, solder sealing, or lacquer linings used for the canning of foods, as well as traces from machinery, cooking vats, from steam used in heat processing, or cutting tools. Contamination may result from the interaction of constituents in food and packaging, or from water, which may contain contaminants present in the source or derived from the piping. Cadmium may be in tin or aluminum cans, from the recycling of metals from cars and airplanes.

Extraction. Nutritional losses result when food is divided into its components by refinement or extraction. When milk is separated from the cream, some of the trace elements (chromium, manganese, cobalt, copper, and molybdenum) remain in the cream and butter, while the magnesium and zinc remain in the skim milk. The minerals in the butter are needed for proper digestion of the skim milk. The refining of raw cane sugar into white sugar removes most of the trace elements (chromium, manganese, cobalt, copper, zinc, and magnesium), which are necessary for the body to metabolize the sugar properly. When lard is rendered from pork, the lard is low in the essential elements magnesium, zinc, and molybdenum.

Hydrogenation. The molecular modification of oils by "hydrogenation" in modern food processing changes some of the desirable fatty acids to less desirable ones, and some are converted into unnatural forms. The new ones do not act in the body in the same way as the natural ones; their presence has been found to be harmful to health. Hydrogenated fats keep far better than natural oils and fats. Because of this, manufacturers use hydrogenated fats in many processed foods, in margarine, and in shortening.

Reconstitution. Many convenience foods, made possible by modern processing techniques, are prepared under severe conditions of temperature, pressure, and agitation that severely deplete the foods of their original nutrients. For this reason they are "fortified" with various vitamins and minerals. Raw potatoes, harvested in October of one year, lost 91 percent of their ascorbic acid after having been processed as reconstituted flakes in May of the following year. The loss of ascorbic acid in dehydrated potatoes is so severe that the U.S. Department of Agriculture requires fortification of the processed potatoes it purchases. As much as 90 percent of vitamin E may be lost in the flaking, shredding, and puffing of grain in the manufacture of ready-to-eat cereals. Substantial amounts of the same vitamin are lost during the processing of cereal for consumption by infants, and recommendations were made to fortify such cereals.

As yet unknown but essential nutrients doubtless exist in foods, but may be lost in food processing. It is most likely that by eating sufficient quantities of whole foods as close to their natural state as possible and that provide adequate amounts of known nutrients, one will be obtaining the needed amounts of unknown essential nutrients, too. Some formerly unidentified substances such as phytochemicals (substances in plants) have been found capable of counteracting the effects of toxic agents, while others appear to be growth promoters or serve in ways that contribute to good health. Although "nonessential" food nutrients are not generally included in food tables found in government pamphlets and textbooks on diet and nutrition, there is growing recognition of their critical importance in determining the biological effects and health-and-growth-promoting values of food.

Food Additives and Pesticide Residues. An area of concern that presently is largely unexplored concerns the nutritional losses incurred from the use of food additives and the presence of pesticide residues. To date, scant attention has been devoted to the potentially hazardous nature of these substances. Many of them are known to be vitamin antagonists and destroyers of enzymes essential for good health.

Food Preparation. Every phase of modern food processing adds to the sum total of nutrient losses. Besides, additional losses will occur in the home, with the storing, peeling, trimming, cleaning, cutting, and cooking of food.

Where does all this leave the consuming public? We should recognize that although many popular food products, both fresh and processed, appear to be attractive and convenient, they may be seriously deficient in nutrients. Presently, perhaps more than ever before, it is imperative to exercise great care in our day-to-day food selections and methods of preparation. The use of highly processed foods needs to be strictly limited, or better yet, eliminated, so far as practicable. Choices, so far as possible, should be made from basic foods, close to their natural state. Such foods offer the best possibilities for obtaining adequate amounts of nutrients. This is a task that demands careful attention of every homemaker, institutional chef, dietitian, and restaurant owner.

OUR NARROWING FOOD BASE: A PERILOUS TREND

In winter, consumers in our northern states can enjoy fresh strawberries. Ice-packed ocean fish can be bought year round by land-locked Americans. Among many imports, Hawaiian pineapple, Icelandic fish, New Zealand lamb, and the Central American banana are commonly available in food stores throughout the country. This bounteous diversity of food has been made possible through a complex network of suppliers and transportation. While the critical issue of energy use makes it important to evaluate this food delivery system, we need to appreciate the fact that the system does offer certain safeguards.

Essential nutrients are likely to be provided in consuming foods grown or raised in different localities with soils of varied composition. Food variety is strongly protective of health. Crops grown on lime-leached soils may be marginally or seriously depleted of calcium. Livestock and humans feeding exclusively on such foods may also develop the deficiency.

If our food choices were limited mainly to foods in the nightshade family, such as tomato, potato, and eggplant, we could be consuming undesirably high levels of substances that interfere with enzymes used to transport nerve impulses. Excessive amounts of certain vegetables such as broccoli and Brussels sprouts, can cause goiter.

Currently, safeguards provided by variety in foods we eat are being weakened by various trends in the food system. Food processing is responsible for narrowing the food base. Instead of real variety from traditional foods, we are being offered many manufactured products that are different in appearance, but are made from a few basic ingredients such as cereal grains, soybean, or cottonseed. Careful label reading shows that, despite appearances, many formulated foods have the same ingredients and differ merely in flavor, color, or consistency. For example, hydrogenated coconut oil may be a main ingredient in such diverse foods as nondairy creamer, imitation cheese, margarine, imitation nuts, and imitation chocolate.

Food stores offer a dazzling assortment of boxed ready-to-eat cereals. The same few cereal grains are the basic ingredients of all these products. Frequently, there is a multiplicity of flavors and other forms of brand proliferation of the same food product, while there is no real diversity. A snack product, for example, boxed separately with almond, caramel, and raisin flavors, is essentially the same product. This technique gains in-store attention but does not offer real variety to the consumer.

Soybean. The soybean appears in many guises, as flour, grits, bran, kernels, oil, margarine, lecithin, isolates (protein fraction), and textured vegetable protein (TVP), the typical ingredient of imitation meats termed "analogs." The average supermarket now sells hundreds of items based on soy protein. Food processors favor its use for many reasons. When soy is used as a meat extender or replacer, soy greatly reduces the ingredient costs. The soy ingredient can absorb and hold moisture and emulsify fat; these properties reduce shrinkage of meat particles in ground meats. Enzyme-treated soy albumin acts as a whipping and foaming agent; in this way it serves as a low cost egg-white replacer. Powdered soy albumin also reduces the cost of egg and oil as ingredients in salad dressing, and substantially reduces formula costs as a partial or total substitute for milk protein. Use of the soybean instead of the traditional ingredients not only narrows the food base, but offers lower nutritional values.

Many "engineered foods" such as imitation meats, poultry, fish, and even "mushroom" slices are made from a soybean base. Soy is a main ingredient in many infant foods and baby formulas, processed meats and fish, pastas and baked goods, snack foods, ice cream, nondairy products, sauces, and gravies.

The first large-scale introduction of the soybean in the American diet occurred in 1973, at a time of rising meat prices. A soy extender was combined with chopped beef. Success was short-lived. When, by 1974, the price-differential between the regular and extended meat dropped to the point that use of the extender was no longer attractive, most shoppers stopped buying the ground beef with extender. Food serving institutions, however, continued to increase their use of soy extenders, and ultimately as a total replacer of meat. One survey showed that from 1971 to 1976, textured vegetable protein was used by 64 percent of schools, 26 percent of nursing homes, 22 percent of hospitals, 10 percent of full-service restaurants, and 17 percent of fast-food restaurants.

At present, a blend of 20 percent hydrated soy (moist form) and 80 percent frozen ground beef is permitted in the federally subsidized school lunch program. The Department of Defense has approved the same ratio for feeding military personnel. Foods such as tofu (bean curd), are used in the school lunch program. Such cost-saving efforts ignore long-term nutritional deficiencies.

More than a hundred new tofu factories were opened in the United States between 1977 and 1981. Soy delis, a new breed of fast-food outlets, serving and catering to persons wanting take-out soy foods, feature such items as tofu and tempeh burgers, sloppy joes, cutlets, and club sandwiches; soy shakes, yogurts, and ice creams; tofu dressings and dips; and strawberry tofu cheesecakes.

Soy also enters the food supply indirectly. It has long been used in animal feed. A more reprehensible practice is to pump soy isolates into some whole cuts of fresh and cured meats by injection and massage. This treatment, which is not indicated on meat labels, should be regarded as an economic cheat. The shopper pays for inexpensive and nutritionally deficient soy at expensive meat prices. Also, in such treated meats, soy is a hidden allergen for many persons who need to avoid it. Because of the extensive use of soy, it has become a major allergen.

Cottonseed. Extension of the use of cottonseed in food products is also narrowing our food base. Defatted, glandless cottonseed flour is used in cereals and many bakery products, in pastas, in snack foods, gravies and sauces, puddings and whipped toppings, and soft ice creams. Cottonseed can be "texturized" in extrusion machinery and it can replace soybean flour as a meat extender. Further processed into concentrates, it has been suggested for use in certain carbonated and citrus beverages, in order to add protein to drinks that are poor in nutrients. Processes have already been developed to produce edible cottonseed kernels. Simulated nut products contain the dehulled portion of the cotton plant and whole kernels have been made into clustered candies. A "butter" has been made from roasted kernels, and a novelty product, said to resemble black-eyed peas, has been made from cottonseed kernels. As with soybeans, processors are exploiting cottonseed to produce a variety of manufactured food products that may look different, yet fail to offer real, needed variety.

Restricted Menus. Restaurant practices, too, make major contributions to a narrowing food base. Fast-food places with extremely limited menu selections restrict the choices of nutritionally valuable edibles. Such food is consumed daily by many children, not only on fast-food premises but at school cafeterias ranging from the elementary school grades through universities, and even at some children's hospitals and museum restaurants. Coffee shops, drugstores, pancake, crepe or doughnut eateries, and vending machines limit choices.

Even in full-service restaurants, certain menu restrictions are developing. For example, increasingly, restaurants depend on "fish farms" to supply their fish. Fewer species are available on menus. Most restaurant-served trout and salmon are raised at fish farms, which also produce catfish and shrimp.

Variety, balance, and moderation must remain valid criteria for good nutrition. Factors that interfere with a broad base of food sources make it difficult to achieve good nutrition and its accompanying benefits for health. . . . It is more important than ever to choose from a variety of basic foods (such as meat, fish, poultry, eggs, fruits, and vegetables) coming from different localities, to achieve a broad food base.

The millions of vegetarians narrow their food base voluntarily. Within recent decades, vegetarianism has escalated dramatically. There are degrees of vegetarianism that form a continuum. The range goes from those who abstain from red meat, to those who use eggs, milk products, poultry, and fish, all the way to extreme fruitarians and vegans who limit their food base solely to plant foods. All vegetarians have chosen to limit variety and to narrow their base. The base is precariously narrow for the fruitarians and vegans. Anyone whose diet is strongly dependent on grains and legumes will find it difficult, if not impossible, to achieve optimum nutrition. In the history of humankind, no culture has survived based on total vegetarianism.

Certain agricultural practices contribute their share in narrowing the food base. The genetic stock for livestock, poultry, and crop seeds has become limited.

Variety, Balance, and Moderation. Variety, balance, and moderation are three interlocking ideas that form the basis of traditional nutrition education. While lip service is being given to these three concepts, our food supply is being pulled strongly in the opposite direction. Instead of variety, the food supply is becoming increasingly dependent on relatively few food materials (such as soybean, cottonseed, wheat, and corn). Instead of balance, there is imbalance as many foods are stripped of nutrients, and others are drastically modified by harsh processings of heat, pressure, restructuring, or treatment with chemicals. Consumers are stimulated by advertising and restaurant menus to gorge on foods high in added sugars, refined starches, fats, salt, emulsifiers, and preservatives, instead of practicing moderation.

Variety, balance, and moderation remain valid criteria for good nutrition. Factors that interfere with a broad base of food sources make it difficult to achieve good nutrition and its accompanying benefits for health. As food processors continue their rapid development of fabricated, restructured, synthetic, and overly processed food products, it is important to shun those foods that narrow the food base, such as imitation foods (for example, imitation orange drink) and foods that are extremely deficient in essential nutrients (such as pies, cookies, etc.). It is more important than ever to choose from a variety of basic foods (such as meat, fish, poultry, eggs, nuts, seeds, fruits, and vegetables) coming from different localities, to achieve a broad food base.

OPTIMAL NUTRITION

What is the optimal diet for humans? This intriguing question is raised repeatedly, and a definitive answer remains elusive. Two recent reports from medical journals are of general interest and also deal with the question. Both describe preindustrial diets. Although we cannot return to the lifestyle of our ancestors, study of their dietary habits might contribute some insights into our own best decisions concerning diet.

Hunter-gatherer Diet. In one recent experiment, ten Australian aborigines with diabetes agreed to return to their hunter-gatherer lifestyle. Previously, while in an urban setting on the outskirts of Melbourne, they had maintained Western lifestyles, partaking of meals that consisted, in part, of fatty meats, carbonated soft drinks, and alcohol. They had become obese and had developed high blood pressure and diabetes.

Returning to the wild, they consumed only what they could obtain by hunting and fishing: kangaroo, turtle, and crocodile, for example. With much activity expended in the search for food and consuming only about 1,200 calories daily, they lost their excess weight within several weeks. After two months in the wild, their blood sugar levels fell. There was significant improvement in their bodies' ability to remove sugar from the blood after eating, and they experienced a partial, and in some cases complete reversal of adult-onset diabetic abnormalities.

These findings confirm results of other studies showing that, in cases of adult-onset diabetes, normal functioning of the insulin-secreting cells in the pancreas can be partially restored if high blood sugar levels are reduced. According to the researcher conducting the aborigine study, the main finding was that "a low-fat, low-calorie diet is an effective diet for control of diabetes. . . . The low-fat content of the diet may be one of the most important therapeutic components, particularly for reducing the vascular complications of diabetes." This conclusion is remarkably similar to many of the present-day dietary recommendations for achieving and maintaining general health.

Stone-age Diet. Elsewhere, the dietary habits of Paleolithic humans have come under renewed investigation. Researchers have noted that humans today "are confronted with diet-related health problems that were previously of minor importance and for which prior genetic adaptation has poorly prepared us. Chronic illnesses affecting older, post-reproductive people could have had little selective influence during evolution, yet such conditions are now the paramount cause of morbidity and mortality in Western nations." The food of "Stone Age" humans is regarded as having "the nutrition for which human beings are in essence genetically programmed."

Differences between the diet of our remote ancestors and that of present industrialized society have important implications for health. Increasingly, physicians and nutritionists are convinced that the dietary habits adopted by Western civilization over the past century contribute to coronary heart disease, high blood pressure, diabetes, and some types of cancer. These conditions, which have become dominant health problems only recently, are virtually unknown among the few currently surviving hunter-gatherer populations whose food habits resemble the Stone-age diet. How did some of these differences develop?

Affluent Malnutrition. The introduction of agriculture, a mere 10,000 years ago, radically changed human nutritional patterns. With growing populations and dwindling supplies, the proportion of meat in the diet declined drastically, while plant food came to comprise up to 90 percent of the total diet. As a result, people became considerably shorter than they had been in preagricultural times. Their skeletal remains show suboptimal nutrition, both from protein-calorie deficiency and the interactions between malnutrition and infection. Since the Industrial Revolution, the animal-protein content of Western diets has become more nearly adequate. Once again, we are nearly as tall as the early, biologically modern humans. However, our diets still differ markedly from theirs, and these differences are crucial in what has been termed "affluent malnutrition."

For example, the animal protein eaten by Paleolithic populations (deer, bison, horse, mammoth, etc.) differed considerably from the meat available to us in the modern supermarket. It had less total fat, more essential fatty acids and a much higher ratio of polyunsaturated to saturated fats than ours does. The fat of wild animals contains an appreciable amount of one particular long-chain unsaturated fatty acid, now being investigated for its possible property of preventing the development of atherosclerosis. Domestic beef contains nearly undetectable amounts of this valuable nutrient. Meat from free-living animals contains fewer calories and more protein per unit of weight than meat from domesticated animals. Our Paleolithic ancestors consumed more structural fat and less depot fat.

Our diets still differ markedly from theirs [early, biologically modern humans], and these differences are crucial in what has been termed "affluent malnutrition."

Foods from the vegetable kingdom reflect another difference between our ancestors' diet and ours. As foragers, they ate a wide range of roots, beans, nuts, tubers, fruits and, at times, even flowers and edible gums. We have a relatively narrow variety of domesticated crops produced by horticulturists and traditional agriculturists. Furthermore, many of our domesticated plant foods have higher ratios of starch to protein than do their wild counterparts.

The Paleolithic diet not only differed substantially from the typical Western diet today, but it also differed somewhat from the recommendations currently advocated by nutritionists and federal agencies. The foods we eat are classified into four basic groups: protein foods, fruits and vegetables, dairy products and grain products. We are encouraged to have two or more daily servings from each group to achieve balance. But our ancestors, who lived prior to the development of a stable agriculture of domesticated crops and animals, derived all their nutrients solely from the first two food groups. Dairy foods were nonexistent, and cereal grains were rare. Yet various estimates, using modern standards, reveal that the Paleolithic diet was adequate in animal protein, iron, vitamin B_{12} (cyanocobalamin), and folate. In this century, agricultural populations in the world's underdeveloped countries suffer from widespread deficiencies of all these nutrients. It is believed that the Paleolithic diet offered the health benefits of much more fiber than is now contained in a typical Western diet, and the sodium intake of our remote ancestors was only one-sixth of that present in the typical salt-laden American diet.

Of what value are these findings? The extent to which some major chronic diseases of industrialized society are related to the typical Western diet is now being analyzed critically. Evidence of linkage is accumulating steadily. Medical researchers in diverse fields are beginning to formulate a generally preventive diet against such conditions as atherosclerosis and cancer. The diet of our remote ancestors cannot be duplicated by us, but it can serve as a reference standard for modern nutrition as we continue to strive toward that elusive goal: achieving an optimal diet.

APPRECIATING INDIVIDUAL DIFFERENCES

"One man's meat is another man's poison." "Jack Sprat could eat no fat, his wife could eat no lean. " Such adages acknowledge individual differences. Every human has distinctive finger and voice prints. DNA typing—termed DNA fingerprinting—reveals that everyone's blood pattern is unique. Also, the chemistry of one's saliva is unique. The individual body odor is so distinctive that a bloodhound can identify and track it.

Variation in Physiology. Individual differences need to be considered in nutrition. For example, human digestive organs differ in shapes, sizes, and efficiency. At least a dozen different stomach sizes are found in any large group of people. The size of the human liver may vary from one individual to another by a factor of four. The human pancreas produces insulin from as few as 250,000 specialized cells in one person, to ten times that number in another.

Individuals differ in their frequency of eating, amounts of food consumed, and time required to eat. These differences may be imposed by a physical characteristic—such as a narrow esophagus or a small stomach—or by a metabolic difference, such as the amount of available gastric juice.

Human digestion is not uniform, but differs according to an individual's chemistry. Pepsin and hydrochloric acid in the stomach, which help digest protein, vary from person to person by a factor of 1,000. The levels of these two substances strongly influence the efficiency of protein digestion, but may not be taken into account in recommendations for protein requirements.

A small meal for one person may be an overload for

another. Circulatory differences may dictate how large a meal may be tolerated. During eating, blood is diverted to the digestive tract. Those with small blood vessels, low cardiac output, and reduced circulation to the heart may need to eat small meals.

Variation in Nutrient Needs. Wide variations have been found in the requirements for various nutrients. In tests, a fourfold variation in thiamine needs was found within a group of as few as fifteen individuals.

Animal studies showed extreme variation in growth and weight gains for a group of sixty homogeneously bred rats fed the same diet. One rat was able to gain only 2 grams (g) of weight, another, 212 g—more than a 100 times as much. The weight gains of the rest of the rats were all distributed evenly between these two extremes.

The study showed that even homogeneously bred rats may have highly individual nutritional patterns. Heterogeneous humans may have a far wider range of individual differences.

The U.S. Recommended Daily Allowances (RDAs) represent an attempt to establish nutritional requirements for the heterogeneous American population. The stated purpose is "to provide for individual variations among most normal persons as they live in the United States under usual environmental stresses." The recommended allowances are divided for males and females, and further divided into ten age groups. To estimate the nutritional needs of the elderly, only suggestive evidence is used, by extrapolation from studies with fifty-year old adults. Such estimates may be unreliable. Also, requirements of centenarians may be quite different from those of septuagenarians, in addition to individual differences within all age groups.

Nature and Nurture. Both nature and nurture appear to play roles in individual differences. Some individuals may be sodium-sensitive due to their genetic inheritance, while others are not. Some may retain whatever sodium is consumed, while others may consume high levels and excrete it.

Individuals may respond differently to dietary fiber intake as a result of lifetime nutritional patterns. Amounts of fiber that provide adequate roughage for some may result in gastrointestinal upset for others,

How much one's cholesterol level changes may depend on genetics, as well as the fatty acid composition of one's diet. Although the average cholesterol level of a group of individuals may increase somewhat by consumption of saturated fats, individual levels can have no, low, or high increases. The individual liver may be acting as the controlling factor. Some livers will remove cholesterol as rapidly as it is manufactured, regardless of how much saturated fat is consumed. Other livers cannot remove cholesterol from the blood as rapidly, in which case high levels of consumed saturated fats will lead to elevated blood cholesterol levels.

Responses of healthy human adults to fat-modified diets showed wide variations, attributed largely to genetic fluctuations of serum cholesterol within a person, rather than to systemic between-person differences in response to dietary change.

Individual differences need to be appreciated in other areas of health. Often, the amount of a drug necessary to bring about the same effect in different people may vary as much as tenfold. Also, an individual may not always react consistently, and may be far more sensitive at certain times. Levels must be established high enough to be effective, but not high enough to be toxic. Such risk assessments need to take into account the individual differences, especially those at extreme ends.

Chapter 2

Special Food and Health Concerns throughout Life

MOTHERS' MILK: A UNIQUE FOOD

"What we now know about human milk is just the tip of the iceberg," remarked Dr. W. Allan Walker, a researcher at Massachusetts General Hospital, in 1979. By the late 1970s, researchers had discovered that human milk is far more complex than formerly appreciated. To date, more than 100 components have been identified in human milk. And surprising findings continue to be made.

For instance, there is growing recognition that, in addition to meeting the human infant's specific nutritional needs, human milk provides other subtle but important factors for growth and development—factors that could provide for well-being into the adult years.

A Lifetime of Health Benefits. The newborn goes from a sterile womb into a world filled with infectious microorganisms. Immune responses in the infant are, however, incompletely developed. Human milk contains many antibodies, lymphocytes and certain proteins that help protect the newborn from immunologic and infectious complications.

One such antibody, termed IgA, protects against intestinal infections. Infants are unable to produce their own IgA antibodies until months after birth. It is found in abundance in mothers' milk. The lymphocyte found in breast milk can prevent necrotizing enterocolitis (see page 39), the prime killer of babies in need of blood transfusions.

Lactoferrin, an iron-building protein found abundantly in colostrum (the first milk produced after delivery), seems to be involved in the killing of bacteria by phagocytes (cells that surround foreign bodies, kill and remove them).

Human milk also has a natural ability to inhibit the growth of *Escherichia coli,* a bacterium commonly found in the intestines. Macrophages are other potent immunological substances found abundantly in breast milk.

In laboratory tests, mothers' milk has killed *Giardia lamblia,* a common pathogenic intestinal parasite in humans, and *Entamoeba histolytica,* a dysentery amoeba.

Human milk also contains growth-stimulating substances. In the late 1970s, a powerful substance was discovered to be present in milk in high concentrations immediately after birth. It is present in mothers' milk for at least six months after delivery.

The substance, epidermal growth factor (EGF), might play a significant role in the growth and development of digestive enzymes in infants.

It is believed that EGF helps an infant resist certain gastrointestinal problems. Breast-fed infants, for instance, suffer fewer intestinal diseases than bottle-fed babies, even after weaning. Colostrum contains fifteen times as much EGF as milk produced two months after colostrum. In addition to EGF, breast milk might contain other growth factors that stimulate different cell types.

Mothers' milk contains many substances that protect the infant from allergies for months, until the infant's own defense mechanisms are developed more fully. Breast-fed infants suffer fewer allergy problems than bottle-fed infants, especially if they are fed exclusively on breast milk for the first six months following birth. IgA antibodies can block the entry of foreign substances and other allergy-provoking substances through the infant's immature intestinal wall. A common source of allergy in infants comes from cows' milk protein found in bottle formulas.

Substances identified recently in breast milk might benefit the infant's developing brain as well. They might even prevent health problems in later years, such as inflammatory bowel disease, obesity, and heart disease.

The fat composition of mothers' milk changes to meet the needs of the infant. The milk becomes creamier, for example, toward the end of the meal, and the fat composition changes during the first three weeks after birth. Cholesterol and phospholipids (two families of fat molecules) decrease rapidly during that time.

There is evidence that substances in breast milk can enhance the body's later ability to handle fats. Experimental studies show that animals fed breast milk are less likely to develop arteriosclerosis, or hardening of the arteries, even when given high-cholesterol diets. Is this true for humans, too? One study, begun in 1931, continues to monitor 129 men and women fed exclusively on breast milk for more than two months as infants. As adults, they have lower than average cholesterol levels—even when their adult diets have been high in fat.

Parallel studies, conducted at three other centers, involving over 420 adults, showed similar results.

The ample supply of cholesterol in breast milk might be important for the development of the infant's brain and nerve tissues. Also, adequate cholesterol might be necessary to produce enzymes that will lower the cholesterol level in later life.

As *Medical World News* notes, "New facts about mothers' milk keep turning up that suggest Nature, in instance after instance, is best left to her own devices."

Nutritional Benefits of Mothers' Milk. Mothers' milk is the food best suited to meet the nutritional needs of an infant. It is species specific—just like cows' milk, which best suits the calf, and sows' milk, the piglet, etc. The following explains the nutritional benefits of mothers' milk in terms of proteins, amino acids, fats, vitamins, and minerals.

In human milk, whey accounts for about 70 percent of the protein, and casein the remainder. In cows' milk, whey accounts for only about 20 percent, and casein the remainder. These differences in protein ratios are reflected in the curds formed in milk during digestion. Because curds formed by human milk are soft and flocculent (with loosely aggregated particles), they are easily digested by an infant. Unprocessed cows' milk forms large, firm curds that are difficult for infants to digest. For this reason, cows' milk is modified to reduce the size of the curds before it is used in infant-feeding formulas.

Mothers' milk is the food best suited to meet the nutritional needs of an infant. It is species specific–just like cows' milk, which best suits the calf, and sows' milk, the piglet, etc.

The human baby, dependent on its mother, has little need to develop muscle size and mass (unlike the calf, which becomes independent early in life). Instead, the infant needs high-energy foods and fatty acids to promote development of its central nervous system, and small amounts of protein to increase its body mass slowly. Human milk contains only one-fourth as much protein as cows' milk. Even so, protein from breast milk is still better absorbed by the infant because the larger stools formed by the modified cows' milk carry out some of the nutrients. Some scientists have even suggested that the infant fed modified cows' milk has been started along a path of large body mass and obesity.

The amino acid levels in human milk meet nutritional

needs particular to the human baby. These levels differ from those in cows' milk: human milk contains more cystine and taurine. The infant's ability to manufacture taurine is limited, and this amino acid might play a vital role in the transmission of nerve messages and in brain development. The newborn infant also has a limited ability to metabolize the amino acids methionine and phenylalanine, which are found in lower levels in human milk than in cows' milk.

Fat from mothers' milk is well absorbed in the intestinal tract of the human baby, whereas the same is not true of the butterfat in cows' milk. The two fats differ in composition and arrangement. Human milk is rich in polyunsaturates and their long-chain derivatives, as well as other substances vital for brain development. Cows' milk contains only traces of these nutrients, but is rich in saturates and monounsaturates. Lipase (a fat-splitting enzyme), which helps an infant utilize fatty acids for energy, is amply provided in human milk. There is four to five times more linoleic acid, an essential fatty acid, in human milk than in cows' milk. A diet deficient in linoleic acid retards an infant's growth rate and produces dry, scaly and thickened skin.

Human milk also has three times as much vitamin A as cows' milk. It supplies all the vitamin B needed by the infant and contains two to three times as much vitamin C as cows' milk. Moreover, the ascorbic acid in cows' milk is destroyed by heat treatment of feeding formulas. Human milk contains about twice as much vitamin D as cows' milk, although both vary in composition according to the diet of the mother or the cow.

There is some uncertainty regarding vitamin E. It is thought that most humans are born with low levels of this vitamin because it does not pass from the pregnant woman into the developing fetus. However, a few weeks after birth, the breast-fed infant seems to have an adequate supply of vitamin E. Feeding formulas need to be supplemented with this vitamin.

Mothers' milk appears to give complete protection against calcium deficiency during an infant's first three weeks of life. Although human milk contains little iron, it contains nearly twice as much as raw cows' milk. In spite of this, the breast-fed infant generally does not become anemic. Interestingly, the bottle-fed infant is more likely to become anemic—even with an iron-fortified formula. The reason? Adequate amounts of copper are relevant to a program to prevent iron-deficiency anemia. Human milk contains about three times as much copper as cows' milk. Human milk also has a critical ratio of zinc to copper, which is lower than the ratio found in most foods, including cows' milk.

Infants can thrive, whether they are supplied with breast milk, formulas, or a combination of the two. However, the many differences in the nutritional compositions and ratios should be considered by prospective parents as well as health professionals. Immunologic and anti-infective substances afforded by mothers' milk are not present in feeding formulas. (See article below, "Infant-Feeding Formulas: Improved, But Still Imperfect.")

In 1982, the U.S. Department of Health and Human Services announced an official program to promote breastfeeding. Professor Graham Carpenter of Vanderbilt University's School of Medicine commented that ". . . human milk is not duplicated by the industrial products, and . . . our scientific technology is not always able to better or even equal nature."

INFANT-FEEDING FORMULAS: IMPROVED, BUT STILL IMPERFECT

Prior to modern times, there were no infant-feeding formulas. If a mother died in childbirth or was unable to produce milk to meet the infant's needs, a wet nurse acted as surrogate. Or, even an animal might serve as surrogate. Nin teenth-century textbooks on infant care included instructions on the correct tethering of cows or goats and positioning of infants for suckling them.

The major drive toward manufacture of infant-feeding formulas began in the mid-nineteenth century with a decline of wet nursing. The Borden Company developed evaporated milk in 1856, and by 1883, with the discovery of a way to sterilize evaporated milk, infant-feeding formulas were developed. Evaporated milk, now condensed, is still in use. This process modifies the casein curds of unpasteurized cows' milk that otherwise would be indigestible to infants.

By 1930, marketing of formulas had become a highly profitable and aggressively promoted enterprise. Given added impetus by the rise of women employed away from home during World War II, bottle-feeding became the norm in the United States and Western Europe.

From 1930 to 1950, evaporated milk was the most widely used ingredient for home-mixed infant-feeding formulas. By 1960, evaporated milk was used by 80 percent of all bottle-fed babies.

Infant-feeding formulas in powdered form were developed originally for dilution and use in hospitals. At present, nearly all such formulas are in liquid form. Some 40 percent of them are sold as ready-to-feed products. The remainder are as concentrates, to be diluted in water.

Since the 1960s, evaporated-milk infant-feeding formulas have been nearly totally replaced by commercial feeding formulas. Worldwide, there are hundreds of commercial products. Six brand names dominate the American market. Most of the formulas are based on cows' milk. Several have a protein base of soybean isolate, for use with infants who are allergic to cows' milk, or who have difficulties digesting formulas based on cows' milk. In addition, there are special formulas for infants with inborn errors of metabolism, those with other medical problems, and those who fail to thrive normally.

Early Problems. The high concentration of solid matter in infant-feeding formulas has always meant that the relatively inefficient water-conserving power of the infant kidney has little leeway under the impact of a dehydrating illness, such as diarrhea. This problem was compounded in the early home use of dried powders. Some products had imprecise directions for preparation of liquid formulas. There was a widespread practice of adding an extra scoop of powder "for the pot." This well-intentioned action produced high blood concentrations of sodium in infants. When water loss was already suffered from diarrhea or simply from sweating, a serious condition could result with too much salt in the blood, leading to lack of water in body tissues. If this condition was not corrected promptly, convulsions and brain damage could result.

Another effect of high salt formulation on infants in their first few weeks of life was that they tended to put on too much weight. Although many factors may be responsible for babies being overfed, feeding them with improperly prepared formulas containing high sodium levels was an important one. The sodium would create abnormal thirst. The infant would cry for more formula, which would make it more thirsty, and the cycle would be repeated. Also, fat babies might become obese adults.

As a result of this problem, a major change in the composition of infant-feeding formulas was instituted in 1974. In particular, sodium (and phosphate) concentrations were reduced. The newer formulations may have solved some problems. However, more remained unresolved.

Bottle vs. Breast. All mammal milk is highly complex and species-specific. Cows' milk may be ideal for the calf, but not for the human infant, as mentioned earlier.

The combination of sugar and casein, two substances found in most infant-feeding formulas, can cause necrotizing enterocolitis, a potentially fatal disease that affects up to 8,000 infants in the United States each year. In the intestines of premature babies, undigested sugar ferments and becomes acidic. This triggers an inflammatory process that can break down the intestinal lining. Within hours, the infant's developing immune system may be overwhelmed, and the intestine can rupture. Symptoms of necrotizing enterocolitis include a distended stomach, bloody diarrhea, fatigue, loss of appetite, and lowered body temperature. Even with this information, hospitals continue to give premature babies cows' milk-based feeding formulas because, at present, no adequate alternatives exist.

Infant-feeding formulas, based on soy, are marketed for infants known or suspected of being intolerant to cows' milk. Investigators have found that soy inhibits the uptake of iron, is deficient in iodine, and that bone mineralization of infants fed soy-based formulas may be less than that of infants fed cows' milk formula. The Committee on Nutrition of the American Academy of Pediatrics cautions that infants fed soy-protein formulas should be closely monitored for evidence of allergy to soy protein. The Committee reports that soy-protein formulas should not be used "for the routine feeding of premature and low birth weight infants; use should be for limited periods, if at all." The formulas should not be used "in the dietary management of documented clinical allergic reactions to cows' milk protein and/or soy protein formula." Nor should they be used for "the routine management of colic." As soy is being insinuated more and more into the food supply, soy has become a common allergen. (See the article "Our Narrowing Food Base" on page 18.)

Attempts to Fine-Tune Infant Formula. Through the years, with further investigations and newer knowledge about infant nutritional requirements, there has been growing awareness of certain shortcomings of infant-feeding formulas. A chronological sequence of events reflects the various attempts to fine-tune infant formula.

Infants who are genetically or environmentally stressed and fed infant-feeding formulas that contain little or no carnitine, such as soy-based formulas, may be carnitine-deficient. Carnitine is a nutrient that plays a major role in metabolizing fat. In 1985, a manufacturer of soy-based infant-feeding formulas decided to reformulate and add L-carnitine. This nutrient, present in human milk and in milk-based infant formulas, is lacking in soy.

Infants with impaired renal function are especially susceptible to aluminum toxicity. In 1985, *The Lancet* reported the death of two babies dialyzed for kidney disease. Their deaths were traced to aluminum-induced brain damage from aluminum in the feeding formula. As a result, other infant-feeding formulas, both powdered and ready-to-use products, were examined and found to be high in aluminum. Although these high levels might not be fatal to babies with normal kidney function, there is no assurance that the high aluminum levels do not induce subtle but harmful long-range effects.

In 1986, it was reported that cows' milk-based infant-feeding formulas were low in selenium, compared with human milk. Normal breast milk has two to three times as much selenium as in formula. Infants are at great risk of selenium inadequacy. Plasma selenium levels, low at birth, may drop even lower during the first months of life. Infants may be especially at risk due to their dependence on a single food to supply all of their nutritional needs. Supplementation of formulas with selenium was suggested. However, this would have to be done very carefully, because too much selenium is toxic.

In 1986, a national survey of infant feeding evaluated,

among other foods, noniron and iron-fortified formulas. The average intake of iron in infants fed nonfortified formulas was below the recommended dietary allowance. By 1990, the Committee on Nutrition of the American Academy of Pediatrics recommended that all infant-feeding formulas be fortified with iron.

In 1987, it was reported that iron fortification of infant-feeding formulas inhibited copper absorption in infants. It was judged unlikely that healthy full-term babies would become copper deficient. However, pre-term infants were judged to be at risk.

The same year, researchers at the U.S. Department of Agriculture's (USDA) Children's Nutrition Research Center suggested that lactoferrin be added to infant-feeding formulas. Lactoferrin (literally, iron milk), a natural protein in human milk, is known to help infants absorb iron from breast milk, and to protect them against colic, diarrhea, food intolerances, and intestinal infections. Studies suggested that lactoferrin also speeds growth and maturation of the gastrointestinal tract. This rapid intestinal growth may not occur in infants fed formulas, which may also make them prone to chronic diarrhea and other intestinal problems. Infant-feeding formulas are unable to offer the means to suppress the growth of potentially pathogenic enterobacteria.

In 1991, it was noted that serum carotene concentrations are very low in the first six months of life, until the infant begins to eat solid foods that contain carotene. Studies found that breast-fed infants in their first three months showed significantly higher levels of carotene than formula-fed infants.

During the same year, two different risks were reported with infant-feeding formulas. The first, reported by Harvard University scientists, was that the lead content from tap water, used to prepare infant-feeding formulas, might be cause for concern. The second was the discovery that many infant-feeding formulas were overfortified with vitamin D, and could cause hypervitaminosis (toxicity from an overdose of a vitamin).

Inositol is a nutrient present in concentrations several times greater in breast milk than in various infant-feeding formulas. Varying amounts of inositol have been added to some infant-feeding formulas. In 1992, during a three-week test period, it was found that serum concentrations of inositol increased in infants consuming breast milk, but not in those consuming infant-feeding formulas. The investigators suggested that the importance of adequate inositol nutrition in early growth and development previously may have been underestimated.

The issue of fats and oils has long been of concern in attempting to develop infant-feeding formulas. Some mixes may have an imbalance of saturated and unsaturated fats and cause a condition known as steatorrhea (too much fat in the stools due to poor absorption of the fat in the intestines).

When infant-feeding formulas were first developed, various homogenized vegetable oils and animal fats were added to skim cows' milk to approximate the fatty acid composition of human milk.

Recently, the lack of certain fatty acids in some infant-feeding formulas has come under close scrutiny as increased attention is being given to the special attributes of DHA (docosahexaenoic acid), a major omega-3 fatty acid. DHA is found in human milk but, until recently, had not been added to infant-feeding formulas.

It is believed that infants probably can convert linolenic acid to DHA. Liquid formulas made with soybean oil may provide an adequate source of linolenic acid, but some powdered formulas may not. It is thought that DHA is essential for proper brain and eye development. There is increased interest to add linolenic acid or DHA to infant-feeding formulas for both pre- and full-term infants. Unfortunately, at present there are no good natural sources of DHA that are suitable additions. DHA is present in fish oil, but that source would contribute an off-taste to the formula. Also, fish oil contains EPA (eicosapentenoic acid), which might delay weight gain in the infant.

Several Solutions. The dilemma may be solved. One approach is the recent development of a formulation that includes DHA and other fatty acids, in proportions that approximate those found in human milk. The new formulation also contains arachidonic acid (ARA), an omega-6 polyunsaturated fatty acid. ARA is added because it can stimulate other fatty acids to produce DHA. Unlike fish oil, the new formulation does not contain EPA.

Another approach is to make use of microscopic algae that manufacture DHA. By growing the algae in large fermentation vats, future supplies of DHA may become available for infant-feeding formulas.

Two proteins present in cows' milk can cause allergy in infants fed formulas. One of the proteins, beta-lactoglobulin, which is not found in human milk, is chiefly responsible for infant milk-protein allergy. It needs to be minimized when cows' milk is modified for use in infant-feeding formulas.

Cows' milk contains several types of casein proteins. Only one of them—beta-casein—is present in human milk.

Recently, a new process was patented to make cows' milk more like human milk, in terms of proteins, so that infants will digest it easier, and will be less likely to experience milk-protein allergy. The process involves cooling cows' milk to about 39°F for sixteen hours, and then microfiltering it through synthetic membranes. This process keeps the undesirable proteins from passing through. (They are not wasted, but incorporated into cheese or other dairy products.) The milk's proteins are reduced. The beta-casein is separated out, and the beta-lactoglobulin is reduced to four percent or less, by adjusting the pH (acid-alkaline) level and adding salt after filtration.

During the first few days after birth, the breast-fed infant receives colostrum, a watery fluid that contains protein and antibodies that protect from infections. These antibodies are not present in infant-feeding formulas. By means of biotechnology, it may become possible to have plants produce antibodies that could be added to the formulas.

Findings published in Oslo as recently as September 1992 showed that breast-fed babies are intellectually brighter and have better eyesight than those fed on infant feeding formula.

Regardless of how closely formulas approximate breast milk, there are unique properties of human milk that can never be duplicated with formula. For example, the quality of the breast milk when the infant begins a feeding is quite different in its composition from that at the end of a feeding. During the course of a fifteen-minute feeding period, the fat content in human milk increases fivefold, and the protein nearly doubles. These changes in composition probably offer satiety for appetite control.

Breast milk has a variety of immunological properties that cannot be matched by formulas. (See the article "Mothers' Milk: A Unique Food" on page 31.)

Formula-fed babies are prone to "nursing bottle caries syndrome" (rampant tooth decay), otitis media (infection of the inner ear), and other health problems associated with bottle-feeding. Breast-fed babies are spared these problems.

The psychological bonding of mother and infant through breast-feeding cannot be duplicated with bottle-feeding. The bonding is thought to have profound and lasting beneficial effects.

Findings published in Oslo as recently as September 1992 showed that breast-fed babies are intellectually brighter and have better eyesight than those fed on infant feeding formula. The findings depend on the amount of fatty acids the infant receives in the last three months in the womb and, after birth, in breast milk. Only in the last three months before birth does the fetus accumulate its vital supply of long-chain polyunsaturated fatty acids. Maternal milk is rich in these vital nutrients. If the mother is on a well-balanced diet, she will supplement the baby's needs after birth through breast-feeding. Infant-feeding formulas do not contain these fatty acids.

As Dr. Marvin S. Eiger, M.D., director of the Lactation Program at Beth Israel Medical Center, stated: "Human milk is still the nutritionally, immunologically, and emotionally superior product. Make no mistake about it, because nature doesn't!"

NUTRITIONAL PROBLEMS OF CHILDREN: OBESITY AND UNDERNUTRITION

Current concerns about children's dietary habits are directed at overconsumption and the chronic diseases that may result later in life from unhealthy eating habits developed in childhood. This attention is reflected in the policy announced in 1994 by the U.S. Department of Agriculture (USDA) to reduce total calories, fats, cholesterol, and sodium in foods provided in school food programs. During the next few years, planned changes were to be made gradually to try to achieve this goal.

Obesity. Currently, it is estimated that 27 percent of American children are overweight. The problem exists at all economic levels, from the most economically limited to the most affluent. The problem is more common than in previous generations. Over the past two decades, the prevalence of obesity in six- to eleven-year-old children has increased by 54 percent; and in twelve- to seventeen-year-old children by 39 percent. One to five-year-old children now consume more calories, less milk, more soft drinks, and more snack foods than children did in earlier decades.

Some concern has been voiced that low-fat diets may interfere with a child's growth and development by providing too few calories and essential nutrients. A study of nearly 900 ten year olds found that those who ate less than 30 percent of their calories as fat, than those with higher fat intakes, were more likely to consume low amounts of certain nutrients, such as calcium, phosphorous, magnesium, iron, and thiamine (vitamin B_1), riboflavin (vitamin B_2), pyridoxine (vitamin B_6), vitamin B_{12} (cyanocobalamin), and vitamin E. The children on the lower fat diets ate more candy and drank more soft drinks, but had less meat and dairy food intake than children on higher fat diets. This finding shows that food selections must be made carefully, with attention to the diet's composition.

Numerous factors contribute to childhood obesity, including too much food and too many undesirable foods. One feature that has been linked to these factors has been documented extensively: the role of long hours of television viewing, accompanied by sedentariness and overindulgence in snacks containing high levels of calories, fat, cholesterol, and sodium. These are the same food components that already are oversupplied in many American meals. Sodium contributes few calories. But very salty foods provoke thirst, which may be quenched by high-caloric drinks.

On average, children between the ages of two and seventeen have been found to watch between twenty-two and twenty-five hours of television each week. By itself, excessive television viewing may promote obesity by increasing food intake either during viewing, or as a result of seeking foods advertised on television.

At the same time, the "couch potato" has reduced caloric output—either by displacing time that might otherwise be spent in physical activity or by decreasing the metabolic rate from long hours of television viewing. This setting increases the risk of obesity.

The American Academy of Pediatrics encourages parents to limit children's television watching to a maximum of one or two hours daily, and to offer children appropriate snacks, including fresh fruit, raw vegetables, or plain popcorn. Also, family encouragement of physical activity may not only prevent obesity in young children but may reduce the risk of health problems, such as high blood pressure and osteoporosis, later in life.

Surprisingly, few data are available regarding the nutritional needs and dietary intake of children beyond infancy. Most data are extrapolated from adults. Currently, the recommended dietary allowances published by the Food and Nutrition Board of the National Research Council are regarded as the most reliable guide.

By itself, excessive television viewing may promote obesity by increasing food intake either during viewing, or as a result of seeking foods advertised on television.

Compared to the infant, the rate of growth slows dramatically for the toddler and preschooler, and remains fairly constant until the adolescent spurt. Intake of 1,300 calories a day is judged to be sufficient for a one- to three-year-old child, with an additional 500 calories for the four to six year old. These estimates are for the average child engaged in light activity. Individual needs may vary, depending on the metabolic rate and the extent of physical activity.

Obesity may influence cholesterol and this issue has become controversial. Concerned parents question whether toddlers and preschoolers should be screened routinely for blood cholesterol levels. The federal government's National Cholesterol Education Program's Expert Panel on Blood Cholesterol Levels in Children and Adolescents advised screening only for those children identified as at-risk because of a family history of coronary heart disease. The panel concluded that for this group the weight of evidence is sufficient to warrant dietary intervention. This recommendation, too, has become controversial.

Data on children's serum cholesterol levels have been gathered by the federal government's Health and Nutrition Examination Survey, as well as from large epidemiological studies. At least 25 percent of American children and adolescents have blood cholesterol levels above the level defined as acceptable by the panel. Given the present state of incomplete data, some regard these defined levels as arbitrary and not firmly based scientifically.

Undernutrition. In 1993, the USDA's Office of Public Affairs released results of a childhood study showing that more than 12 million American children under eighteen years of age suffer from hunger. Prolonged hunger, accompanied by nutritional deficiencies, increases the risk of many health problems.

Although socioeconomic problems receive the most attention, there are instances of induced undernutrition inflicted on children, due to the lifestyle chosen by the parents. Extreme vegetarianism, such as the macrobiotic diet, is comprised mainly of foods that are high in starch and fiber, but low in quality proteins. This pattern resembles the diet commonly followed in developing countries, not from choice but from necessity. The macrobiotic diet followed in developed countries, such as the United States and Europe, is not associated with poverty, infectious diseases, or other unfavorable circumstances typically found in developing countries. Thus, any health effects on children raised on a macrobiotic diet in a developed country are almost certainly attributable solely to the dietary limitations rather than to confounding factors.

Researchers at the Agricultural University in Wageningen, the Netherlands, studied the growth patterns of children raised on macrobiotic diets. Measurements showed substantial growth retardation, beginning at the age of weaning, with no catch-up growth if the children were kept on a macrobiotic diet. Additionally, the children showed signs of rickets, a nutritionally induced problem. In summer, 28 percent of the children showed ricket signs; and in winter, 55 percent. Iron deficiency was found in 15 percent of the children; major skin and muscle wasting in 30 percent of the infants; low plasma vitamin B_{12} concentrations in infants; and biochemical signs of riboflavin deficiency.

As a result of these findings, all families in the Netherlands who followed a macrobiotic diet were advised to add fat and fish to their children's food. Six months later, the children from families who followed this advice, by increasing the consumption of fatty fish and/or adding dairy products, showed improvement. The children grew in height more rapidly than those without any dietary changes. Improvement was greater in the children fed these additional foods at least three times a week than in those who rarely or never ate them.

In many American homes, breakfasts are skipped by children as well as by adults. This practice may result from a lack of food in the home or from time constraints. Skipped breakfasts place children at nutritional risks.

A study of 467 school children in the Bogalusa Heart Study showed that those who skipped breakfast had lower intakes of several nutrients, compared to breakfast eaters. Overall, the breakfast skippers consumed 200 to 500 fewer calories than the breakfast eaters and had less intake than the recommended daily allowances (RDA) for vitamins A, D, E, riboflavin, and calcium.

The RDA for calcium is 800 mg a day for children up to ten years of age and increases to 1,200 mg daily for adolescents. Low intake of calcium by children is worrisome, because this nutrient is essential for building strong bones and teeth. Adequate calcium intake during the early years is needed to attain peak bone mass that, in later years, helps protect against some health problems, such as osteoporosis.

In many American homes, breakfasts are skipped by children as well as by adults. This practice may result from a lack of food in the home or from time constraints. Skipped breakfasts place children at nutritional risks.

In a three-year study of twenty-two pairs of prepubertal identical twins, bone mineral density was greater in those consuming 1,600 mg of calcium daily than those with 900 mg (which is close to the RDA). Similarly, healthy twelve-year-old girls who increased their intake from 80 to 110 percent of the present RDA for calcium for eighteen months were able to increase the total bone density of their bodies including their spine bones. This suggests that modest increases of calcium above the present RDA during the years of childhood and adolescence may lower the risks of some health problems, involving bones and teeth, later in life. Also, there is some evidence that the benefits may extend to preventing or postponing high blood pressure.

Adequate intake of calcium-containing foods, such as dairy products (if tolerated), broccoli, sardines, tofu, and other commonly available foods, contribute calcium for good bone health in children. Phosphorus interferes with calcium absorption. Hence, it is prudent to have children limit or avoid carbonated soft drinks, which are high in phosphoric acid.

In the Bogalusa study, iron and zinc also were found to be in short supply for many of the children. Iron deficits were greatest in the one-year-old children who were fed cows' milk as the major source of energy. Unless fortified, cows' milk is low in iron. Relative to their weight, children require more iron than adults. Iron deficiency and its more advanced state, iron-deficiency anemia, may result from inadequate iron intake and low iron absorption. Deficits can reduce a child's attention span and learning ability. Good iron sources are red meats, poultry, and wholegrain products.

In the Bogalusa study, about 30 to 50 percent of children and adolescents, respectively, did not meet even two-thirds of the recommended zinc intake. Mild zinc deficiency leads to low-height-to-age ratio in young children. Adequate zinc intake improves growth in such children. Many of the same foods that are good sources of iron are also good sources of zinc. Oysters and clams are especially high in zinc.

Although many food intake data have been collected, they usually aren't analyzed to distinguish between intake of nutrients from animal or plant foods. Yet data show that diets heavily dependent on plant products, but low in eggs, dairy products, meat, and fish, are inadequate to support the normal growth and development of children.

EATING DISORDERS: PERILOUS COMPULSIONS

According to the American Academy of Pediatrics, 30 percent of American school-age children are overweight. Half of them will grow into overweight adults. Obesity is a risk factor in high blood pressure, elevated cholesterol, diabetes, some malignant tumors, and shortened lifespan.

Factors attributed to childhood obesity include poor food choices and sedentary habits. Fast food meals—often favorite choices—typically contain 40 to 50 percent of their calories from fat, but these foods are low in fiber, iron, and vitamins A and C. As for lack of exercise, the title of an article in a medical publication summarized the problem: "Profusion of TV produces plump couch-potato tots." By adolescence, a child has watched 15,000 hours of television, and has been exposed to 350,000 commercials, more than half of which promote highly processed food products and soft drinks.

Linked to this problem of childhood obesity are various attempts to control dietary intake. At times, well-intentioned pressures may lead to unintended and regrettable developments. Eating disorders may develop during the adolescent years, and parents need to be aware of warning signs and symptoms. There is an emerging preoccupation with "healthy eating" and fitness among some adolescents, especially girls, that may lead to eating disorders, according to Dr. David S. Rosen, director of adolescent health at the Medical Center of the University of Michigan at Ann Arbor. According to Rosen, healthy eating for teenage girls parallels the "vilification of fat in the media and the increasing availability and aggressive marketing of low-fat and no-fat food options." Rosen observes that moderately limiting fat intake may be desirable, but when carried to an extreme, "the compulsive avoidance of fat begins to take on the characteristics of an eating disorder and probably requires the same kind of intervention."

Pressure to be thin is increasing. Over the last few decades, *Playboy* centerfold models and Miss America contestants have become leaner, with smaller busts and hips. By contrast, the average female between seventeen and twenty-four has become heavier and heavier.

Despite the plethora of weight-reducing diets, meals-in-cans, pills, low-fat products, noncaloric sweeteners, gym equipment, exercise programs, sweat boxes, and other approaches, young people, as well as other segments of the population, are becoming more and more obese. According to the Centers for Disease Control and Prevention, Americans are more overweight now than at any time since the government began to keep complete statistics in the 1960s.

Risks in Dieting. "Dieting is a chief cause of obesity in America," according to Professor Judith Rodin of Yale University. "Some middle-class parents trying to save their daughters from the stigma of fat insist on severe diets, but depriving children of food may only make them more interested in eating. At some early stage in infancy, people, as well as animals, are pretty well biologically regulated. It takes something to deregulate that system. And one of the things that we know that does that is dieting. That kind of girth control begins to slow down the metabolic rate, and makes the body begin to change in order to protect itself against the reduction in calories. This causes more problems when the dieter returns to eating normally."

Eating disorders are now the third most common illness among adolescent females. More than one in five girls score in the abnormal range on tests of eating attitudes and behaviors . . .

Weight cycling—popularly called "yo-yo" dieting—attracts many young women. Studies have shown that repeated attempts to lose weight, followed by weight gains, greatly increase the risk for developing heart disease. Also, people who diet frequently may develop a preference for high-fat and sugary foods, resulting in increased weight.

Crash diets, which depend on drastic calorie reduction to induce weight loss, often backfire and result in weight gain. Severely restricted caloric intake triggers a body response that slows the rate at which calories are used for daily activities. The body adjusts itself to run on fewer calories, and it becomes more efficient in using the available calories in order to conserve its nutrient reserves. When weight loss plateaus, many dieters become frustrated and return to their previous eating habits. However, because the body has learned to function with fewer calories, it stores more calories from the regular diet in the form of fat. The initial pounds lost on a crash diet are mostly water, released by the metabolic changes that occurred as the system adapted to reduced calories. However, the pounds regained are stored as fat. The weight gain will continue until the body returns to its former rate of processing nutrients. Thus, many crash dieters may gain back more weight than they lost on the diet.

Dieting is especially common among adolescent girls and young women who typically report weight concerns and who attempt to restrict their fat or caloric intake as early as age nine or ten years. In the last few decades, the prevalence of such concerns and subsequent efforts to diet have risen dramatically. Eating disorders are now the third most common illness among adolescent females. More than one in five girls score in the abnormal range on tests of eating attitudes and behaviors, and abnormal scores are noted commonly in girls as young as fourth and fifth graders.

Although these problems are encountered mainly with females, adolescent boys and young men with severely abnormal eating habits are being identified more frequently as well.

Dieting by teenagers, from infrequent to uninterrupted, is a sign of possible eating disorders. Parents should be alert to this. Rosen says that eating disorders occur on a continuum, ranging from mild to serious manifestations.

Anorexia Nervosa. On the continuum of eating disorders, anorexia nervosa is in the extreme of the range. It has long been recognized as a serious health problem, thought to result from emotional or psychological stresses. The typical patient is a white middle-to-upper middle class young woman, but increasingly, cases are reported among some women of other ages, and in males, and in nonwhites.

Typically, an anorexic refuses to maintain weight that is above the lowest weight considered to be normal for her age and height. Her total body weight is at least 15 percent below normal. She displays an intense fear of weight gain, despite the fact that she may be severely underweight. Regarding herself in a mirror, she has a distorted image of her body and is convinced that she is fat. Frequently, she fails to menstruate. She suffers a pathological loss of appetite, accompanied by nutritional deficiency symptoms. Over time, vital organs such as the heart and liver may be damaged. Without intervention, there is emaciation, wasting, shrunken organs, and death.

According to governmental surveys, cases of anorexia nervosa have doubled in the past ten years. Between 0.5 and 1.0 percent of women during late adolescence and early adulthood are thought to be affected. Onset may be triggered by a stressful life event, such as leaving home.

In young males, compulsive running has come to be regarded as a counterpart of anorexia nervosa in young women. Compulsive running is self-destructive and pathological behavior. It is primarily a male manifestation of what is termed an "ascetic disorder." However, there are some young women who are compulsive runners, too, but they are fewer in numbers. Like anorexics, compulsive runners tend to be high achievers from affluent families. Pathological commitment begins at a time of heightened stress. In recent years, its incidence has increased dramatically.

Anorexia is poorly understood. One theory relates this eating disorder to a malfunctioning hypothalamus, an organ

Eating Disorder Information

For more information on organizations that can help you learn more about eating disorders and treatment, contact:

National Eating Disorders Association
603 Stewart Street, Suite 803
Seattle, WA 98101
(800) 931-2237; www.nationaleatingdisorders.org

National Association of Anorexia Nervosa and Associated Disorders
P.O. Box 7
Highland Park, IL 60035
(847) 831-3438; www.anad.org

that controls the release of morphine-like endorphins in response to stress. Emaciated anorexics have abnormally high brain levels of endorphins. The same brain chemistry may play a role in the emotional "high" reported by compulsive runners.

Bulimia Nervosa. Bulimia nervosa is another serious eating disorder of young people, characterized by repeated binge eating and purging. The episodes may be repeated frequently. The person—usually a young woman—consumes excessive amounts of food within a brief period of time, and then induces vomiting or uses a laxative, diuretic, or enema to get rid of the food. When not binging, the bulimic may adhere to a strict dieting or fasting regime, or indulge in vigorous exercise, in attempting to prevent weight gain.

Often, bulimics attempt to hide their problem. They may

eat normally with other people, but binge and purge in private. Many maintain normal weight. Observant family members, college roommates, or school personnel who suspect bulimia, should look for some warning signs: a chronically inflamed and sore throat that bleeds, decaying tooth enamel caused by frequent exposure to stomach acid that results from induced vomiting, and swollen salivary glands in the neck and jaw which makes the face look puffy.

Recent studies by Christopher G. Fairburn and his associates at Oxford University have pinpointed some of the psychological risk factors in early childhood that can contribute to bulimia at a later stage. Frequently, at an early age, the children had viewed themselves with extreme disdain. They had experienced minimal contacts with their parents, or were physically or sexually abused. They encountered parental conflicts or criticisms. The parents, themselves, frequently had suffered from obesity or bouts of depression. Many of the parents had demanded perfection. Many of the children who later developed bulimia had wrestled with obesity early in life, or had other health problems. Early menstruation, accompanied by body-shape changes, spurred dieting. Bouts of depression or other mental conditions often preceded bulimia. Current dieting by other family members or their critical comments about dieting reinforced the problem. In gathering these risk factors together, psychological components become apparent in the origin of this eating disorder.

It is estimated that between 1 and 3 percent of American adolescent and young women are bulimic. Among college-age women, the problem may affect as many as 20 percent.

Little is known about the long-term prospects for recovery from bulimia, either with or without intervention. A statistical compilation of existing data suggests that about 50 percent of all women initially diagnosed with bulimia were free of their symptoms after five to ten years, regardless of whether or not they received treatment. Another 20 percent still had the disorder. The remaining 30 percent continued to binge and purge, but they fell short of being classified officially as bulimic.

According to Pamela K. Keel and James E. Mitchell of the University of Minnesota in Minneapolis, treatment for bulimics could speed the recovery of women who, on their own, stop binging and purging after five to ten years. Nonetheless, Keel and Mitchell reported that in the first four years after the initial bulimic diagnosis, about one-third of those who recover still suffer relapses.

Binge Eating. Binge eating, a related eating disorder, has some features similar to bulimia, but is regarded as a distinct entity by medical doctors. Even less is known about binge eating than anorexia or bulimia. It is estimated that about 2 percent of the general American population is affected. Bingers may comprise about 30 percent of all individuals who attend weight-control programs in hospital settings. An even larger percentage of bingers may exist among some members of the population, such as obese patients who suffer from compulsive mental disorders.

Like bulimics, bingers may consume extraordinary amounts of food in a brief time, but unlike bulimics, they do not attempt to purge. After an episode of binging, the following morning may produce symptoms similar to those of the severe hangover of an alcoholic. The binger is rendered nonfunctional for school activities or in the workplace.

Among college students, group alcoholic binges are popular in some student groups. Mob psychology may be involved in group binging; actions that a person might not take by himself may be taken if an entire group is engaged in the action.

Pica. Pica, a bizarre eating disorder, has long been

known. It was described in the ancient world by Hippocrates. It is known globally. Its name is derived from the Latin word for magpie—a bird known for its voracious and indiscriminate appetite. Persons suffering from pica display persistent and compulsive cravings to eat inedible substances such as buttons, ice, paper, dried paint, cigarette butts, burnt matches, ashes, sand, soap, toothpaste, oyster shells, or even broken crockery. The cause(s) and prevalence of pica are unknown.

Pica is a serious eating disorder that can inflict gastrointestinal problems that may require surgery, dental injury, phosphorus intoxication (from matchheads), or environmental poisoning from lead or mercury that can be contaminants in the ingested substances.

Coping with Eating Disorders. Eating disorders are complex and cannot be treated solely with dietary means. Individual cases may need to address fundamental psychological, familial, societal, and cultural aspects of the disorder. The development of an eating disorder is not necessarily triggered only by a desire to be thin. Although much has been written about the role of Hollywood, professional models, and the media in presenting unrealistic body images to young people, the main cause of eating disorders is not from trying to achieve the perfect body.

According to a nutrition therapist, Amy Tuttle from the Renfrew Center in Philadelphia—a residential center for women with eating disorders—family dynamics often contribute to eating disorders. Tuttle reported that "some people with eating disorders come from enmeshed families where emotional, relational, and physical space boundaries may be blurry. This 'enmeshment' inhibits independence and the development of a separate self." Depression, anxiety, loneliness, stress, anger, troubled personal relationships may all contribute to disordered eating patterns. They need to be regarded as problems of coping, along with other problems such as compulsive gambling, or chronic alcohol or drug abuse.

Findings from recent research suggest that biochemical imbalances should be investigated as possible factors in eating disorders. Neurotransmitters such as serotonin and norepinephrine control appetite as well as mood, alertness, and sleeping patterns. Low levels of these chemicals may explain the relationship between eating disorders and depressive illness, or abnormal eating patterns.

Many American children are low in zinc, and zinc deficits are known to reduce the appetite. Some researchers believe that low zinc levels from crash dieting may play a role in anorexia nervosa, in addition to the psychological problems associated with that eating disorder.

Hormonal changes that can lead to taste aversions is another suspected factor in anorexia nervosa in some girls. Carl and Joan Gustavson from Arizona State University at Tempe conducted animal experiments over the past decade and found that male rats frequently became nauseated and developed taste aversions after they had been injected with estrogen, the female hormone. Similar reactions were experienced in estrogen-depleted female rats whose ovaries had been removed shortly after birth. The Gustavsons suggested that girls who produce low amounts of estrogen—possibly due to prenatal exposure to toxic substances—acquire a male-like estrogen sensitivity. Later, when estrogen concentrations greatly increase at puberty, these girls become anxious and develop taste aversions to foods. A vicious cycle continues. Dramatic weight loss reduces the nauseating estrogen concentration. Any weight gain from eating will lead only to increased estrogen concentration. In turn, this leads to anxiety and food aversions.

Currently, medications—especially antidepressants—commonly are prescribed for eating disorders. They should be regarded only as adjunct treatments to the more basic ones that address the multiplicity of factors. It is to be hoped that various areas of research may yield better understandings of the factors that cause eating disorders, and produce improved treatments.

PEANUT ALLERGY: NO TRIVIAL MATTER

Food allergies are more common than formerly, according to Steve L. Taylor, codirector of the Food Allergy Research and Resources Program at the University of Nebraska in Lincoln. The mechanisms behind food reactions are similar to those with hay fever, bee sting, or allergic reactions to pharmaceuticals. More consumers die yearly from food allergy-induced anaphylaxis than from bee stings, reports Anne Munoz-Furlong, of the Food Allergy and Anaphylaxis Network. Just one bite of an offending food can induce a reaction. There is no known cure for food allergy. The best help is to avoid the offending food.

Normally, our bodies develop a tolerance to most foreign proteins. The body's immune system provides protection against foreign proteins (antigens), including those in food. But the bodies of people with food allergies mount an inappropriate immune response to these antigens, and generate immunoglobulin E (IgE) antibodies. These antibodies latch onto the antigen and to the surface of the immune system's mast and basophil cells. These cells then release "mediators," such as histamine, that lead to the symptoms of allergic reactions such as stuffy nose, breathing difficulty, and rash.

Two groups of genes have been identified as responsible for inducing the inappropriate immune response and overreaction, and confirm the innate sensitivity of some people to allergens. One gene codes for an amino acid chain that is involved with an IgE receptor. Some variants of this gene tend to make individuals susceptible to asthma and allergies. Another identified gene alters a receptor chain in some allergy-prone people. It is thought that this alteration affects the receptor's functioning. Although the change may be subtle, its effects can be profound.

Some food allergies are based on a different mechanism, which can be traced to reactions mediated by sensitized T lymphocytes in the gastrointestinal tract. This type of food allergy is not well understood, and is difficult to test.

Less commonly, some food allergies are induced by exercise, performed before or after eating a specific food.

Medical reports attribute 90 percent of food allergies to a list of the "big eight": milk, eggs, fish, crustacea (crabs, shrimp, and lobster), peanuts, tree nuts, soybeans, and wheat. The remaining 10 percent consist of 160 other foods.

If a person becomes sensitized, the amount of an allergen needed to induce adverse reactions can be exceedingly small. In 1997, Fred Shank, Director of Food Safety and Applied Nutrition at the Food and Drug Administration (FDA) reported that the agency determined that if something can cause an allergic reaction, there is no insignificant level. This point is well taken. A spatula, used to remove peanut-containing cookies from one pan, and then to remove nonpeanut-containing cookies from another pan, can render the latter cookies hazardous to peanut-allergic individuals. Similar cross contaminations can occur with shared ice cream scoops, utensils, and machinery used with peanut and nonpeanut-containing products. The problem of peanut allergy deserves better recognition by health professionals and the general public.

Peanut Allergy. In the early 1990s, major allergy centers began to note a rise in peanut allergy. According to Professor Gary A. Bannon, of the Department of Biochemistry and Molecular Biology at the University of Arkansas for Medical Sciences at Little Rock, peanuts are responsible for "one of the most severe food allergies."

How Extensive?

The extent of peanut allergy—or for that matter, any food allergy in the general population—is unknown. Estimates are uncertain and varied. Some allergens are lifetime; others may disappear. Real allergies, with discernible effects on the immune system as well as on other systems of the body, may be confused with intolerances and sensitivities that are nonimmune system responses. Their mechanisms, as yet, are unclear.

Information about peanut-allergic individuals was collated in a United Kingdom questionnaire of 622 self-reported peanut-allergic subjects. Two-thirds of the group reported symptoms experienced on contact with peanuts. Ninety percent reported adverse reactions after eating less than one peanut; 50 percent, even after touching a peanut. For 93 percent, symptoms occurred in less than a half hour after exposure by ingestion, inhalation, or touching peanuts. The most severe symptoms experienced were collapse and cyanosis. Symptoms were experienced most frequently in adults. Peanut-allergic reactions were associated significantly with abdominal symptoms. Individuals with a history of asthma were more likely to develop severe reactions to peanut exposure. Due to extreme reactions, 13 percent required hospitalization. Sixty-five percent carried some form of adrenaline (epinephrine) with them. One-third of the group reported that with each episode, their reactions became more severe.

James D. Astwood, manager of Monsanto's Protein Characterization and Safety Center, reports that only a handful of peanut proteins—out of thousands of different proteins present—are allergenic. Although proteins usually are digested rapidly in the gastrointestinal tract, major food allergens such as those in peanuts, are indigestible. They remain in the gastrointestinal tract, causing the body to mount an immune response.

A spatula, used to remove peanut-containing cookies from one pan, and then to remove nonpeanut-containing cookies from another pan, can render the latter cookies hazardous to peanut-allergic individuals.

As little as one milligram of exposure to a peanut allergen can provoke immune system responses in individuals who are peanut-allergic. A few well-documented medical cases demonstrate the problem:

- In December 1995, a thirty-three-year-old woman with peanut sensitivity read the contents on the label of a container of split pea soup. Peanuts were not listed. She consumed part of the soup, and within minutes experienced severe systemic allergic reactions. At an emergency room in a hospital, she was treated with intravenous fluids, corticosteroids, and diphenhydramine (an antihistamine). The woman had a lifetime history of peanut sensitivity. Her reactions were so intense that she developed welts on her face if her husband kissed her after he had eaten a peanut butter sandwich.

  As follow-up after her hospitalization, the split pea soup was analyzed and found to contain peanut flour as a component of the "flavoring" ingredients, but not listed on the label. The soup manufacturer discontinued using peanut flour in the product. This case, and others, prompted the FDA to consider a requirement for declaring known allergens used in spices, flavorings, and colors added to food products.

- A young boy, highly allergic to peanuts, had been trained

by his parents to read labels carefully and avoid peanut-containing products. A neighbor offered the boy some ice cream. They read the label ingredients on the package. Peanuts were not listed. The boy ate the ice cream, went into anaphylactic shock, and died. The product actually contained peanuts, but they were not listed.

- In 1986, a Providence, Rhode Island college student ate some restaurant chili, went into anaphylactic shock, and died. Unknown to her, the creative cook had added peanut butter to the chili. The young woman had been peanut-allergic. Subsequently, Rhode Island state health officials requested that restaurateurs list any "highly unusual ingredients" in dishes. Also, they encouraged patrons with allergies to question ingredients used in restaurant dishes. The city of Providence instituted a policy of requiring ambulances to carry adrenaline so that persons in anaphylactic shock can be treated promptly.
- Recently, peanut-allergic individuals traveling on airplanes have complained of experiencing allergic reactions to peanut protein released into the cabins when other passengers eat mid-flight peanut snacks. Allergic reactions can occur through inhalation as well as through consumption or skin contact.

The 1986 Air Carrier Access Act guarantees airline access to the disabled. Citing this Act, the U.S. Department of Transportation (DOT) issued guidelines for major airlines to provide "buffer zones" to accommodate passengers who, in advance of the flight, present medical documentation of peanut allergy. However, the buffer zone extends only to the passenger's row and the rows immediately in front and in back of this row. Passengers in these three rows are not to be offered peanut snacks. Although DOT promised to comply with the "buffer zone," in the catch-all spending bill approved by Congress in October 1998, regulators were directed not to spend any funds to enforce the policy. In any case, this arrangement may be ineffective. A study, conducted in 1996 by the Mayo Clinic, showed that peanut allergens are not filtered efficiently out of the air by the airplanes' ventilation systems. The peanut dust is carried in the recirculated air.

To date, at least one airplane had to make an emergency landing because a peanut-allergic passenger reacted to the peanut dust released when other passengers opened peanut snack bags.

One airline has banned peanuts from being served on any flight after a peanut-allergic passenger gives proper advance notice. Other airlines have substituted nonpeanut snacks such as pretzels.

Peanut-Allergic Children. Allergic reactions to peanuts have increased in the United States by 95 percent over a recent ten-year period. This rise parallels the common practice of offering the seemingly benign jelly-and-peanut butter sandwich to very young children.

This finding is worrisome. Unlike some food allergies, peanut allergy generally persists into the adult years. Peanut allergy is thought to be the leading cause of life-threatening anaphylaxis caused by food allergies. (See "Anaphylaxis: A Violent Reaction" on page 68.)

In 1993–1994, at Addenbrooke's Allergy Clinic in Cambridge, England, peanuts were found to be the most common cause of allergy in sixty-two patients, ranging in age from eleven months to fifty-three years. Peanuts were responsible for all allergies in children sensitized by the age of three years. In many cases, a single allergy to peanut butter in very young children progressed to multiple allergies, including tree nuts, cat dander, pollen, and dust mites as the children grew older. The Addenbrooke staff advised that peanuts should not be given to children before the age of three years, and in cases where allergies were common in families, to hold off until seven years.

Dr. Hugh Samson, a renowned pediatric allergist at Johns Hopkins Medical School, also has been concerned about the increased numbers of children with peanut allergies. Samson advised breast-feeding mothers with family histories of allergies to eliminate peanuts and other potential food allergens from their diet.

Samson's advice was repeated in 1998 by Chief Medical Officer Kenneth Calman of the United Kingdom, who warned pregnant women and breast-feeding mothers to avoid eating peanuts in order to prevent peanut allergy in their offspring. The warning was issued after receiving a report by the government's Committee on Toxicity, citing a rise in the number of British children who were peanut-allergic. Scientists had reported that about one in 200 people are peanut-allergic. Calman reported that the warning was precautionary and based on evidence that the developing fetus and the breast-fed infant, exposed to peanuts from the mother's diet, are at an increased risk of developing peanut allergies. The warning extended to women whose partners had peanut allergies, as well as to pregnant women who had already given birth earlier to children with peanut allergies. The government estimated that the warning was applicable to about one in every three women of childbearing age.

The National Jewish Center for Immunology and Respiratory Medicine in Denver, Colorado, recently conducted a long-term follow-up of children previously found to have severe peanut allergies. Although all of the children had been instructed about the need for peanut avoidance, including information about the variety of disguises in which peanuts could appear, only one-fourth of the children succeeded in avoiding peanuts completely. The staff conducting the follow-up was concerned about the frequency of accidental peanut ingestion, and none of the children demonstrated any evidence that they outgrew peanut reactivity.

Strategies by Food Manufacturers to Minimize Food Allergens. Increasingly, food manufacturers have become aware of the potential problems created by inadvertent

Anaphylaxis: A Violent Reaction

Anaphylaxis is a violent allergic reaction that involves a number of parts of the body simultaneously. Like less serious reactions, anaphylaxis occurs after a person is exposed to an allergen. However, in this case, the severe reaction occurs only after having had previous experiences with the same allergen.

According to the FDA, as little as $\frac{1}{5}$ to $\frac{1}{5,000}$ of a teaspoonful of an offending food has caused death from anaphylactic shock. Peanuts have been implicated in numerous cases of anaphylaxis, and many have been fatal.

Anaphylaxis can produce severe symptoms within five to fifteen minutes, although its life-threatening reactions may progress over a period of hours. Warning signs include itching; swelling of the lips, mouth, and throat; and difficulty in breathing. There may be a sense of impending doom, drop in blood pressure, and loss of consciousness.

The sooner anaphylaxis is treated, the greater the chance for survival. The person who is suffering from anaphylactic shock should be hospitalized immediately, even if the symptoms appear to be subsiding on their own without any intervention.

There is no specific test to predict the likelihood of anaphylaxis. Persons at greatest risk are those who have a history of gastrointestinal and respiratory symptoms, hives, or swellings immediately after eating an offending food.

introductions of allergenic ingredients in their products. Many manufacturers have extended the concept of HACCP (Hazard Analysis Critical Control Points), devised to improve food safety, to include allergenicity.

The Allergen Protection Plan, developed by scientists from the National Food Processing Association, General

The American Academy of Allergy and Immunology suggests that a person who has experienced anaphylaxis and fortunately survived should carry at all times injectable epinephrine (adrenaline) to treat any future reactions promptly, and to wear a Medic Alert bracelet that identifies the allergy(ies).

Epinephrine works directly on the cardiovascular and respiratory systems, causes rapid constriction of blood vessels, reverses throat swelling, relaxes lung muscles to improve breathing, and stimulates heartbeat.

For emergency home use, epinephrine is available in a traditional needle and syringe kit and provides two doses. Also, there is an automatic injector system, which resembles a pen. The person removes the safety cap and pushes the automatic injector tip against the outer thigh until the unit activates and provides a premeasured dose. The person holds the device in place for several seconds, and then discards it. These medications have expiration dates.

The incidence of fatal anaphylactic reactions to foods has been increasing yearly. Some causes are from the widespread use of protein additives in many commercially prepared foods; increased consumption of foods prepared by others who may be unaware of allergic problems created by their "creative" recipes; inadvertent food contamination; and undeclared ingredients on labels that may be present in the food products.

Mills, and Campbell Soup Company, was created in 1997 to identify potential areas of contamination and to build a preventive strategy similar to HACCP.

There is general consensus that trace amounts of peanut contamination are a major problem, and among the most difficult allergens to control. Raw materials may be intermingled by a supplier before being delivered to a food processing plant. Or, in a large factory where breakfast cereals are extruded, peanut dust released from a peanut-containing cereal being manufactured can contaminate a non-peanut-containing cereal being extruded in the same area. Sometimes, a simple printing error can result in mislabeling an entire production run.

Manufacturers have become aware of the need to mark clearly any allergenic ingredients, and to store them away from nonallergenic ones. "Reworked" products—a combination of batches produced at different times—should be in containers separated from others, and marked by distinguishing labels or color codes.

Major food processors have hot lines and/or toll-free numbers for consumer inquiries or complaints. Thomas Trautman of General Mills reported that allergy-related inquiries increased tenfold from 1988 to 1998. The Kellogg Company reported that hot-line requests for information about allergens tripled from 1991 to 1994. Other companies also report large increases of inquiries about allergens.

Food manufacturers recognize their responsibility to label products adequately to meet the needs of allergic consumers. The Grocery Manufacturers Association (GMA) agrees with the FDA that "proper labeling of foods that contain allergenic substances is a vitally important public health issue." GMA established a Food Allergy Task Force and reported that food manufacturers "understand the necessity and value of good manufacturing practices and strongly oppose the use of precautionary, or 'may contain' labeling of allergens in lieu of applying good manufacturing practices." However, even with good manufacturing practices, "certain manufacturing processes present the potential for 'cross contact' of ingredients from product to product, resulting in the potential presence of an undeclared allergen in a food product." GMA recommends that the FDA formulate a uniform method to state, in the simplest way possible, that allergens may be present in foods.

Some manufacturers use "prophylactic labeling," by including in the ingredient listing those substances that, unavoidably, may be present. An example is the declaration "may contain traces of peanuts due to manufacturing." Some groups oppose prophylactic labeling, and cite the Federal Food, Drug, and Cosmetic Act which provides that the list of ingredients are those included, not those that might be in the product. However, this control is weakened by FDA's tolerance of the phrase "may contain . . . " for listing specific fats or oils that may or may not be present in a food product. (This policy was instituted to allow manufacturers to choose ingredients of the least cost with fluctuating market prices, before the time of increased awareness of the problem of allergenicity of undeclared ingredients.) It is argued that if this tolerance is extended to cover unintended but potential allergens, manufacturers may not follow quality control procedures that can reduce, if not eliminate, this problem.

Ultimately, if the phrase "may contain" is used extensively, consumers with allergies will find that their food choices are narrowed still further. Often, food allergies are multiple, and may not be only from peanuts, but may extend to allergens in other foods, too.

Most often, allergen contamination in food plants is due to incomplete cleaning of equipment, failure to declare ingredients, use of reworked mixtures, and unknown ingredients in a raw material. For example, black pepper was adulterated with dry mustard and wheat germ. Another risk may be created when the research and development group of a company modifies a well-established product that previously had been allergen-free, or develops one product in a line of products that contains an allergen. Also, there are human errors, with mixups on labels or packaging.

At times, manufacturers may become aware of a problem and conduct a voluntary recall. At other times, the problem is caught by the FDA, a state agency, an inspector, or a consumer report. Recalls due to allergenic ingredients in food products have increased. In 1996, there were thirty-five Class 1 recalls (those most serious as imminent health threats) involving fifty-seven products; in 1997, thirty-five recalls of seventy products; and in 1998, fifty-eight recalls of 240 products.

The FDA has become more aggressive in recalling foods with allergenic components. A frequent focus is on ice cream containing undeclared peanuts.

Strategies by Organizations to Minimize Food Allergens. The Food Allergy and Anaphylaxis Network, established as a nonprofit organization, provides educational materials for parents and children with food allergies, as well as for health professionals and educators. The organization issues newsletters and "Special Alert Notices" to members, which caution readers about hidden allergens in specific food products. For further information, contact The Food Allergy and Anaphylaxis Network, 10400 Eaton Place, Suite 107, Fairfax, VA 22030; (800) 929-4040; www.foodallergy.org.

The National Institute of Allergy and Infectious Diseases, a branch of the National Institutes of Health, publishes free materials about allergies, including food allergy resources, the immune system and how it works, and allergens. Some publications are intended for the general public; others, for health professionals. Request a list of publications from NIAID Office of Communications, NIH Bldg. 31, Room 7A50, 31 Center Dr., MSC 2520, Bethesda, MD 20892-2520; www.niaid.hih.gov.

LACTOSE INTOLERANCE

Seventy percent of the world's population cannot, to some degree, digest lactose, the main carbohydrate in milk and milk products. To break down lactose, the enzyme lactase is needed, and, in most individuals, this enzyme declines quickly after early childhood. But in those who are genetically or culturally predisposed, the decline is gradual, allowing normal digestion of lactose.

For the lactose-intolerant, consumption of dairy products is often followed by discomfort, including abdominal pain, bloating, flatulence and diarrhea. Until now, these sufferers have been advised to shun dairy foods. But recent studies suggest that total avoidance might not be necessary.

Two studies recently published in the *American Journal of Clinical Nutrition* reported that a number of factors can determine how tolerant a person is to lactose. Also, there are different ways to deal with lactose intolerance.

Milk Consumption. The more slowly lactose is presented to the intestine, the more readily it is digested and absorbed. Consuming milk with solid foods, for example, delays gastric emptying (when food leaves the stomach and goes into the small intestine) and thereby favors lactose absorption.

In one of the studies, when lactose-intolerant people consumed one- and one-half cups of milk (containing 18 grams of lactose) along with solid foods, such as breakfast cereal, bananas or hard-cooked eggs, the rate of lactose fermentation in milk was cut by about half. Another strategy is to consume milk periodically in small amounts, rather than in large amounts all at one time.

Gastric emptying is also delayed by the presence of fats

and amino acids, among other things. For this reason, whole milk—with its fat—is tolerated better than skim milk. Likewise, chocolate-flavored milk is tolerated better than unflavored milk (due to the fat in the chocolate).

Fermented Milk Products. Although fermented dairy products such as cheese, buttermilk, and yogurt have been recommended for lactose-intolerant individuals, it has been found that not all of these products are equally well tolerated.

Some fermented milk products, such as aged cheddar or Swiss cheese, are significantly reduced in lactose because the whey, not the remaining curd, contains most of the lactose. On the other hand, the lactose level of other fermented dairy products, such as yogurt, cultured buttermilk, and sweet acidophilus milk might be just as high as that of whole sweet milk. The lactose content of these products varies according to the processing techniques. And, while added nonfat milk solids might increase the nutritional values, it also raises the lactose content of the product.

Yogurt, with its bacterial beta-galactosidase (lactase), is tolerated better than sweet milk. Yogurt's bacteria survive gastric digestion and are active in the gastrointestinal tract. Hence, the bacteria can substitute for the individual's own lactase that might be low or missing. A word of caution: these benefits are bestowed only with unpasteurized yogurt. Presumably, the heat from the pasteurization process, which is used to prolong shelf life, destroys yogurt's beneficial lactase.

Cultured buttermilk does not change the extent of lactose digestion significantly because only a small amount of lactose is metabolized by its bacteria. For the same reason, the action of sweet acidophilus milk is equivalent to that of sweet milk. (Earlier claims held that sweet acidophilus milk improved lactose absorption. But more recent studies show that sweet acidophilus milk does not alleviate the distressful symptoms for lactose-intolerant people.)

Enzyme Preparations. Commercial food-grade lactases (beta-galactosidase enzyme preparations from microbial organisms) are used to produce lactose-hydrolyzed milk and other reduced-lactose products, which can be used instead of sweet fluid milk. These products, though sweeter than regular sweet fluid milk, contain from 40 to 90 percent less lactose. They are tolerated by many people who would otherwise need to avoid dairy products. Reduced-lactose dairy products are available in some areas.

Lactose-Reducing Products. Another approach to making sweet fluid milk more tolerable is to buy lactose-reducing products, such as Lactaid®, sold in different forms, which can be added at home. However, such products add about six cents per cup to the cost of milk. They are also inconvenient to use: they require a twenty-four-hour incubation period to be fully effective. Lactose-reduced milk is available.

Efforts are ongoing to make lactose digestion more possible by adding beta-galactosidases in different forms to milk at mealtimes. Results of preliminary studies show that the addition of such lactase enzymes is easy to do, improves lactose absorption, and decreases undesirable colonic hydrogen production.

Furthermore, when added at mealtime in appropriate amounts, these lactase enzymes can hydrolyze milk lactose even if solid foods are eaten at the same time.

Determining Whether You Are Lactose-Intolerant. If you suspect that you are lactose-intolerant, two diagnostic tests are available: an oral lactose tolerance test, based on routine laboratory procedures and readily available in hospitals; and a breath hydrogen test, which is considered more reliable and useful in evaluating lactose digestion.

MIXING FOODS AND DRUGS

Certain foods and drugs interact, changing the effects of the medications. The presence of food in the stomach and intestines can influence a drug's effectiveness by slowing down or speeding up its passage through the intestinal tract, and to send it to where it is needed. Also, certain foods contain natural constituents or chemical additives that react with some drugs and make them ineffective, dangerous or even fatal. For this reason, certain medications need to be taken on an empty stomach; others must be taken before meals and others, during meals.

Certain foods can increase or retard absorption of drugs into the bloodstream. For example, if an individual eats fatty foods before taking griseofulvin (Fulvicin, Grifulvin, Grisactin, Gris-PEG), which is used to combat fungal infections such as ringworm, the blood level of griseofulvin rises significantly.

Food and Drug Interactions. More commonly, however, food impairs absorption of drugs. One well-recognized interference comes from antibiotics. If dairy foods are used during tetracycline therapy, the calcium in the milk, cheese, yogurt, or other dairy product, will impair absorption of tetracycline. So will sardines. Other antibiotics, such as penicillin, ampicillin, and erythromycin, should not be taken with fruit juices, citrus fruits, tomatoes, vinegar, pickles, or cola drinks.

If drugs need to be swallowed with liquid, it is safest to drink plain water. Soft drinks or acidic beverages, such as fruit or vegetable juices, can result in excessive acidity and cause certain drugs to dissolve in the stomach instead of later in the intestines, where they can be absorbed more readily into the bloodstream.

Alcohol, a drug itself, can interact with a wide variety of medications. A good general rule is to avoid all alcoholic beverages when taking any prescription medications—or even over-the-counter medications. Alcohol can combine with antihistamines, tranquilizers or antidepressants and lead to excessive drowsiness. This state can be especially hazardous for individuals who are engaged in any activity that requires mental alertness, such as driving a car or operating machinery.

Individuals taking monoamine oxidase (MAO) inhibitors, prescribed at times for depression or high blood pressure, need to exercise great care in food and beverage selections. Foods and drugs that contain high levels of tyramine (a natural component) can interact with MAO inhibitors and force blood pressure to dangerous levels, causing severe headaches, brain hemorrhages, and even death. Tyramine-rich foods and beverages include aged and fermented items (such as sharp cheeses, yogurt, sour cream, pickled herring, salami, pepperoni, soy sauce, active yeast preparations, beer, Chianti wine and sherry), as well as livers from beef and chicken, broad beans, canned figs, bananas, and avocados. Other items suspected of reacting adversely with MAO inhibitors include cola beverages, coffee, chocolate, and raisins.

Individuals who take thyroid medication need to restrict their intake of those foods known as goitrogens. Under normal circumstances these foods are beneficial. But they inhibit the body's production of the thyroid hormone, which can lead to goiter. Such foods include soybeans, rutabaga and purple-topped turnips, Brussels sprouts, kale, mustard greens, cauliflower, and cabbage.

Persons who have been placed on anticoagulants need to restrict consumption of foods that are rich in vitamin K, the blood-clotting nutrient. Under normal circumstances, blood-clotting is beneficial. For example, it stops a cut's bleeding. However, anticoagulant drugs are used to prevent clotting, and foods rich in vitamin K work in opposition to this action. Foods rich in vitamin K include green leafy vegetables, broccoli, Brussels sprouts, asparagus, beef liver, and bacon.

Individuals on diuretics need to avoid foods containing the so-called flavor enhancer monosodium glutamate (MSG), which may eliminate too much sodium from the body. Protein hydrolysate, also known as hydrolyzed protein (HVP), also contains MSG.

Aspirin and aspirin-containing medications do not mix with acidic foods such as fruit juices, citrus fruits, pickles, tomatoes, vinegar, or cola drinks. These items only intensify the irritating effects on the stomach and may result in ulcers or serious gastric bleeding.

Levodopa (Laradopa), a drug used with Parkinson's disease, should not be taken with foods rich in pyridoxine (vitamin B_6) such as liver, pork, beef or wheat germ. These foods block the drug's effects and make the medication less efficacious.

Drug and Nutrient Interactions. Just as some foods can affect the way certain drugs behave in the body, some drugs can affect the way the body uses certain nutrients. Drugs can impair proper nutrition in different ways. They can interfere with the body's ability to convert nutrients into usable forms. They can hasten the excretion of nutrients before they are absorbed and utilized. They can compete with vitamins for the sites of actions. Some drugs, such as broad-spectrum antibiotics, can interfere with the synthesis of vitamin K, which normally is manufactured in the body by microorganisms naturally present in the colon.

For individuals who need to take medication over long periods of time, nutrient depletion may be gradual. The groups at greatest risk are the chronically ill, children, the elderly, and individuals with poor dietary habits.

Perhaps the most common long-term drugs that profoundly affect nutrients are the estrogen-containing oral contraceptives. Women who have low stores of folate (a B vitamin component) are at risk of a clinical folate deficiency. Oral contraceptives inhibit absorptive enzymes and increase the synthesis of folate-binding macroglobulin, which can lead to megaloblastic anemia. Moreover, certain oral contraceptives reduce levels of pyridoxine, which may be associated with the mental depression commonly experienced by women on the pill. Oral contraceptives also can adversely affect other B vitamins, notably B_{12} (cyanocobalamin), riboflavin (B_2), and thiamine (B_1). Oral contraceptives decrease the absorption of vitamin C and alters its distribution into various tissues. Many users of oral contraceptives are found to have low vitamin C levels.

Long-term use of cholestyramine (LoCholest, Questran), which is used to treat individuals with high fat levels, can reduce folate absorption by forming complexes with the molecule, impair vitamin B_{12} status, and lower the levels of fat-soluble vitamins A, D and K by binding the bile salts. These depletions can lead to osteomalacia (softening of the bones due to impaired mineralization), unless nutritional supplements are supplied.

Long-term therapy with isoniazid (Laniazid, Nydrazid, Rifamate, INH, and others), a drug used with tuberculosis, depletes the body of pyridoxine (B_6). Before this became recognized, patients often developed neuropathies. Now patients are given pyridoxine supplementation along with the drug. This drug also decreases the body's supply of niacin, which, if uncorrected, can result in frank pellagra.

Mineral oil, an ingredient still used in some over-the-counter laxatives, was the first agent found to cause malabsorption. It forms an insoluble complex in which the fat-soluble vitamins (A, D, E, and K) pass through the gut before they can be absorbed. Mineral oil is still widely used in nursing homes and by the elderly. Over a period of time, users of the oil risk developing rickets as a result of malabsorption of vitamin D. As little as four teaspoons of mineral oil twice daily is enough to interfere with the absorption of vitamins D and K, as well as carotene (a precursor of vitamin A). (See "Over-the-Counter Drugs" on page 126.)

A number of drugs affect specific nutrients. Both hydralazine (Apresazide, Apresoline, Ser-Ap-Es), a drug used to control high blood pressure, and isoniazid, a drug used with tuberculosis, can inhibit the production of an enzyme necessary to convert pyridoxine into a form usable by the body, or can combine with the vitamin to form a compound that is not utilized, and excreted. Both actions deplete the body of pyridoxine.

Similarly, anticonvulsives (drugs used to control epilepsy) increase the turnover rate of folic acid and vitamins D and K, and create vitamin deficiencies. Unless supplemented, these deficiencies can lead to megaloblastic anemia or rickets, or hemorrhage in the young infant.

Long-term use of many other drugs, including colchicine (ColBenemid) used with gout, oral antidiabetic agents, potassium chloride (a table-salt substitute), and the antibiotic neomycin (Ak-Spore, Bacticort, Minims, Neo-Cortef, and others), can all impair vitamin B_{12} absorption and, unless supplemented, ultimately cause vitamin B_{12} deficiency.

Long-term use of diuretics, or "water pills," to treat conditions such as congestive heart failure can lead to serious potassium depletion. Heart patients who take digitalis need to prevent potassium loss to keep the heart from becoming more sensitive to digitalis. Foods that are good sources of potassium include oranges and orange juice, tomatoes and tomato juice, bananas, cantaloupe, figs, white and sweet potatoes, winter squash, figs, dried apricots, raisins, and prunes.

The above are among the commonly recognized drug-induced nutrient deficiencies. Doubtless, many other drug-nutrient interactions occur, both in short-term and long-term therapy, but to date remain unrecognized.

HOW FARE THE ELDERLY?

Knowledge has been scanty regarding the nutritional requirements of the elderly. It was long assumed, falsely, that their needs were quite similar to those of younger adults. In recent years, with interest and funding, researchers have begun to discover distinct and substantial differences of the elderly's nutritional needs. Their physiological status and overall health tend to differ from younger adults. Yet, in dietary guidelines up to the present, these two groups have been lumped together in one broad classification, as if the requirements were the same.

For the first time, the forthcoming dietary reference intakes that will update and expand the existing U.S. Recommended Daily Allowances (RDA) from the last edition (1989) will have a separate category for the elderly.*

Recent scientific findings indicate that, to meet elderly needs, the current RDAs may be too low for many nutrients, and too high for a few. There is growing consensus that the goals of the RDAs should be not only to prevent nutrient deficiencies, but to reduce major chronic diseases, for example, osteoporosis in the elderly. Reduced energy needs in aging result from the decline in functioning of the metabolic rate, and the lessening of physical activity. At the same time, there is increased need for certain nutrients, and the diet of the elderly needs to be nutrient-dense.

---

*The growing recognition of differing needs for specific groups may establish another classification. At present, there are RDAs for female teenagers, and for lactating women. New guidelines are being considered for teenage nursing mothers. Preliminary research suggests that this new classification would be appropriate.

The following surveys up-to-date information regarding the nutrient needs of the elderly, covering vitamins, minerals, trace minerals, protein, and other dietary nutrients.

Vitamin B_{12}—Serum levels of vitamin B_{12} (cyanocobalamin) decline in aging. Formerly, the prevalence of vitamin B_{12} deficiency in the elderly was underestimated. Although it was recognized that anemia could occur in the elderly who were severely depleted of vitamin B_{12}, those with less severe deficiencies were not recognized. Over time, even milder vitamin B_{12} deficiencies can lead to various neurological symptoms, such as a burning sensation in the tongue, tingling or numbness in the hands or feet, impaired balance, mental confusion, and dementia. Symptoms may appear even before vitamin B_{12} levels drop below the lower limit of the normal range.

The physiological status and overall health of the elderly tends to differ from younger adults. Yet, in dietary guidelines, these two groups have been lumped together in one broad classification, as if the requirements were the same.

It is estimated that about 30 percent of the elderly are deficient in vitamin B_{12} due to atrophic gastritis, an inability of the stomach to secrete enough gastric acid and pepsin to digest food. The "intrinsic factor" is a substance secreted by the stomach that binds vitamin B_{12} to the intestinal wall and prepares it for transit into the bloodstream so that vitamin B_{12} and other nutrients—such as folate, calcium, and iron—can be absorbed and utilized. If vitamin B_{12} deficiency remains uncorrected, bacterial growth, too, can contribute to vitamin B_{12} malabsorption.

Many cases of atrophic gastritis result from chronic *Helicobacter pylori* infection, which is associated with stomach ulcers. People with this type of gastritis may absorb unbound vitamin B_{12} normally, but are unable to absorb protein-bound B_{12} from foods. In such cases, a vitamin B_{12} supplement may be helpful.

Intramuscular injections (shots) of vitamin B_{12}, or nasally administered, or tableted vitamin B_{12} have been given regularly to some vitamin B_{12}-deficient elderly persons. Such supplementation may be helpful in the early stage of atrophic gastritis, because the crystalline form of vitamin B_{12} in a supplement actually may be absorbed better than vitamin B_{12} present in food. However, if the atrophic gastritis is allowed to progress, unattended, even the supplement may not be absorbed.

Some drugs reduce vitamin B_{12} absorption. A drug used for ulcers and heartburn, omeprazole (Prilosec), reduces vitamin B_{12} absorption dramatically. Other drugs commonly used for ulcers, such as ranitadine (Zantac) and cimetidine (Tagamet) also reduce vitamin B_{12} absorption.

Vitamin B_{12} may influence bone metabolism. Osteoarthritis is common in the elderly. Some studies suggest that osteoarthritic patients given vitamin B_{12} and folate treatment improved hand-grip. Unlike NSAIDs (nonsteroidal, anti-inflammatory drugs) commonly used as palliatives for osteoarthritis, vitamin B_{12} and folate are inexpensive and do not produce undesirable side effects.

Determining the amount of vitamin B_{12} needed by the elderly is complex. The 1989 RDA lowered vitamin B_{12} levels by one-third for all adults. With present knowledge, this recommendation appears to have been unwise. The action was based on two assumptions that have proved to be wrong. First, it was assumed that although serum vitamin B_{12} levels decline in the elderly, they still fall within a normal range. Now, we know that the lower limit of the normal range should be higher. Thus, with revised calculations, larger proportions of the elderly population—actually

Undernutrition and Malnutrition

Undernutrition in the elderly results from different causes. Gum disease and poorly fitted dentures can reduce the total food intake, with inadequate consumption of nutrient-dense and fibrous foods. With multiple health problems, many elderly people are on numerous medications. As the numbers of medications increase, the risks increase for drug-nutrient interactions that interfere with nutrient absorption.

Undernutrition can result from lifestyle factors. Lack of transportation may present a problem for food shopping, and low income may limit selections of nourishing but costly foods. Those who live alone or are isolated socially may lack the incentive to plan and prepare nutritious meals. Preparation may be difficult due to disabilities such as arthritis or poor vision. Impaired mental ability, confusion, or depression are important risk factors for malnutrition. Multiple nutrient deficiencies and protein-calorie malnutrition are prevalent among the elderly in nursing homes and other long-term care facilities.

Setting appropriate nutritional standards and dietary recommendations for the elderly is complicated by the all-too-common presence of disease processes and impaired reserves of nutrients in many organs of the body. A lowered metabolic

as much as 25 percent of women and 50 percent of men—may be B_{12} deficient. Second, it was assumed that vitamin B_{12} malabsorption in adults cannot be corrected by diet, and must be done with injections. This assumption appears to be incorrect, too. Dietary supplementation can be helpful.

Folate—Folate is associated closely with vitamin B_{12}. In 1989, the folate RDAs were lowered. This was another rate is associated with reduced muscle mass. As the body ages, it digests, absorbs, and utilizes nutrients less efficiently. Glucose tolerance and kidney function may be impaired. Age-related physiological changes, including a decline in smell and taste acuity, can impair food selection and consumption, and may fail to alert individuals to moldy or otherwise toxic substances consumed.

Even for the otherwise healthy, aging can impair the ability to match food intake with energy needs. In studies of over- or under-feeding, older men could not adjust their caloric intake automatically to lose weight gains, or to regain weight losses, as did younger men. The elderly do not shed extra pounds readily, and can be at increased risks for high blood pressure, diabetes, and heart disease. Or, a prolonged illness may cause an elderly person to lose weight significantly, and fail to regain it readily. This results in decreased resistance to infectious diseases.

Older people do not process fat as well as do younger adults. They have significantly more fat circulating in their blood after a fat-rich meal than do younger adults. The fat may be moved out of circulation at a slower rate, and may account for added pounds in aging. The elderly are unable to break down and use large quantities of fat. As a result, instead of fat being burned as energy, it is deposited in the tissues.

unwise decision. More recent data indicate that a return to the older higher values is justified. Folate deficiency in the elderly may be related to poor absorption and utilization of nutrients, leading to malnutrition and anemia.

Pyridoxine—The 1989 RDA for pyridoxine (vitamin B_6) was lowered substantially for adults. The elderly were included in this grouping. The actual needs of the elderly were not known, yet the elderly appear to need more pyridoxine than previously assumed, in order to maintain glucose tolerance and normal cognitive functions. Numerous studies suggest that marginal pyridoxine deficiency may be widespread in the elderly, resulting from poor dietary intake, chronic illness, or poor absorption. Some forty drugs are known to alter the metabolism or bioavailability of pyridoxine, which is apt to affect many elderly people.

Pyridoxine deficiency rarely occurs alone, and it is most commonly found in people who are deficient in other B complex vitamins. This finding is reflected by research in recent years on homocysteine, an amino acid normally present in the blood. Deficiencies of pyridoxine, vitamin B_{12}, and folate are all involved in high homocysteine levels that relate to many health problems experienced by the elderly. High homocysteine levels are linked to cardiovascular diseases, atherosclerosis, diabetes, high blood pressure, obesity, and elevated cholesterol levels. Elevated homocysteine can harm brain function and damage blood vessels.

Pyridoxine deficiency in the elderly may be reflected in low blood levels of this vitamin, as well as in impaired tryptophan metabolism and malfunctioning of the immune system. Severe pyridoxine deficiencies may lead to dermatitis, epileptiform convulsions (resembling epilepsy or its manifestations), and anemia.

In a study, a group of hospitalized elderly individuals benefited from pyridoxine supplementation. The researchers recommended that the current RDAs of pyridoxine for elderly men and women probably are insufficient, and should be reevaluated.

Thiamine—Some of the elderly, especially those institutionalized, have been found to have low levels of thiamine (vitamin B_1). They may be at increased risk for thiamine deficiency because of reduced food intake, decreased variety of food, consumption of grain products made largely from refined flours, increased use of medications, decreased ability to absorb nutrients, alcohol abuse, prolonged hemodialysis, and gastric partitioning surgery.

Thiamine deficiency has been reported among the elderly both in free-living as well as in institutionalized settings. Early signs of marginal thiamine deficiency are difficult to recognize clinically because they are nonspecific and may have other causes as well. The symptoms include loss of appetite, disturbed sleep, nausea, and peripheral neuropathy. Signs of more severe thiamine deficiency include mental confusion, loss of eye coordination, loss of fine motor control, and general weakness.

Riboflavin—The RDAs for riboflavin (vitamin B_2) were lowered for adults over fifty years of age because it was assumed that they eat less than younger adults. However, research conducted with people in their sixties and seventies showed that the elderly need more rather than less riboflavin as they age.

Vitamin C—The elderly appear to need more vitamin C (ascorbic acid) than the current RDAs. Due to impaired physiological function, poor diets, or prescription drugs, many are low in vitamin C. This is especially true for those who are chronically ill or institutionalized.

Numerous studies show that serum vitamin C levels decrease in aging both for men and women. Men have consistently lower levels than women. There may be a gender difference in how the kidneys process vitamin C.

Adequate vitamin C may be critical for favorable outcomes of health problems that require hospitalization or surgery. In recent years, adequate vitamin C intake has been found to reduce the risk of cataract formation—a common problem for the elderly—as well as other problems of deteriorating eyesight.

In aging, as the immune function declines, the elderly are more prone to disease and infection. Adequate vitamin C intake has been shown to benefit cellular immune responses. The elderly appear to be at greater risk for developing symptoms of vitamin C deficiency than are other age groups. Their lower plasma and cellular levels of vitamin C indicate decreased body stores of this vitamin. This may be caused by changes in physiologic and metabolic functioning, as well as various factors associated with aging, such as changes in food intake and economic status. Body stores of vitamin C may be depleted further by acute or chronic illnesses that are prevalent among many of the elderly.

Vitamin E—"Our knowledge about vitamin E needs in old age is distinguished by paucity of data. Clinically evident deficiency of vitamin E is extremely rare in the elderly. However, metabolic and cellular considerations indicate that vitamin E requirements may be greater in old age compared with that in younger groups," reports Dr. Ranjit Kumar Chandra, at the Memorial University in Newfoundland, Canada.

Commonly, the elderly do not obtain adequate vitamin E from food. Studies at the Human Nutrition Research Center on Aging at Tufts University showed that vitamin E supplementation, at far greater doses* than could possibly be obtained from the diet, might help limit the age-related decline in immune function.

---

*Although vitamin E is generally regarded to be of low toxicity, high doses must be used cautiously, and should be closely monitored by a health professional. High doses antagonize the functions of other fat-soluble vitamins and can lead to decreased bone mineralization, reduced liver storage of vitamin A, coagulation disorders, and an impaired immune system. Nausea, gastrointestinal upset, headache, fatigue, muscle weakness, and double vision have been reported from high vitamin E doses. Individuals with liver disease, kidney dysfunction, or those using anticoagulants, including aspirin, may suffer adversely from high vitamin E doses.

Vitamin D—The elderly may require more vitamin D than younger people. The main source of vitamin D used by the body comes from exposure to sunlight. Many of the elderly spend little time outdoors. Some are housebound, and others are institutionalized. In addition, they have impaired vitamin D synthesis through the skin. The amount of serum vitamin D depends more on sunlight exposure than from food intake. Foods make a relatively small contribution of vitamin D unless one eats inordinate amounts of fatty fish such as cod, mackerel, and sardine. The elderly have poorer intestinal absorption of vitamin D from foods, and decreased kidney function handles vitamin D less efficiently.

Vitamin D, along with vitamin A, prevents long-term bone loss and fractures such as those commonly experienced in the elderly. Vitamin D deficiency may also contribute to post-menopausal osteoporosis, glucose intolerance, and increased risk of adult-onset diabetes.

A single large dose of an intramuscular injection of vitamin D every six months in the elderly was found to be effective in treating osteomalacia—a softening of the bones due to impaired mineralization resulting from vitamin D deficiency. For other health problems resulting from vitamin D deficiency, low daily dose supplementation has been found safe and effective. The present RDAs for vitamin D are deemed inadequate for many of the elderly, especially those who are sunlight-deprived. Current recommendations are being reconsidered and may be increased substantially.

Vitamin A—Current RDAs for vitamin A may be too high for the elderly. Due to an age-related delay in clearing vitamin A by the liver and other tissues, its absorption increases in the elderly. As a fat-soluble vitamin, too much vitamin A can be toxic.

Calcium—Calcium, along with vitamin D, is important to prevent long-term bone loss and fractures, especially in the elderly. Calcium supplements have been shown effective in reducing bone loss in elderly women even when calcium intake from food is close to the current RDA level. New recommendations for calcium are expected to be substantially higher than the current ones—perhaps nearly double.

Concern about postmenopausal bone loss has been focused on calcium, somewhat neglecting other nutrients involved. Mature bone matrix (the formative cells or tissues) also depend on copper and other trace minerals such as manganese and zinc. Studies showed that the risk of bone loss in calcium-supplemented elderly women could be decreased further by intake of these trace minerals.

Trace Minerals, In General—Trace minerals, needed only in thousandths or even millionths of a gram daily, are important nutrients disproportionate to their small requirements. National surveys show that even apparently healthy elderly persons have suboptimal intake of trace minerals.

Poor trace-mineral intake among the elderly in nursing homes may be even higher than in the free-living elderly. This finding may reflect the poorer general health status of the institutionalized group.

The requirements for trace minerals are affected by many chronic diseases prevalent among the elderly, and also by possible drug-nutrient interactions. Also, trace mineral supplementation is potentially toxic for the elderly, due to slower metabolism and impaired organ functioning. For many trace minerals, the amount between too little and too much is quite small.

Although much still needs to be learned about major mineral nutrients such as calcium, phosphorus, and magnesium, far more information is needed about trace minerals. The RDAs for one, selenium, were established only as recently as 1989. Only estimated safe and adequate intake ranges have been added for copper, manganese, fluoride, chromium, and molybdenum. Too little information was available in the 1989 RDAs to make any recommendations for silicon, vanadium, nickel, boron, or arsenic.

One study with healthy elderly persons showed that supplementation of all known essential trace minerals, in physiological doses, improved immune responses and reduced the incidence of infection. The supplementations given daily consisted of iron, zinc, copper, selenium, iodine, calcium, and magnesium, in addition to beta-carotene, vitamins A, C, D, and E, and B vitamins, including folate.

Iron—It had been assumed that iron stores in the elderly generally are adequate, because men have had a lifetime of iron accumulation, and women have accumulated iron after menopause.

However, recent surveys show that this assumption is wrong. Iron deficiency is not uncommon among the elderly who, in other respects, appear to be healthy. Possible contributing factors are low dietary intake or iron consumption in poorly absorbed forms. Low iron intake may exacerbate malabsorption of folic acid and vitamin B_{12}, and contribute to nutritional anemia. Other factors in low iron stores may result from various health problems such as gastric intestinal bleeding, arthritis, kidney failure, or cancer.

High serum iron levels are associated with reduced risks of coronary artery disease. Low levels could be a marker for increased cardiovascular risk.

Copper—At present, no RDAs have been established for copper. Surveys indicate that the majority of American diets contain less than adequate amounts of copper. Copper deficiency is thought to be linked with aging, because copper-deficient diets are known to produce several symptoms common to aging, including anemia and damage to the heart muscle. Copper deficiency is associated with many health problems that are especially prevalent with the elderly, including immune dysfunction, frequent infections, diseases of the intestines and kidneys, diabetes, elevated cholesterol, heart enlargement, aneurysm (a sac formed by localized dilation of an artery or vein), damage to heart tissue from free radicals, and coronary heart disease. Patients who receive nutrients solely from tube feeding may become copper deficient.

Several animal studies showed that a copper-deficient diet produced many health problems also encountered by elderly humans. One study demonstrated that a copper-deficient diet, combined with too much sodium, increased the risk of kidney failure; with adequate copper, the animals were able to excrete the extra sodium and fluid. Another study showed that a diet with high levels of fructose (a sugar found in table sugar and in corn sweeteners) depressed copper-containing enzymes that function as antioxidants. Still another study showed that copper deficiency, combined with stress, raised blood pressure.

Zinc—A zinc deficiency in the elderly can delay wound healing, disturb taste and smell acuity, and impair immune functions. Senile purpura, a well-recognized condition affecting some elderly people, is characterized by skin bleeding, accompanied by reddish or purplish blotching. This condition reflects zinc deficiency (and possibly deficiencies in other trace minerals). Zinc is needed for tissue repair in senile purpura.

Protein Intake. Although the current RDAs call for the same amount of protein for adults of all ages, a growing body of scientific evidence indicates that the protein needs of the elderly may be higher than those of younger adults. The elderly may utilize protein less efficiently, and their protein requirements may be greater due to body composition, physical functional capacity and activity, food intake, and disease.

About 50 percent of the free-living elderly and 25 percent of the institutionalized elderly habitually fail to consume even less than half of the low amount of protein presently recommended. At this time, the consequences of consuming low amounts of protein by the elderly are unknown, but are thought to impair the immune system as well as to retard recovery from illness or surgery. Researchers recommend that future RDAs for protein intake of the elderly should be based on studies actually conducted with this group, and not depend merely on extrapolations from studies with younger adults.

Fluid Intake. Water is a vital (see the article "Water: Missing in the Diet" on page 137), yet potentially problematic, nutrient for the elderly who may have difficulties in meeting fluid requirements. Water balance depends on water intake and output, regulated by thirst as well as kidney function. In aging, both may decline.

Some elderly people purposely restrict their water intake to cope with incontinence, or bathroom trips during the night. Others may not drink enough water because of impaired mobility. Other dehydration risk factors in the elderly include blunted thirst sensation, laxative abuse, overuse of diuretics, depression, and dependence on tube feeding.

The elderly are at risk of serious dehydration when faced with water losses due to physical illness or hot weather. Although the elderly may be physically less active than when they were younger, their water requirements may still be high. Often, dehydration as a health problem is overlooked because the symptoms are not dramatic. Severe dehydration can have grave consequences, such as increased toxicity of medications, both hyperthermia (greatly increased body temperature) and hypothermia (greatly decreased body temperature), and impaired cognition. Dehydration combined with heat exhaustion can cause loss of consciousness and heat stroke. Often, dehydration in the elderly is associated with hospitalization. If untreated, dehydration mortality may exceed 50 percent.

Future RDAs and the Elderly. Obviously, the nutritional requirements of the elderly should not be based on false assumptions of the past. This age group deserves study for its actual needs. Some researchers even think that the needs may differ between the elderly and the very elderly.

For various reasons, nutritional deficiencies appear to be widespread in the elderly. However, greater understanding of the risk factors can lead to solutions. In the past, food fortification had been accepted readily, but supplementation was met with strong resistance. With newer findings, this resistance is weakening.

Dr. Ranjit Kumar Chandra reported: "The era of nutrient supplements to promote health and reduce illness is here to stay. In selected groups such as the elderly, there is overwhelming evidence of immunologic enhancement following such an intervention. . . . Deficiencies of vitamins and trace elements are observed in almost one third of all elderly. . . . Since there is no evidence to suggest that physiological amounts of vitamins and trace elements given for prolonged periods have any toxic or adverse consequences and given the high prevalence of deficiencies of several micronutrients in old age, it would be prudent to opt for a suitable micronutrient supplement in modest amounts for all elderly individuals in order to achieve the maximum physiological and health benefits with the least risk of toxicity. A reduction in illness and suffering would be a laudable goal of any nutritional intervention in the elderly. After all, this is what preventive medicine is or should be all about."

Chapter 3

Form and Function: The Body Knows Best

SMALL, BUT BIOLOGICALLY SIGNIFICANT

Anton van Leeuwenhoek, a seventeenth-century Dutch scientist, was astonished by what he saw through a microscope when viewing red corpuscles, body tissues, and various "animalcula"—his term for tiny organisms. By using sophisticated techniques and instruments, the modern counterparts of van Leeuwenhoek can measure various substances at extremely low levels. These substances may be small but are often powerful and may enlarge our understanding of many disciplines, including nutrition, physiology, biochemistry, agriculture, and food science.

Nutrition. A substance in humans, if present in amounts less than 0.01 percent of the body, is considered to be a trace element. Intake of nutrients such as trace minerals and vitamins is vital to our well-being in amounts sometimes as low as micrograms (millionths of grams).

In the case of the trace mineral iodine, the difference between a normal and a severely retarded child may depend on 70 micrograms (mcg) or fewer daily (about two millionths of an ounce). To appreciate how small this amount really is, consider that the same child consumes a billion mcg of food and water daily.

The amount of copper contained in a single penny is enough to supply our needs of this trace mineral for four years.

Other biological systems also may be profoundly affected by trace minerals. As little as one part per billion (ppb) of selenium can exert biological effects on some aquatic organisms. Concentrations of one ten-trillionth part of cobalt increases the dry weight of soybeans by 69 percent.

Some vitamins are needed at exceedingly low levels, too. Adults need only three mcg of vitamin B_{12} (cyanocobalamin) daily—or three millionths of a gram. (One gram would barely fill one-fourth of a teaspoon measure.) Yet, over time, a lack of this important vitamin can lead to serious health problems, including neuropsychiatric disorders.

On the other hand, as little as 1/5,000 of a teaspoon of an offending food has been known to cause death from allergic reaction.

Biochemistry. Prostaglandins (hormonelike substances manufactured in our bodies) are biologically very potent. As little as one nanogram (a billionth of a gram) per milliliter of fluid causes an animal's smooth muscles to contract. Detection methods sensitive to picograms (trillionths of a gram) are needed to identify the presence of prostaglandins in body tissues.

The size of some biological organisms can be very tiny, yet they can exert powerful effects. A human sperm measures only about 3,000 nanometers (billionths of a meter) across its head. The acquired immunodeficiency syndrome (AIDS) virus measures only 100 nanometers, and the flu virus is 1,016 nanometers in diameter.

Less than one mcg of the toxin that produces botulism can kill an adult. Experimentally, the mold aflatoxin B_1 at a level as low as 0.000000001 percent of the total diet was found to induce liver tumors in rats.

Agriculture. Agriculture also experiences profound effects from some substances at very low levels. Systemin, a plant peptide, is so potent that as little as one part in ten trillion can trigger a plant stress hormone.

Triacontanol (a simple alcohol compound derived from alfalfa) is a plant growth stimulant. Used in a concentration of only 4 milligrams (mg) per acre (roughly equivalent to 1.0 ounce being spread over 7,000 acres) results in a spectacular stimulation of plant growth.

Corn plant roots generally grow straight down. But when one side of a root is warmer than the other, it bends toward the warm side. The corn roots can detect differences in temperature as small as 0.09°F.

Our senses can be acute at extremely low levels. Our sense of smell is the most sensitive, being at least 100 times more discerning than our sense of taste.

Food Science. Generally, flavor components in foods are present from one to 100 ppb, but some are as low as parts per trillion (ppt). Of eight aromatic chemicals responsible for the pleasant flavor of tomato paste, we can detect one aromatic chemical (beta-damascenone) at less than 100 ppb. This potency is equivalent to a single pinch of salt to season 1,000 tons of potato chips.

Modern-day van Leeuwenhoeks . . . widen our boundaries of understanding of the infinitesimally small, in contrast to the explorations of the outward vast reaches of the universe.

We can smell the volatile compound pyrazine in bell peppers at levels as low as one ppt, and the rancidity of fatty acids at a level of about one mg per quart of water.

Chocolate contains some 400 flavor compounds, and we can taste two of the most important classes of these compounds at parts per million (ppm). Slight differences in their concentrations give different chocolates their distinctive flavors.

The sweet, light flavor of good-quality fresh pineapple depends mainly on nine aromatic compounds. One (ethyl-

2methylbutanoate) is so potent that our noses detect it at 6 ppt—a level equivalent to six grams of sugar in an Olympic-size swimming pool.

Physiology. Time may be brief yet also result in profound effects. Catacholamine (a group of amino acids that have important physiological effects) can erupt from the surface of a single cell in a millionth of a second. Chemical bonds, such as those with free radicals, break and form in femtoseconds (quadrillionths of a second). Pulsar lasers can produce pulses that last 150 femtoseconds. Atoms shift positions in picoseconds (trillionths of a second), and quarks (subatomic particles) are thought to last only one billionth of one billionth of a second!

Modern-day van Leeuwenhoeks, in probing substances at ever-lower levels of activity, size, and time, widen our boundaries of understanding of the infinitesimally small, in contrast to the explorations of the outward vast reaches of the universe. As well as instructing many academic disciplines, knowledge of low levels has affected the regulation of food additives, pharmaceuticals, pesticides, environmental pollutants, and industrial chemicals.

WATER-SOLUBLE VITAMINS

Nutrients can have many different forms. Some are biologically more active than others. It is necessary to know how the body uses the different forms. Water-soluble vitamins are those that dissolve in aqueous solutions; fat-soluble ones, in fat.

Some forms are more bioavailable than others. Bioavailability is defined as "the proportion or the amount of an element in a nutrient medium that is potentially absorbable in a form that is metabolically active." Simply put, bioavailability measures the amount the body absorbs and utilizes. Not all nutrients are absorbed totally in the body.

Riboflavin (vitamin B_2). Laboratory tests, using U.S.

Pharmacopeia standard stomach intestinal juice, showed that pure synthetic riboflavin went into solution ten times faster than the same amount of riboflavin from yeast or liver. The sudden high serum value derived from a rapidly soluble substance such as synthetic riboflavin does not necessarily result in higher tissue absorption of the vitamin. It may exceed the kidney threshold, with the riboflavin merely excreted in the urine.

Niacin (vitamin B_3). In nature, niacin exists as the amide in nicotinamide adenine dinucleotide (NAD). Pure nicotinamide and niacin can be synthesized from the nicotine in tobacco. When nicotine is simplified by cracking open one of the rings, it becomes the valuable niacin.

Niacin, as nicotinic acid, has a cholesterol-reducing effect. It reduces triglycerides, total serum cholesterol, the undesirable low-density lipoproteins (LDLs), and increases the favorable high-density lipoproteins (HDLs). However, another form of niacin, niacinamide, is active as a vitamin but does not produce a cholesterol-reducing effect.

Two forms of niacin used to treat high cholesterol differ in their reactions, both in effectiveness and safety. The sustained release (SR) preparation is helpful in reducing total serum cholesterol and LDLs, but an immediate release (IR) preparation is favored for increasing HDLs.

At high levels, both SR and IR forms of niacin can lead to significant adverse effects. IR products are reported to have more side effects, possibly because the SR form has a slower absorption rate and lower peak serum values of niacin. However, the SR form of niacin can be toxic to the liver.

Niacin is used in schizophrenic therapy because, with this condition, there appears to be a failure to deliver sufficient NAD to the brain. For this purpose, nicotinic acid in niacin is useful; the niacinamide form is not. Also, the former form causes flushing; the latter does not.

Pyridoxine (vitamin B_6). Foods from animal sources have higher bioavailability of pyridoxine than those from plant sources. The active form of pyridoxine is pyridoxal phosphate.

Cyanocobalamin (vitamin B_{12}). Vitamin B_{12} probably has the most complex chemical composition of any vitamin. To date, the vitamin has defied attempts to be duplicated in the laboratory. However, it can be synthesized by means of fermentation, a process similar to that used in making antibiotics.

Cobalamins are related, structurally, to hemoglobin in the blood. A deficiency of vitamin B_{12} can cause anemia that, in turn, causes neurological disease, depression, and premature aging. Now, a specific cobalamin, the methylcobalamin form, is found effective against these health problems.

Folic Acid. The generic term "folate" represents different forms of this water-soluble component of the vitamin B complex: folic acid, folacin, and folinic acid. Folate is a complex chemical form of which the simple form—folic acid—is readily available in the body. Theoretically, folic acid can be obtained from foods rich in folates. However, studies show that blood concentrations in women who take folic acid supplements rise more than from those who depend on folic acid from folate-containing foods. About 85 percent of folic acid from supplements and fortified foods is absorbed by the body; only about 50 percent is absorbed from folates in foods. Much folate is lost from foods due to long storage, processing, and preparation. Also, folate-containing foods, especially vegetables, lose some folate due to exposures to light and heat.

Folic acid is well absorbed from the human gut, but the metabolic conversion process to the active form is fairly complex, and requires the presence of other B complex fractions: niacin and pyridoxine.

Oral folic acid generally is regarded as a nontoxic form for normal humans, but may cause neurological injury to

THE IMPORTANCE OF FORM

The importance of vitamin form was emphasized by Alexander Berglas from the Pasteur Institute: "In spite of the therapeutic value of synthetic vitamins in the treatment of certain diseases one should not believe that the mere ingestion of the pure synthetic vitamins, even if identical in chemical structure to the natural vitamins, necessarily has the same effect on our bodies as the consumption of vitamins in combination with their natural concomitants. The latter are not to be dismissed as 'excessive baggage' but must be thought of as the result of millions of years of evolution of optimal combinations."

patients with undiagnosed pernicious anemia. Synthetic folic acid can provoke allergic responses and epileptic convulsions, whereas folates from foods do not.

Folacin, or folic acid, is found in many kinds of food, but may be most bioavailable in milk. Milk contains folic acid, both in a free form and in a complex, with folate-binding proteins that mediate the absorption of folic acid in the intestine. Bound folic acid is absorbed more efficiently than free folic acid.

Folinic acid is the most stable of reduced folates. It is transported more readily into the central nervous system than folic acid. Also, folinic acid seems to be more efficient in enlarging body stores of the vitamin than folic acid. In human studies, red cell folate, regarded as a reliable indicator of folate body stores, was significantly higher in people given folinic acid than in those given folic acid.

Vitamin C. Frequently, "ascorbic acid" and "vitamin C" are used interchangeably. However, they differ in form and activity. Ascorbic acid consists solely of an isolated pure crystalline substance. Vitamin C, derived from foods, has accessory factors as well, including other vitamins, minerals, trace minerals, enzymes, coenzymes, and other nutrients. In combination with ascorbic acid, as well as with each other, these substances can exert marked effects and determine the degree to which the ascorbic acid in vitamin C is bioavailable. Some doctors have reported that naturally derived vitamins such as vitamin C are not likely to over-stimulate the glandular system as would the same amount from concentrated synthetic ones.

FAT-SOLUBLE VITAMINS

Previously, naturally derived vitamin E was rated 30 percent more active than synthetically derived vitamin E. A report, issued jointly in July 2000 by the Antioxidant Panel of the Food and Nutrition Board of the Institute of Medicine, and the National Academy of Sciences, noted that the difference is even greater than previously stated. Naturally derived vitamin E supplements have been found to be *twice* as potent as the synthetically derived ones.

Natural sources, from plants, are fully recognized and utilized by the body. Synthetic sources, from petroleum, contain some substances that the body does not recognize as vitamin E, and does not utilize.

The two different sources are distinguished on supplement labels: "D-alpha tocopherol" denotes that the product contains naturally derived vitamin E; "DL-tocopherol" denotes synthetically derived vitamin E. An easy way to remember the difference is to think that "D" delivers and "DL" delivers less.

One key difference is the structure of the two types. Natural vitamin E is a single stereoisomer.* Synthetic vitamin E is a mixture of eight stereoisomers in equal amounts, and only one is the same as the single stereoisomer found in natural vitamin E. The other seven stereoisomers have different molecular configurations, and less biological activity.

Maret Traber, Associate Professor at Oregon State Univeristy, found that natural vitamin E is 100 percent more bioavailable than the synthetic form. Also, Dr. Traber found something new. The body seems to discriminate between the two types, and favors retaining the natural form to use within the body, and excreting the synthetic form. In Traber's study, people given natural vitamin E retained about *twice* as much plasma tocopherol concentration as synthetic vitamin E.

Human urine shows significant differences. Almost three times as much of a degradation product of vitamin E was found in urine excreted from people who had been given a synthetic vitamin E supplement as those given a natural one. This finding suggests that the body prefers to bind the natural form to a tocopherol-binding protein in the liver before releasng it into circulation, but chooses to metabolize the synthetic form at a higher rate in order to excrete it rapidly from the body. Thus, the natural form is more efficient and effective, and preferred by the body.

Also, there are specific-binding proteins for natural vitamin E, but none for synthetic vitamin E. The binding proteins, present in the liver, bind the vitamin and help to transport it between membranes. This transfer protein binds to d-alpha-tocopherol, the natural form, in preference to other stereoisomers of vitamin E, and results in beneficial activity.

The two major forms of natural vitamin E are alpha and gamma tocopherol. They may have complementary antioxidant activity. The two forms differ only by the presence of

---

*Isomers are two or more substances, composed of the same elements in the same proportions, but different in properties due to the differences in their arrangement of atoms. Stereoisomers consist of a group of isomers whose molecules have the same number of atoms bonded to each other, but differ in the way the atoms are arranged in space.

The Body Can Distinguish

Studies show that the human body has the ability to distinguish strongly between natural and synthetic forms of vitamin E. Robert Acuff, Director of the Center for Nutrition Research at East Tennessee State University, reviewed numerous published studies comparing the two forms. Acuff concluded, "In the case of vitamin E, the natural form is clearly the one our bodies were designed to use."

• *Animal Studies with Vitamin E.* Numerous animal studies suggest the superiority of natural forms of vitamin E over synthetic ones. For example, in one study, six to twenty-four hours after rats were given natural vitamin E, they had four times as much tocopherol in their red blood cells as rats given the same quantity of synthetic vitamin E. (Tocopherol measurement in red blood cells indicates its amount in biological membranes.)

After rats were given natural vitamin E in acetate form (liquid form), the alpha tocopherol levels in red blood cells were four to six times higher than in rats given a similar amount of synthetic vitamin E in acetate form. There were favorable ratios, too, in all other tissues of the rats given natural vitamin E.

In studies with rainbow trout, tocopherol in the liver, kidney, spleen, and heart increased six to eighteen times more within the first four hours after administration, and were two to three times more, even eight to sixteen hours after the fish were fed natural vitamin E than fish given similar doses with synthetic vitamin E.

Other animal studies have also shown a greater and longer retention of vitamin E in certain tissues, with natural rather than synthetic forms of vitamin E. In one study, rats were fed a mixture of natural and synthetic vitamin E. The ratio of the natural form in the rats' bodies shifted rapidly to favor the natural form.

After ninety-six hours, the ratio of natural to synthetic vitamin E in body tissues was 3.2 greater in the heart muscle, and 1.9 greater in the liver. When the two types were given separately, after ninety-six hours, there was a 2.3-fold greater retention of the natural form of vitamin E in the liver, and a 2.6-fold greater retention in the heart muscle. In another trial, although the synthetic vitamin E was absorbed readily in the rats, over twenty-four hours it was excreted three times faster than natural vitamin E. In other rat studies, the tocopherols from natural sources were retained in tissues far longer than from synthetic sources. After thirty-two days, the ratio of the two types favored the tocopherols from natural sources, in the lung, liver, and brain, by 1.9, 1.2, and 3.2, respectively.

• *Human Studies with Vitamin E.* In humans, the relative bioavailability of natural versus synthetic vitamin E showed a twofold higher plasma concentration of the former than of the latter. This finding confirms earlier studies that showed the effects of various levels of natural vitamin E given to male adults who, intentionally, had been fed diets low in vitamin E for a period of fifty-four months. When synthetic vitamin E (also in acetate form) was given as a supplement to these vitamin E-depleted men, the supplement showed only half the biological potency displayed by a natural vitamin E (in acetate form) supplement given to the men.

Humans excrete a normal metabolite of vitamin E in urine. In studies, after ingesting equal amounts of natural and synthetic forms of vitamin E, the average total quantity of the metabolite from the synthetic form was approximately 2.7 times more than from the natural form. This finding was similar to those in animal studies, and demonstrates that the body attempts to excrete, rather than to use, the synthetic form.

an additional methyl group (an organic compound) in the alpha form. Of the two, the alpha form is the more potent antioxidant against free radicals in the body, and is present at much higher levels in blood plasma. It is the main form used in naturally derived vitamin E supplements. However, the less potent gamma form is the principal one in poor diets. Studies show that the two forms react differently with inflammatory agents. The alpha form is more helpful. (See "The Body Can Distinguish" on page 104.)

Vitamin D. Similarly, another fat-soluble vitamin, namely vitamin D*, differs, depending on its form. Two types of vitamin D are found in nature. Vitamin D_2 is found in plants, and vitamin D_3 in animal foods. Both forms have been used successfully in treating rickets and other conditions related to vitamin D deficiency.

The molecular structure of synthetic and natural forms of vitamin D_2 and D_3 are identical. Both can be toxic if consumed in excessive amounts. However, vitamin D, obtained from foods or by sunlight through the skin, is accompanied by various metabolites or isomers that may have biological benefits. As many as a dozen of these substances have been identified in the vitamin D present in animal foods. (Metabolites are substances produced by metabolism. Isomers are two or more substances, composed of the same elements and in the same proportions, but that are not the same, due to different atomic arrangements.)

Vitamin D is essential for the efficient use of calcium in

---

*Classifying vitamins A and D as vitamins is controversial. Vitamin A (retinol) is synthesized in the body from beta-carotene, a photosynthetic plant pigment in food. Some contend that beta-carotene is the vitamin. Regarding vitamin D, its action is more like that of a steroid hormone than of a vitamin. It is synthesized in the body from cholesterol and activated by sunlight.

the body. But vitamin D supplements are ineffective if the body has lost its ability to convert them to an active form.

Vitamin D may be activated by more than twenty different plant sterols, substances closely related to cholesterol. The major precursor, sterol-7-dehydrocholesterol, is synthesized in the body. The precursor sterol is found on the skin. When the skin is exposed to shortwave ultraviolet light—such as sunlight—the sterol manufactures vitamin D. The irradiated sterol-7-dehydrocholesterol must be chemically modified further in the liver, and later in the kidney, to form 1,25,dihydroxy-7-dehydrocholesterol. Actually, this compound is the active form of vitamin D, which acts on the tissues in the body.

Vitamin D_3 (cholecalciferol) is produced in humans in layers under the skin's surface. It is absorbed by the body after exposure to sunshine. Also, it is found in activated animal sterols and in eggs, fish, and fish oils.

Synthetic vitamin D (calciferol) is prepared by irradiating ergosterol, a vegetable sterol, to develop vitamin D activity. This form of vitamin D is recognized on labels by the phrase "irradiated ergosterol."

After vitamin D was synthesized in the 1920s, food processors began to fortify many products. Because the body can store all forms of vitamin D for long periods and accumulate them to toxic levels, such fortification was dangerous. This vitamin must be consumed in moderation. Infants are especially at risk of developing hypercalcemia (excessive calcium in the blood) from too much vitamin D. During the period of uncontrolled food fortification with vitamin D, numerous cases of infant hypercalcemia were reported.

By 1957, food fortification with vitamin D was reduced substantially in Great Britain.

In the 1960s, the Food and Drug Administration (FDA) reviewed the issue. Finally, in 1972, the agency proposed to limit the level of vitamin D in products in order to prevent toxicity.

Vitamin A. Vitamin A is also fat-soluble. (See footnote on page 106.) When this vitamin is taken into a cell, it is oxidized to retinic acid, and then diffuses into the cell's nucleus, where it binds to one of several specific receptors.

The term "vitamin A" is used for retinoids that exhibit the biological activity of retinol. Although adequate amounts of vitamin A are vital for health, excessive amounts are toxic. Yet its precursors, carotenoids, are not toxic even if they are consumed in large amounts from foods.

Retinol from animal products is stored in the liver, from which it is distributed as a protein complex to various organs. Also, vitamin A is formed from pro-vitamin carotenoids.

Nearly all retinyl esters (from animal tissues) are converted enzymatically to retinol in the intestinal lumen (the inner open space) before they are absorbed by the intestinal walls. Carotenoids are converted partially to retinol before they are absorbed.

A synthetic vitamin A-like substance (13-*cis*-retinoic acid) has been found helpful to prevent certain types of cancers. This substance is in a family of compounds called retinoids, which may help prevent cancers by slowing the growth of premalignant cells.

PROTEINS, FATS, AND CARBOHYDRATES

The plane of a beam of polarized light rotates in all natural substances, either to the left (L-form, from the word "levorotary") or to the right (D-form, from the word "dextrorotary"). A substance composed of equal D- and L-forms (DL-form) is optically inactive. (See "chirality" on page 118.)

Protein. Food proteins as well as proteins in the human body contain only L-forms of amino acids, the building blocks of protein. The body possesses only L-enzymes to metabolize the amino acids. L-form amino acids are absorbed immediately in the digestive system by the L-enzymes, but delayed if the D- or DL-forms are consumed. The body cannot utilize DL- amino acids efficiently. Under certain conditions, the body may split the DL-form of amino acids, use the L-form, but have difficulty using the D-form. Problems arise in the intestine in trying to absorb and utilize the wrong amino acid form. The body attempts to get rid of it as quickly as possible. The correct form is transported by enzymatic reactions; the incorrect D-form requires some diffusion process. Thus, the L-form is relatively active and selectively absorbed by the body. The D-form forces its way by means of osmosis. Despite this problem with the DL-form of amino acids, some food processors use it to boost protein foods of low biological value, and it is used in animal feed supplements.

Another distinction between amino acids is whether they are in a bound form or a free form. For example, the amino acid, glutamate, acts differently when it is bound to proteins in foods such as mushrooms, beef, or tomatoes, from when it is in a free state, such as in monosodium glutamate, the flavor enhancer. This amino acid, in bound form, is benign. In its free form, it is a neuroexcitor of the brain and central nervous system. At a high level, it is a neurotoxin.

Some foods, such as soybeans, contain the amino acids, lysine and alanine. Treating soybeans with heat and alkali causes the amino acids to crosslink into a structurally different form, lysinoalanine (LAL). This new form is unnatural and toxic, especially to the kidneys. LAL in a free state is even more toxic than when it is bound to protein. LAL forms in the proteins extracted from soybeans and made into numerous soybean analogs used in meat substitutes, baby formulas, corn chips, nondairy creamers, and nondairy whipped toppings.

Genistein, an isoflavone (a plant constituent with estrogenlike activity) found in soy, acquires different chemical forms, depending on its soy source. Not all forms are absorbed the same way in the digestive tract. Soy foods such as full-fat soymilk and tofu, processed in a hot water leaching step, contain different genistein conjugates (substances paired together) than other soy products. Because of their different conjugations, different forms of soy produce different effects. Genistein is absorbed in different places within the digestive tract, depending on the conjugations. These differences are crucial. For example, soy's reported role in preventing stomach cancer may depend on whether the chosen form of soy is one that is not absorbed in the upper gut.

Fat. The distinct differences in forms of fat is best illustrated by comparing the fatty acid composition of butter and margarine. The *cis* form of fatty acids, naturally present in butter, is converted to *trans* form in margarine. This conversion is achieved by the hydrogenation process.

As early as 1957, Dr. Hugh Sinclair, from the Laboratory of Human Nutrition at Oxford University, reported that hydrogenated fats induced a deficiency of essential fatty acids (EFAs) by destroying them or by producing abnormal, toxic, fatty acids with an antiEFA effect.

Shortly after, Franklin Bicknell, M.D. (co-author of the prestigious book, *The Vitamins in Medicine,* Lee Foundation for Nutritional Research, 1953), described how hydrogenated fat forms new molecular structures that are inappropriate in the human diet. The atoms of the molecules of EFA are arranged in space in a particular manner. Hydrogenation produces a different spatial arrangement, and a completely abnormal fatty acid. Bicknell compared the different spatial arrangements to ordinary handwriting and mirror handwriting. Although identical, they differ spatially. At best, reading the latter is difficult; at worst, serious mistakes may be made. Using this analogy, Bicknell suggested that, similarly, mistakes are made by the body when abnormal EFAs are presented. Not only does the body fail to benefit from them, but it is deluded by their similarity to normal EFAs, and attempts to use them. The body attempts to incorporate the wrong EFAs in biochemical reactions, but discovers that their shape is wrong. Unfortunately, the reaction has gone too far to jettison them. They are not only useless, but they prevent the use of normal EFAs.

Hydrogenation produces a different spatial arrangement, and a completely abnormal fatty acid.

Carbohydrates. Carbohydrates differ. Simple ones are found in fruits and vegetables, as well as in table sugar; complex ones, in potatoes and whole grains.

The normal geometric arrangement of sugar is "right-rotating" (D-form). During evolution, humans developed enzymes capable of metabolizing right-rotating sugar molecules, but not left-rotating ones. Although right- and left-rotating sugars may have identical components, the former is digested and caloric; the latter is not digested and noncaloric. These differences are being examined for the possible creation of a left-rotating product that would be a noncaloric sugar.

Some nutrients are obtained more readily and efficiently by cooking them rather than eating them raw. For example, raw broccoli was found to be 20 percent less effective in raising vitamin C levels in the blood than when the vegetable was cooked. The high-fiber contents of vegetables such as broccoli, cauliflower, and carrot are locked into a matrix of fiber and protein that are not broken down readily by chewing. Brief cooking breaks down their protein and fibers, and makes the nutrients more readily absorbed and utilized. At the same time, brief cooking retains other valuable nutrients present in the vegetables.

Fiber is a general term for a variety of substances of different chemical and physical forms and functions. The physical form of the fiber may be especially important. When fiber is cooked, pureed, or otherwise broken up or softened, it loses some of its characteristic effects on the human body.

Knowing the effects of food on blood sugar metabolism is important for maintaining good health. It is especially important for diabetics. The glycemic index rates foods according to their benefit for managing glucose. The lower the foods appear on the list, the more desirable they are in managing glucose. Whole grain foods are low on the list. When grains are ground into flour, they are higher on the list. For example, ground rice flour produces a far greater glucose and insulin response than does whole rice. Wheat in bread or cereal is lower on the list than wheat in pasta.

MINERALS

Minerals have many forms. It is important to recognize the differences, especially in choosing supplements. Calcium, for example, may appear in supplements as calcium ascorbate, citrate, carbonate, gluconate, lactate, or tricalcium phosphate. How do they differ?

Calcium. Calcium carbonate contains the highest amount of elemental calcium, which makes it possible to concentrate calcium in a small pill. By contrast, calcium lactate requires a larger number of pills to get the same amount of elemental calcium. However, the latter form is well absorbed. Calcium citrate is readily absorbed, and frequently is used to fortify fruit juice products. Calcium gluconate requires a large number of pills to obtain sufficient elemental calcium. Generally, calcium from bone meal or dolomite should be avoided because of possible contamination with lead and other toxic metals.

Regardless of the calcium supplement form, its degree of bioavailability depends on the individual's calcium status. The more calcium taken in from the diet, the less calcium will be absorbed from a supplement.

All calcium preparations are similar in their solubility at the level of pH in the stomach. They have high absorption, from 85 to 90 percent. At the higher pH level in the small intestine, differences in absorption depend on the form. Calcium gluconate and tricalcium phosphate are 40 percent bioavailable. Both calcium phosphate and calcium carbonate are only 20 percent bioavailable.

Magnesium. Among various forms of magnesium in supplements are magnesium alginate, carbonate, chloride, citrate, gluconate, malate, orotate, oxide, and sulfate. The human body absorbs the chemical form of magnesium in water more readily than magnesium in food. Magnesium chloride is highly soluble and absorbable. So, too, is magnesium citrate. Both magnesium carbonate and magnesium oxide are relatively insoluble and not as readily absorbed by the body.

Commonly used products, especially over-the-counter medications, contain various forms of magnesium, such as milk of magnesia, Epsom salts and other laxatives, and antacids. Intake of such forms of magnesium needs to be limited in order to avoid excessive magnesium intake from various forms other than from foods.

Iron. Iron is in many forms, and they vary in the degree to which they are absorbed. The ferrous forms are absorbed more efficiently than the ferric forms. Also, the ferrous forms do not react unfavorably with vitamin E, as do the ferric forms.

About 50 percent of iron is absorbed from ferrous chloride, ferrous gluconate, and ferrous sulfate; 40 percent from ferrous orthophosphate; 10 percent from ferric phosphorate; and only 5 percent from ferric orthophosphate.

Heme and nonheme iron are the two major forms of iron in foods. The heme forms are ferrous and ferric. The nonheme forms are ferritin and hemosiderin.

All of the iron found in plant foods (grains, seeds, legumes, and produce) is *solely* in the nonheme form. Plants contain *no* heme iron. Animal foods contain heme iron. About 13 to 30 percent of heme iron is absorbed by the body; only about 3 to 8 percent of nonheme iron is absorbed.

Lactoferrin, a milk protein, helps maintain iron solubility in the intestinal tract, and increases the concentration of bioavailable iron. A protein, duadenal cytochrome b, can reduce dietary iron into a form that can be transported across the gut wall.

During digestion, the two separate iron pools of heme and nonheme iron are used. They are absorbed differently, and at different rates. The amount of iron absorbed is not so much affected by the iron present in the food, as it is regulated by the individual's needs. Individuals with adequate iron stores absorb less iron than those whose iron stores are low or deficient. Heme iron is absorbed much faster than nonheme iron.

Selenium. Selenium, an essential mineral, has different forms. Selenomethionine, present in grains and some meats, is converted, by a long and complex process, to methyl senenol. It is easier to convert selenium salts—the forms used in supplements. However, at high levels, selenium salts can be toxic.

Different forms of selenium offer various types of protection against disease. The inorganic forms—sodium selenite, sodium selenate, and selenium dioxide—help protect against tumor development. The organic form, selenomethionine, does not. However, this form is effective in raising human blood levels of selenium.

Foods contain selenium in different biochemical forms,

and the body uses them differently. Garlic, broccoli, and Brussels sprouts store selenium methyl selenocysteine (SeMSC). The body snips off the end of this amino acid to produce an anticancer agent, methyl selenol. Broccoli, grown in selenium-containing soil, can accumulate substantial amounts of SeMSC. At present, California broccoli may have up to fifty times more selenium than average broccoli because the water used to irrigate California broccoli is naturally high in selenium. Plant breeders are trying to produce selenium-containing broccoli with 100 to 200 times more selenium than that found in the California broccoli.

Chromium. Inorganic chromium compounds must be converted by the body to a biologically active form in order for chromium to perform its functions. Hexavalent chromium is toxic; trivalent chromium is useful and essential for both humans and animals.

Plants can absorb the toxic form and convert it, mainly in their root system, to the nontoxic form within only a few hours. By the time the chromium enters the shoots and leaves, it is in the nontoxic form. Plants that have been shown to take up the chromium and convert its form include broccoli, cauliflower, cabbage, lettuce, spinach, cucumber, radish, tomato, and cantaloupe. The mechanism of plant biotransformation insures a safer supply of essential trace minerals such as chromium than does ingesting inorganic salts of this mineral, found in commercially available supplements.

TOXIC ELEMENTAL METALS

Some essential nutritional elements such as arsenic, chromium, iron, cobalt, molybdenum, and selenium are toxic at high levels or in different forms. Other elements, widely distributed in the environment, do not appear to have nutritional value, but can enter the human body through food, water, or air. The degree of toxicity may depend on form.

Methyl and Tetraethyl Forms. When a metal is methylated (combined with a methyl group) it becomes more toxic. The metal also can be ethylated (combined with an ethyl group). Tetraethyl lead, the gasoline additive, is at least 100 times as toxic as elemental lead. Tetraethyl tin is highly toxic, whereas elemental tin is not. Methyl mercury is fifty times more toxic than elemental mercury. Methyl mercury is only slightly water-soluble but remains in fat and nerve tissues, as well as in the brain, fourteen times as long as elemental mercury. Methyl and ethyl mercury can damage the brain permanently when food is contaminated with these forms, at levels of 20 to 40 parts per million (ppm) of mercury.

An incident in Minamata Bay, Japan, was a dramatic example of the toxicity of the methyl form of mercury. Mercury wastes from industry were spewed into the bay. The mercury, converted by bacteria, formed methyl mercury. Fish became contaminated with the toxic form. People who ate the fish were damaged severely, especially the offspring of pregnant women.

Organic and Inorganic Forms. Organic lead is more toxic than inorganic lead.* Inorganic compounds of tin are not toxic, but alkyl tin is highly toxic. Inorganic nickel shortens the lifespan of rats.

Plutonium, an extremely toxic man-made fuel for nuclear power, is converted in soil to a more soluble form that concentrates in plant roots. Plutonium metal, exposed to air, oxidizes slowly to form plutonium oxide. Particles from this form can lodge in the lungs, enter the bloodstream, and become deposited in bone or liver. Plutonium oxide is weakly soluble in water. Ingested in food or water, a small

*The terms "organic" and "inorganic," as used here, are not related to farming practices. They have chemical meanings. Organic is matter made mainly from carbon, hydrogen, oxygen nitrogen, sulfur, and phosphorus. Inorganic matter is mineral. It is neither animal nor vegetable.

fraction is absorbed into the gastrointestinal tract. Over time, as little as a few millionths of a gram can cause cancer.

Arsenic is present in organic and inorganic forms. Organic arsenic is excreted rapidly by the kidneys, with no excessive accumulation. It has low toxicity. The inorganic form accumulates in the body and is highly toxic.

Some bacteria, yeasts, fungi, and molds can reduce elemental arsenic to toxic arsene gas.

Inorganic arsenic is a naturally occurring element in the earth's crust and is released into groundwater. It is the form thought most likely to cause human cancers of skin and lungs.

Iron and aluminum in the soil bind and detoxify inorganic arsenic. Inorganic arsenics have no value as growth stimulants in feeding poultry or swine, and they are not permitted in feeds.

Inorganic arsenic is used as a wood preservative, and in lead arsinate and lead arsinite insecticides.

Arsenic at levels of 20 ppm does not seem to have an appreciable effect on aquatic life. Anaerobic (able to live without air) bacteria may convert part of it to a gaseous state (hydride arsine) or to an organic gas (methylarsine). Everywhere, seafood contains 2 to 8 ppm of arsine, so the fish must be storing it in a nontoxic form in their phospholipid fatty tissues.

Methyl mercury is only slightly water-soluble but remains in fat and nerve tissues, as well as in the brain, fourteen times as long as elemental mercury.

Natural concentrations of arsenic in foods usually are absorbed rapidly, but also excreted rapidly. What is absorbed is transported to various organs in the following order: first, to the blood; then, to the kidneys, liver, spleen, skin, and hair; and last, to the nails. Some arsenic may remain in the tissues long after it is out of the blood, urine, and feces. Accumulated arsenic becomes a source of physiological dysfunction.

In medieval times, assassination by poison was a frequent occurrence. Bezoar stones—calcified masses of partly digested hairs in goats' digestive tracts—were placed in wine to remove any arsenic that might have been added, deliberately to poison. The bezoar was supposed to render the wine harmless.

Phosphates and Arsenate Forms. Studies at the Scripps Institute of Oceanography found that bezoar stones actually do make arsenic harmless. The finding may offer a clue to control arsenic pollution and poisoning of marine algae. These microscopic plants, in tropical waters, have evolved resistance to arsenic because the water in which they live contains similar amounts of phosphates and arsenates. Algae that need to absorb phosphates absorb the arsenates along with the phosphates. The phosphates buffer the toxicity of the arsenates. Cooler waters are much richer in phosphates than in arsenates, so the algae are not forced to absorb the arsenates present. Arsenates and arsenites are the two forms usually found contaminating ground waters.

PHARMACEUTICALS AND PESTICIDES

Chirality has become an important feature in the manufacture of pharmaceuticals and pesticides. Chirality can be understood simply. Look at your hands. The left one is similar to the right one, but is not the same spatially. They are mirror images, or chiral forms. In chirality, the structural characteristics of a molecule make it possible to superimpose it on its mirror image.

Louis Pasteur discovered molecular chirality. He found that life is based on L (left) form rather than D (right) form proteins, and D-form rather than L-form sugars. He noted that, with tartaric acid, the isomers (chemically identical substances) had remarkably different optical properties as a result of seemingly insignificant differences of structure. The two crystal forms were D- and L-tartaric acid.

Pasteur found that in fermentation, certain yeasts metabolized only right-handed tartaric acid. He concluded that the left- or right-handedness of the biosphere derived from a fundamental chiral force in nature.

How Life Acquired Chirality. Since then, we have learned that natural sugars are almost exclusively right-handed; natural amino acids, left-handed. Also, we now recognize that DNA normally spirals to the right. These findings confirm Pasteur's idea about a fundamental chiral form in nature and have caused much speculation by scientists who attempt to explain how life acquired chirality. Various hypotheses suggest astronomical, electromagnetic, or nuclear forces. One popular idea relates chirality to rays of circularly polarized light from supernovae (exploded stars that are short-lived, very bright, and produce much energy). Their light waves fly in a corkscrew pattern and spin either clockwise or counterclockwise. Such spinning skews chemical reactions and produces one chiral molecule at the expense of its twin.

Another suggestion is that a weak nuclear force governs the radioactive decay of a neutron (a subatomic particle) in the nucleus of an atom into a proton (a stable, positive, electrically charged subatomic particle) and an electron (a stable, negative, electrically charged subatomic particle), and the force has handedness. The decay always produces an electron with a left-handed spin. Because the weak nuclear force is the only fundamental chiral force in nature, it is linked to the handedness of bio-molecules.

A modern version of Pasteur's idea is that a nonsymmetric property of matter, discovered by particle physicists, accounts for the customary inclination toward a preference for certain enantiomers over others. Enantiomers are pairs of molecules that are mirror images of each other, but not identical. They are the different chiral forms. However, many biochemists believe that the appearance of specific "enantiomers" emerged by chance at some critical point in evolution.

Pharmaceuticals. Chirality has practical applications in drug manufacture. By 1998, of the top 100 drugs sold worldwide, half were single enantiomers. By 2000, 40 percent of all dosage-form drugs were single enantiomers. They include drugs for cardiovascular and central nervous system disorders (anxiety, depression, attention-deficit), digestive disorders (irritable bowel, heartburn), pulmonary disorders (asthma, emphysema, chronic obstructive pulmonary disease), noninsulin-dependent diabetes, urinary incontinence, benign enlargement of the prostate gland, erectile ejaculatory dysfunction, and obesity, as well as antiviral and anticancer drugs.

Sometimes, drug activity is present only in one enantiomer; the other is inactive. Or, one has side effects. An example is the left-hand form of albuterol (used by asthmatics), which does not have the side effects inflicted by the right-hand form. Another example is dopamine. Only its left-hand form is useful for Parkinson's disease. Or, take thalidomide, the drug that had been banned because of its tragic teratogenic (capable of causing malformations in a developing embryo or fetus) effects in infants. More recent research showed that thalidomide's safe enantiomer may have several beneficial applications. The drug can decrease concentrations of a molecule in the blood that aggravates conditions such as rheumatoid arthritis, tuberculosis, and AIDS. In AIDS patients, thalidomide helps prevent weight loss, canker sores, and inhibits AIDS virus replication. Other studies show thalidomide curbs the growth of blood vessels that nourish malignant tumors and lessens inflammation and flareups in the skin of patients with Hansen's disease (leprosy).

Single enantiomers are not always safer. For example, sepracor, the single right-handed isomer of the antidepressant, fluoxetine (Prozac), is metabolized at a very different rate from fluoxetine. The right-handed isomer is only 25 percent as effective as fluoxetine circulating in the blood. When tested to achieve an equivalent response to fluoxetine, Sepracor affected the heart adversely. The manufacturer terminated licensing and development agreements to manufacture the single-isomer version of Prozac.

Pesticides. Pesticide manufacturers, too, are using chirality to produce more efficient and safer pesticides by using single enantiomer versions of some pesticides. Manufacturers can select the active form and eliminate its inactive mirror image in the final product.

Currently, about one-fourth of all commercial pesticides are chiral. One form may kill pests but leave nontargeted biological organisms unharmed. Studies showed that soils from warmed sites harbor pests that prefer one pesticide twin, while those from adjacent unheated sites prefer the other form. In some cases, organic fertilizer triggered a breakdown of the twin that previously it did not, due to altered environmental conditions. This change was found especially in soils treated with long-lasting insecticides and herbicides. These findings show that studies, if conducted with a mix of enantiomers, may yield unreliable results. More studies are needed with chirality in pesticides.

Investigations of environmental carcinogens, too, have shown that different enantiomers can have radically different biological effects. For example, the polycyclic aromatic hydrocarbons (PAHs) have about two dozen different structures, which may explain the vast differences in the carcinogenic potential found in this class of compounds. Mirror-image isomers of many PAH metabolites actually bind to DNA so that the adducts (chemical additional products) point in opposite directions. An example is the metabolite of benzo(*a*)pyrene, an important and widespread environmental carcinogen found in many substances, including automobile exhaust, cigarette smoke, and heavily grilled meat. The molecule is metabolized in the body to different forms. One enantiomer induces tumor formations; its mirror image does not.

HOW WELL DO WE ABSORB NUTRIENTS?

Nutrients from foods are not absorbed entirely. Actually, there is a wide range of absorption, determined by many factors. The amount absorbed may depend on the form of the nutrient, or other nutrients present that either increase or decrease its absorption. Or nutrient absorption may depend on factors such as efficient functioning of the gastrointestinal system, lifestyle, medications, supplements, health problems, or age. The extent of nutrient absorption may differ if food is consumed raw or cooked, or if the nutrient is derived from food or from a nutritional supplement.

The official recommended intake of nutrients acknowledges the fact that a nutrient may not be released readily from food during digestion, or may not be absorbed efficiently. The bioavailability (the degree to which a substance is absorbed and utilized) of vitamins and minerals varies greatly from food to food. To establish official recommendations for intake from the limited information available about most nutrients, an estimate is made, and then an average value is established for the bioavailability of a nutrient from the major food sources in the diet. To compensate for low bioavailability, the recommended intake is increased.

Differences in estimating bioavailability result in a lack of uniformity in official recommended intakes in different countries. Human requirements do not differ from place to place, but food availability and food habits differ. An example is dietary iron. In many Western countries, much of the iron intake is in the form of heme iron (from meat and other animal foods) that is well absorbed. Heme iron absorption is estimated to be about 20 to 25 percent. In countries where most of the iron is in the nonheme form from plant foods such as beans, iron absorption may be as low as 2 to 8 percent. Because of this disparity, there may be a two-to-three-fold difference in the recommended allowances for iron in different countries. For example, in Canada, where heme iron intake is high, 14 milligrams (mg) of iron daily are recommended for women. In India, where nonheme iron intake is high, 32 mg of iron daily are recommended for women.

Currently, there is much interest in carotene. Even with normal diets, its absorption from foods is limited. The carotene in green leafy vegetables is far better absorbed than from red or yellow vegetables. Yet even with good absorption more than half is excreted, unabsorbed.

Any condition that impairs fat absorption also impairs absorption of fat-soluble vitamins, such as vitamin A, as well as carotene. Adequate bile levels may be necessary for carotene absorption.

Some Nutrients Increase Absorption. Nonheme iron from plant foods consists mainly of iron salts. Its absorption is influenced by its solubility in the upper part of the small intestine, which in turn depends on how the composition of the entire meal affects iron solubility. For example, nonheme iron absorption from a meal containing some animal protein foods, such as meat, fish, or poultry, is about four times greater than if the major protein source is from equivalent portions of milk, cheese, or eggs. Iron absorption tends to be poor from meals in which whole grain cereals and legumes (beans) predominate. However, the addition of even relatively small amounts of a heme iron source of food substantially increases iron absorption from the total meal.

Another nutrient that increases iron absorption is vitamin C (ascorbic acid), which keeps the mineral soluble and available for absorption in the duodenum where the pH (acid-alkaline balance) is normally alkaline. For example, orange juice consumed with other foods increases nonheme iron absorption.

Additional beneficial nutrient relationships follow:

- Magnesium helps to convert thiamine to its biologically active form.
- Phosphorus intake strongly enhances the metabolism of vitamin B.
- Copper absorption averages only about 30 percent of the intake. Absorption is increased by acids. Copper is absorbed in the stomach and the duodenum.
- Selenium and vitamin E enhance each other. Their respective mechanisms of action are closely related. A deficiency of one may be relieved by the other.
- Absorption of vitamin A is improved when emulsified. Vitamin A is well absorbed in milk because the fat is emulsified in the liquid.
- Vitamin D promotes calcium absorption and facilitates magnesium absorption in the intestine.
- Calcium absorption requires the presence of bile salts, bile, and adequate but not excessive dietary fat. Calcium must be soluble to be absorbed. Acids, such as the stomach's hydrochloric acid, as well as ascorbic and citric acids, and some amino acids, such as glycine and lysine, can increase calcium's solubility and thus increase its absorption. Lactose, the milk sugar, also helps the absorption of calcium from milk.

Some Nutrients Decrease Absorption. Some nutrients, especially if taken in excess, can decrease the absorption of other nutrients. For example, excessive calcium decreases the absorption of iron, phosphorus, magnesium, zinc, and manganese. Excessive calcium also may interfere with vitamin K synthesis and/or its absorption.

- High intake of phosphorus-rich foods, such as meats, grains, potatoes, and soft drinks or other manufactured foods to which phosphorous compounds are added, decrease calcium absorption.
- Inorganic iron is antagonistic to vitamin E. The inorganic iron combines with vitamin E in the gut and renders the vitamin inactive. This form of iron is found in fortified cereals, enriched flours, and in mineral supplements.
- Zinc absorption can be decreased by excessive calcium, copper, folic acid, iron, and phytates.
- Copper absorption can be decreased by excessive zinc or calcium. Copper availability is inhibited by molybdenum in combination with sulfate, which blocks absorption and/or increases its excretion.
- Excessive dietary fiber decreases the absorption of calcium and zinc.
- Oxalates and phytates, naturally occurring compounds present in many plant foods, decrease the absorption of minerals, such as calcium and zinc.
- Iron absorption is decreased by soy, coffee, or tea.
- Excessive sugar consumption decreases calcium absorption and increases the urinary loss of chromium.
- Excessive fat consumption decreases calcium and magnesium.
- A high intake of vitamin E may reduce the intestinal

absorption of vitamin K, and decrease the effectiveness of this vitamin in its role as a blood coagulant.

Lifestyle Factors. Caffeine intake decreases absorption of calcium, magnesium, phosphorus, potassium, and sodium. Increased excretion of these minerals is in the urine.

Alcohol intake is especially damaging to the mucosal lining of the intestine and contributes to deficiencies of many nutrients. In the alcoholic, absorption, especially of thiamine and folic acid, is impaired due to decreased intestinal function. Other depleted nutrients include other vitamin B fractions, such as riboflavin (B_2), niacin (B_3), pyridoxine (B_6), and vitamin B_{12} (cyanocobalamin), as well as vitamin C, fatty acids, and electrolytes.

Smoking reduces calcium absorption. Also, it reduces substantially the possibility of absorbing calcium from a nutritional supplement.

Undue physical and emotional stresses can reduce calcium absorption and result in unexplained dumping of calcium in the intestinal tract. In times of worry and tension, fecal calcium excretion may be twice that of the dietary intake. Ascorbic acid, too, is lost by undue stress.

Over-the-Counter Drugs. Mineral oil, used to relieve constipation, hinders the absorption of fat-soluble vitamins A, D, E, K, as well as beta-carotene. In tests, mineral oil, given in large doses along with vitamin A, interfered with absorption of the vitamin. Much of the vitamin A was dissolved in the mineral oil, rendered unavailable, and excreted. Beta-carotene, too, dissolves in mineral oil and becomes unavailable for absorption. Other laxatives may cause calcium and vitamin D losses.

Antacids, from magnesium and aluminum hydroxide compounds, can impair calcium absorption. The pH of the small intestine is altered by antacids and, in turn, decreases absorption of folic acid and vitamin B_{12}.

A Special Case

Vitamin D has a unique method for absorption. By exposing the human skin to the sun, this vitamin can be absorbed, provided ample time is allowed for the fat on the skin to help absorb the vitamin. Swimming or showering directly after exposure to sunshine, for example, interferes with vitamin D's absorption from sun exposure.

In the animal kingdom, birds obtain vitamin D by preening themselves with oil from the preen glands of their beaks and spreading it over their feathers that have been exposed to the sun. Removal of the preen glands makes birds more susceptible to rickets, a vitamin D deficiency disease. Similarly, the fur of animals appears to be a place where vitamin D is formed. Rats prevented from licking their fur become deficient in vitamin D. The incessant washing of cats for cleanliness, or the practice of monkeys grooming each other to hunt for fleas, also may provide a means of obtaining enough vitamin D to meet their requirements.

We absorb vitamin D, too, from foods of animal origin, and from fortified foods. Vitamin D has been shown to be well absorbed from nutritional supplements.

Prescription Drugs. Drugs can affect nutrient absorption in different ways, by absorbing the nutrient, impairing its absorption, or changing its characteristics. The nutrient may be rendered insoluble, or have its pH altered. These changes may result in nutrient malabsorption by producing maldigestion, or impair the functioning of the mucosa lining. (See the article "Mixing Foods and Drugs" on page 75.)

Health Problems. Some diseases may decrease or delay absorption of nutrients. For example, evidence of decreased absorption of vitamin A is based on its level found stored in the blood of a living patient, or measured in the liver after death.

Chronic constipation impairs absorption of vitamin A and carotene.

Vitamin C is absorbed from the small intestine. A number of foodborne pathogens, such as *Salmonella* and *Escherichia coli,* not only result in food poisoning, but also decompose vitamin C. In patients with gastrointestinal problems, such pathogens prevent vitamin C absorption.

Abnormal conditions in the intestinal tract, such as diarrhea, decrease arterial absorption of ascorbic acid, even when this vitamin is administered in high dosages. Also, vitamin C absorption may be impaired in patients with achlorhydria (an absence of a normal supply of hydrochloric acid from gastric secretions).

Any health condition that impairs fat absorption also impairs absorption of vitamin A and carotene.

Riboflavin is not absorbed readily by patients with gastrointestinal diseases. This vitamin is absorbed from the intestine and requires hydrochloric acid for its absorption. However, injected riboflavin is utilized by patients with gastrointestinal diseases. Given intravenously, most of the riboflavin goes into the small intestine, especially the duodenum, from where it can be reabsorbed. Most riboflavin is destroyed in the large intestine and in its passage through the kidney.

Individuals who lack bile in the intestine due to poor secretion of bile salts or obstructive jaundice (due to stones, cancer, or abnormal narrowing of a duct or passage) may have poor intestinal absorption of vitamin K.

Age. The age of an individual may play a role in nutrient absorption. For example, by examining fecal excretions, it has been found that vitamin A is poorly absorbed in infants, but well absorbed in adults. Also, infants and children absorb or convert carotene very poorly.

The gastrointestinal tract of children differs from adults in permeability, pH, transit time, and enzymatic activity. Children may absorb nutrients well or poorly, depending on the balance of these factors.

Calcium absorption is affected, in part, by the body's needs during different periods. If the need is low, calcium absorption from the intestine may be low. During periods of growth, pregnancy, and lactation, calcium needs are high and its absorption may increase greatly.

Iron absorption, like calcium, is affected, in part, by the body's needs during different periods. If iron stores are low, which is common for most women and children, the intestinal mucosa readily takes up iron and increases the proportion absorbed from the diet. Conversely, high iron stores, typical of men and post-menopausal women, reduce the percentage of iron absorbed, which helps prevent iron overload.

The elderly may experience impaired B_{12} and calcium absorption in the intestine, as well as other nutrients. As people age, many systems may function less efficiently than when they were younger.

Raw vs. Cooked Foods. It might be assumed that more nutrients are absorbed from raw than from cooked foods because the heat and pressure of cooking destroys certain nutrients. This assumption is true for some, but not for all, foods. Antinutrients, present in some raw foods, are deactivated by cooking, and make nutrients available for absorption. For example, tests showed that less vitamin C was obtained from raw than from cooked broccoli.

Years ago, experiments were conducted to determine carotene absorption from carrots. Results were mixed. One investigator found that 20 percent of the carotene in raw carrots was absorbed, compared with only 5 percent in cooked carrots. A second investigator had opposite results. Absorption in the raw carrots was only 1 percent, compared with 19 percent in the cooked carrots. Then, a third investigator showed that about 25 percent of the carotene was absorbed in cooked carrots, regardless of the cooking method employed. The amount of carotene absorbed was doubled if the carrots were pureed. These studies show the difficulty in establishing whether raw or cooked vegetables provide better nutrient absorption.

Foods vs. Supplements. Surprisingly, we largely lack

Supplement Absorption

Generally, for good absorption of nutritional supplements, they should be taken along with foods at meals. However, there are exceptions.

Iron supplements are absorbed best if taken on an empty stomach. Iron absorption is impaired if hydrochloric acid is deficient in the stomach. Iron supplements should not be taken at the same time as vitamin E supplements; iron and vitamin E are antagonistic to each other.

Zinc supplements, if taken with egg, milk, or cereal, are not as well absorbed as when they are taken with other foods.

Inorganic forms of minerals may not be well absorbed. To improve absorption, manufacturers may "chelate" mineral supplements. This technique binds the mineral to an organic chelating substance that mimics the absorption process in the body. Examples of inorganic forms of minerals are carbonate, chloride, hydroxide, iodide, oxide, phosphate, selenate, selenite, and sulfate. Examples of organic chelated forms of minerals are ascorbate, aspartate, citrate, gluconate, glycinate, lactate, orotate, and any substances that are followed by the comparison data for nutrient absorption from foods with that from supplements.

A study conducted by researchers at the USDA's Human Nutrition Research Center in Beltsville, Maryland, compared the absorption of vitamin C from foods with that from vitamin C supplements. Sixty-eight men were placed on a diet designed to be very low in vitamin C to deplete them of this nutrient. After one month, the diet was supplemented with vitamin C-containing foods or supplements. Both foods and

word "chelate." The chelated form of a mineral supplement may be a more expensive product than the inorganic form. However, it may be more cost-effective because of its improved absorption.

Calcium supplements cannot be absorbed unless they disintegrate and dissolve. In 1988, Dr. Ralph F. Shangraw, chairman of the Department of Pharmaceutics at the School of Pharmacy, University of Maryland, reported results of experiments he had conducted with calcium supplements. He found that many calcium tablets had poor disintegration and dissolution, which would indicate that the product might be absorbed poorly, if at all. As a result of Shangraw's findings, some manufacturers reformulated their calcium supplements to improve disintegration and dissolution of their products.

A simple test roughly simulates how effectively a calcium supplement is apt to disintegrate and dissolve in the presence of hydrochloric acid, in the normally functioning stomach. Place a calcium tablet in vinegar and stir occasionally. After a half hour, at least three-fourths of the tablet should be dissolved. If this has not occurred, the result suggests that the supplement will be absorbed poorly, if at all.

supplements were equally effective in restoring plasma vitamin C levels, with the exception of raw broccoli. In a raw state, broccoli was at least 20 percent less effective in raising plasma vitamin C levels than other foods that contain significant amounts of vitamin C.

Unlike vitamin C, it is far more difficult to obtain extra vitamin E from foods. According to Orville A. Levander, from the Beltsville Center, it is virtually impossible to obtain more than 25 International Units (IUs) of vitamin E per day solely from the diet. The U.S. Recommended Daily Allowance (RDA) is 15 IU of vitamin E for men and 12 IU for women. Levander reported that the average intake is about 10 to 15 IU. In recent years, higher levels have been suggested for health maintenance or treatment of diseases.

Levander and his colleagues studied sixty-five men for a comparison of how diets and supplements contribute to plasma levels of vitamin E. The group of men depending on vitamin E absorption solely from food showed no significant differences in their blood levels. The average daily intake was less than 20 IU of vitamin E from dietary sources. However, the group of men who added a multivitamin supplement at least every other day were able to obtain an extra 15 to 60 IU of vitamin E daily. In the third group, the men who took daily vitamin E capsules were able to obtain at least 100 IU of vitamin E above their dietary intake.

Compared with the group that did not take supplements regularly, plasma vitamin E levels averaged 14 percent higher in the group taking multivitamin supplements. However, the levels were more than twice as high in the group taking vitamin E capsules daily.

The researchers suggested that persons who desire to increase their vitamin E plasma levels substantially need to take supplements.

At times, a nutrient may be absorbed more effectively

from a supplement than from a food source. In a study of the Human Nutrition Research Center on Aging at Tufts University, as well as from other studies, it was found that 20 to 40 percent of the elderly lose their ability to absorb the protein-bound nutrient, vitamin B_{12} from food. However, they were able to absorb the crystalline form from a supplement.

The answer to the question "how well are nutrients absorbed?" is far from simple. The basics of good nutrition offer the best possibilities. These basics, stated frequently, bear repetition. Eat a wide variety of basic foods, avoid excesses to minimize imbalances, and improve lifestyle factors related to health. All these factors contribute to better nutrient absorption.

Chapter 4

Basic Foods and Beverages with "New and Improved" Uses

NUTS: HIGH-FAT FOODS FOR HEALTH?

The conventional wisdom has been that all high-fat foods contribute to cardiovascular risks, promote arteriosclerosis, and contribute to obesity. As with many oversimplifications, this is wrong. All fats are not equal.

Foods rich in monounsaturated fats, such as nuts and olives, and the oils pressed from these foods, defy the dictum. Numerous studies indicate that diets high in monounsaturated fats actually can lower the risk of cardiovascular diseases, and in some cases, do so even more effectively than the officially recommended low-fat diet.

Some studies have demonstrated that people who eat nuts regularly experience significantly less heart disease and heart fatalities than those who rarely eat this fat-rich food. Nuts eaten slowly release their fat in a healthful way. All nuts have similar oil-encapsulating structures, so their fat-delivery system is similar. Alpha-linoleic acid (an omega-6 essential fatty acid) in nuts is thought to prevent ventricular fibrillation.

Cardiovascular Benefits. Studies conducted jointly in California, Canada, and Italy demonstrated that the substitution of almonds and almond oil for other fats in a diet could lower both total and low-density lipoprotein (LDL) cholesterol (the harmful form of cholesterol). The same research team conducted a five-week period study comparing diets with fat components from olive oil, almonds, and dairy-based fats. During the first week, participants were instructed to select high-fiber, low saturated-fat meals. At the beginning of the second week, each volunteer was assigned to a similar diet, but with different fat components. The diets increased each person's caloric intake from fat to 35 percent in the olive oil and fat groups, and to 39 percent in the nut group. Although these percentages are above the official recommendation of a maximum 30 percent calories from fat, they reflect actual percentages consumed by many Americans (but from fats that are predominantly saturated).

By the end of the fourth week, the blood cholesterol of the volunteers consuming almonds had dropped by 11 percent, and olive oil, by 4 percent. But the blood cholesterol level rose 5 percent in those in the dairy-fat group. The three groups showed comparable changes in the undesirable LDL cholesterol levels. The LDL fell 17 percent in those on the diet with almonds, and 8 percent with olive oil. But the LDL rose 2 percent in the dairy-fat group.

Why did the almond eaters enjoy more blood lipid benefits? Studies indicate that some people move consumed fat into their blood a little faster than normal, and out of their blood much slower than average. As a result, their fats circulate in the blood longer than in other people, and place them at much higher risk for heart disease. The timing of a nut oil's absorption and processing is similar to other oils. But, when consumed as a nut, the nut's oil enters the bloodstream more slowly, peaks in about an hour, and is flushed out rapidly. Whole nuts deliver the fat differently than if the nut oil is used as part of prepared foods, such as in salad dressing.

All nuts contain high amounts of fat. For example, macadamia nuts derive about 95 percent of their calories from fat. Yet nuts are useful for cholesterol benefits. In one study, a diet rich in macadamia nuts was compared to a typical American diet, or one that was developed to meet low-fat guidelines. For thirty days, fifteen men and fifteen women participated. Total cholesterol levels dropped 5 percent in both the macadamia-containing diet and the low-fat diet. Triglyceride levels fell 1 percent in the macadamia-containing diet. Triglycerides are a neutral fat that is the usual storage form of fat in the body. Yet, when the volunteers switched to the low-fat diet, triglyceride blood levels rose from 10 to 20 percent above those of the typical American diet. The study demonstrated the importance of the overall ratio of monounsaturated to saturated fats.

Weight Loss Benefits. Although it sounds like an oxymoron, fat-rich nuts are useful in weight reduction. A high monounsaturated-fat-diet from nuts and nut oils is appealing and tasty. It is far more agreeable than the Spartan low-fat diet. People are also more apt to comply with a diet that is palatable.

In light of the known health benefits, nuts (and seeds such as sunflower and pumpkin) have been maligned, regarded improperly, and underutilized.

In an eighteeen-month study of 101 overweight people, mostly female "hard core" dieters who failed repeatedly in weight-reduction regimes, entered the study. Most of them weighed about 200 pounds. Half of the volunteers were given a high monounsaturated diet (from nuts, olives, or nut oils) with 35 of the calories from fat; the other half, with only 20 percent from fat.

Within three months, both groups lost from five to thirty pounds. After six months, 62 percent of those on the high-monounsaturated fat diet continued to comply and improve, compared with only 42 percent in compliance on the low-fat diet.

In light of the known health benefits, nuts (and seeds such as sunflower and pumpkin) have been maligned, regarded improperly, and underutilized. Although they are "high-fat" foods, their fatty acid composition is desirable, with a high proportion of monounsaturated fat, and lesser amounts of polyunsaturated and saturated fats. Also, they are good sources of minerals, vitamins, fibers, and beneficial phytochemicals. Being dense in nutrients, nuts may satisfy hunger pangs on fewer calories than other less desirable snacking foods.

WATER: MISSING IN THE DIET

Repeatedly, we are told to drink at least eight glasses of water daily. Yet, many people ignore this advice. They drink only when they feel thirsty and thirst is not a reliable indicator. Inadequate water intake is all too common. Chronic dehydration has many health risks.

Adequate water intake is emphasized in a newly devised Food Guide Pyramid for Americans seventy years of age or older. In the graphic, eight glasses of water are at the base of the pyramid. Similarly, in a nutritional graphic used in Israel, a chalice emphasizes the importance of adequate water intake for overall health. Water, placed at the top of the chalice, forms the largest segment in the vessel. Thus, new emphasis is being given to old advice.

How the Body Uses Water. Adequate water is essential throughout the body. Tissues need water. About 60 percent of the water in the body appears inside the cells of every type of body tissue: blood, bone, muscle, and fat. The remainder of the water is between cells in the gastrointestinal tract, eyes, spinal column, blood plasma, and joints such as knees and elbows.

The body uses water in many ways. Water dissolves many chemical compounds so that the body can utilize them.

Water serves, too, as a medium in which chemical reactions constantly occur. The fluid in blood transports glucose to working muscles, and carries away byproducts. Fluid in the urine helps eliminate metabolic wastes from the body.

In aging, the thirst mechanism (as well as other senses) may decline. If water intake is inadequate, the blood thickens and reduces circulation, which makes the brain more susceptible to senility.

A study of active older men, sixty-seven to seventy-five years of age, deprived of water for twenty-four hours, found they were less thirsty and voluntarily drank less water than younger, active adult men. For this reason, it is especially important for the elderly to acquire a habit of drinking water frequently, even if the body is not signaling thirst. Also, because of incontinence, some elderly people purposely avoid fluid intake before social activities or prior to bedtime. Such avoidance may lessen inconvenience, but can contribute to chronic dehydration and health problems.

Unfortunately, by the time a person has a thirst signal, the body already has become partially dehydrated, and as much as 3 percent of the body's weight may have been lost in water. Both the elderly and children are groups at highest risk of dehydration. Both groups are apt to be somewhat insensitive to thirst signals.

With inadequate water intake, the body slows down. This is true in the dead of winter as well as during the sweltering hot summertime. Signs of inadequate water intake include a general sense of malaise, fatigue, lassitude, dizziness, and irritability. Signs of extreme dehydration may include heartburn, stomachache, noninfectious recurring or chronic pain, headache, depression, and water retention. The last outward sign of dehydration may be thirst.

Chronic dehydration is thought to play a role in some health problems, including asthma, arthritis, high blood pressure, and aging. With asthma, for example, the body has increased histamine production. Histamine helps regulate water metabolism and distribution. Also, it constricts the bronchial muscles in an effort to conserve the water that is lost during the act of breathing. Frequently, the lung tissues of asthmatics contain high histamine levels.

Adequate fluid intake may reduce the risks of certain types of cancer. Increased water intake is thought to be an important factor in reducing colon cancer risk by decreasing bowel transit time, or by decreasing the concentration of carcinogenic compounds through dilution. High fluid intake may also lower the risk of bladder cancer, the fourth leading type of cancer among American men. The American Cancer Society reports that the risk of bladder cancer decreased by 7 percent for every one-cup increment of fluid intake daily. Men with the highest amount of fluid intake (more than ten 8-ounce cups daily) were found to have only about half the risk of bladder cancer as men who drank less than five cups of fluid daily.

The Best Thirst Quencher. Of all fluids, water is the best thirst quencher. Fortunately, water is contained in many other beverages and foods, which contribute to the total daily intake. Milk is about 87 percent water, and fruit juices are high in water. Most fruits and vegetables are comprised of 85 percent to 95 percent water. Very juicy vegetables include cucumbers and tomatoes; and very juicy fruits, watermelons and grapes. Soups and stews contribute some water intake. Starchy vegetables, such as potato, are about 75 to 80 percent water. Eggs, 75 percent water, and cooked meats and fish, are about 50 to 60 percent. Even bread averages 36 percent water; and cakes, from 25 to 35 percent; and a cookie, 5 percent.

All beverages are not good hydrators. The caffeine in regular coffee, tea, and cola drinks is diuretic, and dehydrates by increasing urine excretion. The greater the amount of caffeine consumed, the greater is the need for more non-caffeine fluid intake. Nor do alcoholic beverages count as hydrators. Beer, on a hot summer day, dehydrates rather than hydrates the body, even though it may seem to quench the thirst.

Water is more vital than food. People who fast and do not eat any food can survive for a number of days. But, they cannot live without water for more than a few days.

If you do not habitually drink adequate amounts of water, there are several helpful aids. Plan to take a bottle of water with you whenever you travel. In buildings, drink whenever you pass a water cooler; in parks, use the drinking fountains. If you work at a desk, have a carafe of water nearby. If you work outdoors, take a thermos of water. At home, go to the kitchen faucet frequently.

REFASHIONED EGGS

We associate the phrase "new and improved" with reformulated food products or other consumer goods that have been well established in the marketplace. The phrase is applicable, as well, to basic foods that continuously are being refashioned to make good foods even better. Through breeding programs with plants and animals, our ancestors were able to convert wild grains into edible ones; wizened and acrid fruits and berries into tasty ones. Later, they learned to domesticate fowl and animals, and change their characteristics.

Even the modern term "value added" is applicable to early changes, as when it was discovered that fermented grapes could be turned into wine, grains into beer, and yeast into leavened bread. The Vikings discovered that they could transform cabbage into sauerkraut. This fermented food, rich in ascorbic acid, would protect them against scurvy on their long sea voyages. (It would take the British navy centuries to discover that their seamen could be protected from scurvy by providing them with limes, also rich in ascorbic acid.)

"You are what you eat" and "you become what you eat" are familiar phrases that acknowledge the influence of food on human development and health. Also, they acknowledge the influence of feed on animal development and health.

Continuous changes in feeding practices with animals reflect the research findings in animal husbandry. As newer findings are discovered, feeding practices are modified. This pattern is well illustrated in the continuous reformulations of feed for laying hens in order to refashion the egg.

Basic foods are continuously being refashioned to make good foods even better.

Attempts to Reduce Cholesterol in Eggs. The egg is one of nature's most balanced and nutritious foods. Yet, good as it is, during the 1970s it was wrongfully maligned due to misguided concerns over cholesterol. The scare led to numerous attempts to reduce or even eliminate the cholesterol content of the egg.

One technique was to combine beta cyclodextrin (a modified starch) with the cholesterol present in the egg yolks. The mixture was centrifuged out, and then the egg yolks were added back to the egg whites. The mixture, appearing like whipped egg, was pasteurized, packaged in refrigerated cartons, and sold in retail food stores, as well as to restaurants and food processing plants.

Another technique used to remove cholesterol from the egg was supercritical fluid extraction. This is a well-established technology with numerous food applications, including the extractions of caffeine from coffee or fat from foods.

Some drastic measures were tried, experimentally, in attempts to reduce cholesterol in eggs. Lovastatin (cholestyramine), a cholesterol-lowering drug commonly prescribed for humans, was fed to laying hens by researchers at Purdue University. The drug in the feed of laying hens produced eggs with 15 percent less cholesterol.

At Texas A&M University, researchers experimented with an oligosaccharide derived from yeast cell walls. This complex carbohydrate, not digested by hens, was incorporated in their feed. The main function of this carbohydrate in the gastrointestinal tract is to aid beneficial intestinal bacteria, but also results in lowering the cholesterol content of the egg.

At Louisiana State University, attempts were made to reduce the cholesterol and saturated fat in eggs by changing the feed of the laying hens. A patented additive produced an egg with nearly one-third less cholesterol and saturated fat, and with 40 percent more protein than the ordinary egg.

The Emphasis Shifts. As these various attempts were being conducted to lower cholesterol in the egg, researchers at the University of Arizona found that saturated fat—not dietary cholesterol—was the major contributor to elevated blood cholesterol for the general population. The researchers conducted a meta-analysis of more than thirty years of research. Wanda Howell, Ph.D., R.D., spokesperson for the University of Arizona researchers, reported that, "for most healthy people, the cholesterol they eat does not raise their blood pressure. Healthy individuals with normal cholesterol levels should now feel free to enjoy foods like eggs in their diet every day."

After this finding, efforts shifted toward improving the egg's nutritional quality. By this time, research findings were showing that the quality of fat was important, with increasing emphasis on the benefits of long-chain omega-3 fatty acids (essential fatty acids necessary for health). The search began for sources of omega-3 that would be suitable for use in the feed of laying hens.

At Texas A&M University, poultry researchers fortified the diet of laying hens with fish oil, rich in omega-3, to yield egg yolks higher in these fatty acids. However, the fish oil used from menhaden (a marine fish) proved too "fishy" a taste in the eggs.

Marine algae were substituted to produce "nutritionally enhanced" eggs. An added benefit was an intense yolk color, provided from pigment naturally present in the algae.

At the University of Arizona, researchers substituted chia seeds, rich in plant-derived omega-3 fatty acids, to constitute 12 percent of the fat in eggs produced from chia-fed hens. The ratio of saturated to polyunsaturated fats in these eggs was half that in ordinary eggs. The chia seeds did not give the undesirable fishy taste, as did the fish oil, and the chia also bestowed a longer shelf life.

Purslane was also considered. This weedy herb is the richest known source of omega-3 fatty acids in leafy green plants. Purslane was investigated by Norman Salem, Jr., a lipid biochemist with the National Institutes of Health, and Artemis P. Simopoulos, M.D. from the American Association for World Health. The researchers found that the yolks from large-sized eggs, produced on a Greek farm by free-range hens that chose to eat purslane, contained about 300 milligrams (mg) of omega-3 fatty acids. This was the equivalent of a standard fish oil capsule, and ten times the amount that is found in a typical American supermarket egg. The eggs from the purslane-eating hens lacked the fishy taste and smell of eggs from hens feeding on fish oil.

Another source of omega-3 fatty acids considered by Texas A&M University researchers was flaxseed oil. More than half of the oil in flaxseed consists of linolenic acid, an omega-3 fatty acid. Some linolenic acid is changed in the human body to two substances: EPA (eicosapentaenoic acid) and DHA (docosahexanoic acid). These substances are found, too, in fish, and are thought to be beneficial to health, especially in helping to prevent heart disease.

As a result of the flaxseed research, a Texas-based egg producer began to sell eggs from hens fed feed fortified with flax and vitamin E. The eggs had about as much saturated and monounsaturated fats as ordinary eggs, but they contained 10 mg each of linolenic acid and DHA, and ten times as much vitamin E as found in ordinary eggs.

Although fish oil proved too "fishy" for the feed of laying hens, other foods from the sea, marine algae and kelp (seaweed), were examined. Marine algae added to the feed produced eggs high in DHA. Unfortunately, the attempt to use kelp in the feed of laying hens backfired in America.

In the early 1990s, an American poultry company obtained the rights to a Japanese feed made with kelp to feed laying hens a special diet that included a carefully controlled low-saturated fat content. Before introducing the eggs, the poultry company sponsored research and clinical studies at the University of Alabama, the Medical College in Pennsylvania, and the Lankenau Hospital in Philadelphia, as well as at private research facilities. Studies showed that when humans ate as many as a dozen of the eggs produced by hens on this special feed as part of a well-balanced low-fat diet, the serum cholesterol level did not increase. Rather, most of the subjects on these eggs reduced their cholesterol levels about as much as the control group on a low-fat, low-cholesterol diet and with essentially no eggs in their diet. In addition to the benefits from the special feed producing higher quality eggs, the eggshells were thicker and stronger, and the eggs had a longer shelf life.

Despite all this good news, the Food and Drug Administration (FDA) decided that the iodine content in the feed, from the seaweed, was a level sufficiently high to make the eggs a health hazard. This decision was made despite the

WHAT'S THAT IN HEN FEED?

At the same time that some poultry producers have been trying to improve the quality of eggs by improving the quality of the feed, an opposite trend has developed.

In a 1992 *Weekly Market Bulletin,* Stephen H. Taylor, Commissioner of New Hampshire's Department of Agriculture, announced that some poultry farmers in the state soon would produce a line of premium eggs having more vitamin E and iodine, and a lower ratio of saturated fat to monounsaturated fat, than ordinary eggs. Taylor noted that the hens would be fed "a prescribed ration made entirely of virgin feed stocks." Then, with unusual frankness, Taylor added that "no animal byproducts, bakery wastes, or other reprocessed ingredients are allowed. The only fat in the feed is supplied through canola (oil)."

Taylor's candor was matched by Dr. Jeffrey L. Garwin, director of medical and quality assurance for a producer of eggs with less saturated fat than ordinary eggs. Garwin noted that "most hens are fed everything from leftover bakery crumbs to used deep-frying fat from fast food restaurants."

fact that the feed formulation in Japan produced more than four times as much iodine as the formulation for the feed used in America, with no adverse effects reported. (The iodine content in the daily diets in different countries varies considerably, according to data gathered in the 1980s. It ranged from a low average of 0.058 mg/day of female vegans in Denmark to a high average of 23.727 mg/day in Japan.)

The U.S. Recommended Daily Allowance (RDA) for iodine is 150 micrograms (mcg) daily. The daily intakes by Americans exceed this recommendation. It is thought that intake by men is 250 mcg; for women, 170 mcg. Jean Pennington, from the FDA's division for Food Safety and Applied Nutrition, concluded that iodine intake of less than 1,000 mcg daily was probably safe for the majority of the population. However, the FDA contends that even that level may cause adverse effects in some individuals, and there is no way to discern if individuals are sensitive to it.

The FDA ordered the egg producer to halt sales of its eggs because of the high iodine levels. The poultry company reformulated the feed so that the iodine level of the eggs would be well under the RDA, and at amounts that the FDA would deem safe and appropriate.

Vitamin D Fortification in Hen's Feed. In Japan, vitamin D-fortified dried shiitake mushroom powder was added experimentally to the feed of hens, in order to produce vitamin D-fortified eggs. The result was a great increase in the vitamin D content in the egg yolk—about ten times as much as in ordinary eggs. The increase was in proportion to the amount of the mushroom powder in the feed.

At the Agricultural Research Center in Finland, the vitamin D content of eggs was raised sevenfold by tripling the vitamin D in feed for laying hens. The researchers found that the official recommendations for vitamin D could be met by consuming one of these eggs daily. The lead researcher, Pirjo Mattila, reported that "given the importance of vitamin D to human health and the difficulties some people have in getting it into their diets, the possibility of producing vitamin D-enriched eggs is worthy of consideration." Vitamin D is essential for normal bone formation, and may help prevent postmenopausal osteoporosis.

The Egg as a Delivery System. In ongoing research by Mark E. Cook and his associates at the University of Wisconsin, hens are immunized to stimulate them to produce antibodies. The antibodies in the eggs activate peptides in the digestive system of humans who eat the eggs. The peptides are associated with a sense of fullness. Eggs with these appetite-reducing antibodies may provide a healthier, and less costly weight-reduction regimen than those currently in use. Researchers anticipate that the immunized eggs will become available in the marketplace within several years.

Thus, the concept of "new and improved" links the ancients with the advanced laboratories of today. The ingenuity of humans certainly will continue to produce better foods for tomorrow's consumers.

NEW USES FOR SPICES

Spices have long been valued for their ability to preserve foods against rancidity, and to add variety of flavor to an otherwise bland, monotonous diet. In many cultures, the pharmacological properties of certain spices have been recognized, and they have been used therapeutically.

More recently, due to the problems of foodborne diseases, spices are under investigation for their antimicrobial properties. The present interest in dietary supplements and functional foods has sparked activity to identify, isolate, and utilize bioactive ingredients in spices, such as sulfides, thiols, terpenes and their derivatives, phenol, glycosides, alcohols, and aldehydes and their esters.

Professor Daniel Fung and his associates at Kansas State University have been researching spices as antimicrobials. They studied twenty-three different spices with fresh meat (ground beef) and processed meat (salami) that had been contaminated intentionally with the virulent pathogen *E. coli* 0157:H7. Clove had the strongest antimicrobial effect, followed by cinnamon, garlic, oregano, and sage. The inhibiting effect of garlic increased with the rise in cooking temperature. Garlic contains allicin and other sulfur-containing compounds that suppress harmful organisms. Other spices that demonstrated antimicrobial effects against *E. coli* 0157:H7 in ground beef included clove (from its eugenol and caryophyllene); sage (from its picrosalvin, carnosol, and cineole); and oregano (from its thymol, carvacrol, and borneol).

Other spices, too, have been found to possess antimicrobial properties. Hot peppers inhibited *Bacillus cereus* and *Staphylococcus aureus;* ginger, *Bacillus subtilis* and *Salmonella typhimurium;* mustard, *E. coli, Pseudomonas aeruginosa;* pepper, *Clostridium botulinum* and *Lactobacillus micrococcus;* and sage, *Listeria monocytogenes.*

Dr. Fung and his colleagues added cinnamon to pasteurized apple juice that had been contaminated purposely with *E. coli* 0157:H7. The cinnamon showed antimicrobial activity in the juice, even after three days of storage at room temperature, or up to eight weeks of storage at a cooler temperature.

The researchers reported that they did not determine whether foods, spiced at a high enough level to be effective in controlling pathogens, would be palatable. Nor did they consider that spices be regarded as a replacement for safe food practices. However, they concluded that if more spices are added to cooking, both at home and by food processors, the practice will reduce and inactivate pathogens. Spices can be a useful additional protective measure in safe food handling practices.

Allyl isothiocyanate, a compound in horseradish, is a natural inhibitor of pathogenic microbes such as Listeria, *E. coli,* and *S. aureus.* Researchers at the United States Department of Agriculture's (USDA) Agricultural Research Station at Oklahoma State University investigated allyl isothiocyanate, and found that it exhibited excellent antibacterial and antifungal activity. They explored the possibility that this substance could be useful in packaged cooked uncured meats to prevent the growth of food poisoning bacteria.

Rosemary contains antioxidant characteristics, and is being used to prevent rancidity in fat-containing products such as poultry, pork, and beef. The carnosic acid in rosemary accounts for its antioxidant activity. It can replace synthetic antioxidants that have been used to prevent fat-containing foods from turning rancid.

Oregano is being studied because it contains antioxidants and antimicrobials, such as carvacrol, thymol, and rosmarinic acid. These constituents make oregano an excellent food preservative and potential source of natural disease-preventive chemicals that might fight chronic bacterial infections such as urinary tract infections and ulcers.

For many centuries Inca farmers used mint leaves to keep stored potatoes sound. Knowledge of this practice spurred Dr. Stephen Vaughn and his colleagues at the USDA's Agricultural Research Service at Peoria, Illinois to study spice extracts. They discovered that vaporized oils from cinnamon, cumin, or thyme, applied to potatoes, kept them from sprouting for as long as eleven months, and also protected them from storage-rot fungi. The cooked potatoes had no unusual flavor.

If potatoes sprout prematurely, they soften and lose weight. Much of their starch turns to sugar, and when the potatoes are cooked, they turn an unattractive dark brown. They become undesirable for French fries and potato chips, and represent an economic loss. The spice extracts may prove to be effective for stored potatoes, and lead to non-toxic treatment.

Chemist Richard A. Anderson and his colleagues at the USDA's Nutrient Requirements and Functions Laboratory at Beltsville, Maryland, are investigating spices and other plants used in folk medicine. They found a few spices, especially cinnamon, make fat cells much more responsive to insulin, the hormone that regulates sugar metabolism and thus controls the blood glucose level. In test tube experiments, an active compound in cinnamon increased glucose metabolism about twentyfold. If this substance will do the same in people, it might provide a natural remedy against diabetes. These findings are important. Nearly 16 million Americans have diabetes. One-third of them are unaware that they have the condition. Most have type-2 diabetes (adult onset), in which the body cells fail to recognize and respond to insulin as well as they did formerly. This inability results in elevated blood sugar.

As more investigations go forth with spices, many benefits are being discovered. They can be put to practical use.

From Pantry to Medicine Cabinet. On Columbus' second voyage to the New World in 1494, the expedition's physician, Diego Alvarez Chanca, opened a new chapter in the search for useful chemicals from plants. Chanca wrote the first detailed account of a West Indian plant, the chili pepper, which appeared to have many medicinal uses. In Andean cultures, chili peppers were used against severe headaches and strokes. The Aztecs, Mayans, and Incas used chili peppers to suppress the desire for alcohol, to treat poor memory, and to serve as an aphrodisiac. Ground chili peppers, added to milk, were applied externally to reduce swellings.

Five centuries later, capsaicin (cap-*say*-i-sin), the most potent group of compounds identified in chilies, is being examined for its usefulness in a spate of health problems that challenge modern medicine. Depending on the variety of the plant, soil, and climate, chili peppers contain from 0.1 to 1.0 percent capsaicin.

Uses of Capsaicin. Capsaicin can raise the metabolic rate and reduce the body's absorption of fat. In rat studies, it lowered cholesterol. In dog studies, it cured worms. In people, it reduced nicotine craving. But perhaps its most useful role is its ability to relieve pain.

Hundreds of reports are published yearly about capsaicin's use as a pain reliever. Capsaicin-containing topical creams and ointments are available as over-the-counter products to ease joint and muscle pains, and for post-zoster herpes (a painful condition known as "shingles" caused by reactivation in adults of the chicken pox virus experienced in childhood).

Italian researchers in clinical medicine have used capsaicin cream with patients suffering from rheumatoid arthritis. They noted an increased production of collagenase and prostaglandins. Both reduce pain and inflammation.

... capsaicin ... the most potent group of compounds identified in chilies, is being examined for its usefulness in a spate of health problems that challenge modern medicine.

The anti-inflammatory effect of capsaicin was confirmed in Sweden, where external application of capsaicin-containing creams was used to relieve a number of chronic pain syndromes, including post-herpetic neuralgia, post-mastectomy neuroma, reflex sympathetic dystrophy syndrome, diabetic neuropathy, rheumatoid arthritis, psoriasis, hemodialysis-associated itching, and vulvar vestibulitis (inflammation at the entrance of the vagina).

The Capsaicin Study Group at the Scripps Clinic and Research Foundation also found that topically applied capsaicin-containing creams were effective in easing the pain of diabetic neuropathy. The treatment reportedly led to an improvement of the daily activities of the patients, and enhanced the quality of their lives.

At Case Western Reserve University, capsaicin-containing cream used on patients with osteoarthritis gave significant pain relief, and it gave those with rheumatoid arthritis, moderate pain relief.

How Does Capsaicin Work?

Topical capsaicin creams or ointments do not work like many other creams or ointments that redden the skin and create a burning sensation as counter-irritants. Application of capsaicin to the skin relieves the pain by depleting the body's supply of a peptide (a protein-like compound), called substance P. It is thought that substance P is the main neurotransmitter for relaying pain signals to the brain. Neurotransmitters are chemicals that carry nerve signals across the synapses (gaps) that separate one nerve cell from another. Capsaicin, an alkaloid, produces the sensation of heat caused by the irritation of the trigeminal cells (pain receptors located in the mouth, nose, and stomach) that release substance P.

Substance P is produced and stored in certain neurons (nerve cells) including sensory neurons that carry pain signals from the skin, joints, and muscles. If one of these cells senses a painful stimulus, it produces an electric signal that travels along the length of the neuron. When the signal reaches the end of one neuron, it causes the release of substance P, which flows across the gap to the next neuron. Substance P binds to receptors on the next neuron, causing it to generate another electrical signal that continues on, repeatedly, until it reaches the brain where it is perceived as pain. Capsaicin, applied to the skin, disrupts this process. It causes sensory nerve fibers to use up their stocks of substance P, and prevents them from renewing their diminished supply. With fewer neurotransmitters available, neurons are unable to transmit pain signals effectively, and the individual feels less pain. However, the process is reversible. After capsaicin-containing cream or ointment is no longer applied topically, more substance P may be produced. Pain may return.

Capsaicin targets nerve cells involved in pain transmission. Other nerve functions are unaffected.

Capsaicin blocks the ability to feel pain, without producing numbness. It works by killing small-diameter nerve fibers responsible for pain, but does not affect large-diameter nerve fibers. Dr. Richard A. Meyer and his colleagues at Johns Hopkins Hospital injected a capsaicin analog under the inner forearm skin of eight volunteers. They experienced reduced pain and reduced sensitivity to heat and touch.

Because capsaicin can block pain without numbness, it is useful with burn patients and individuals who have tender surgical scars. Researchers at the Mayo Clinic have used capsaicin to relieve burn pain. Ointment applied to patients brings relief from surgical scars from major cancer surgery, such as mastectomies or lung operations, which can damage nerves and produce sharp burning pain for months, or even years. Even when healed, some patients cannot tolerate even the weight of clothing over scars. Ordinary painkillers are ineffective, but capsaicin ointment may bring relief. Future applications may include use with incisions made on individuals who undergo surgery.

Other Uses for Capsaicin. Capsaicin has been used for a variety of other conditions, including asthma, cluster headaches, urinary incontinence, inflammatory bowel disease, psoriasis, and urticaria (hives) caused by cold temperature.

Capsaicin has been used in Switzerland as a nasal spray for nonallergenic nasal rhinitis (inflammation of the nasal mucous membrane), to replace topical steroids or antihistamines. This treatment is not intended for home use, but needs to be administered in a hospital setting, where local anesthesia can be given prior to treatment. The first few doses are reported to burn, with the eyes watering, and the nose discharging fluid. However, with repeated doses, the organs are clear and dry.

Capsaicin has been used to treat fibromyalgia, a painful

and puzzling condition. The cream, applied to tender areas, appears to lessen the tenderness, and increase grip strength.

Doubtless, further investigations will confirm the usefulness of capsaicin for many conditions. Studies of capsaicin might lead, as well, to improved formulation of analgesic drugs.

SPORTS DRINKS AND ELECTROLYTES

Originally, sports drinks were devised to replace vital nutrients lost in sweat by athletes engaged in strenuous activity, and lost through dehydration in hot weather. Presently, they are targeted to those engaged in mild activities, to women (for calcium), to children, and to the general population for hot weather rehydration. These drinks are intended to replace lost electrolytes.

Electrolytes are chemical substances found in the fluids that bathe all of the body's cells, as well as the fluids within the cells. Electrolytes found mainly outside the cells include sodium and chloride; within the cells, potassium and magnesium.

Electrolytes form the body's electrical system, which is interrelated with the cardiovascular, respiratory, nervous, and digestive systems. The electrical system must function properly to maintain normal body functions.

Electrolytes dissolved in the fluids separate into electrically charged particles called ions. The electrical charge held by ions enables them to perform vital functions. They transmit nerve impulses, contract muscles, maintain proper fluid levels, and control the acid-alkaline balance in these fluids.

Some electrolytes are charged positively, and known as cations (pronounced *kat´-i-ons*). The major ones are potassium, magnesium, sodium, and calcium. Others are charged negatively, and known as anions (pronounced *an´-i-ons*). Chloride is a major anion.

Electrolytes are absorbed by the intestines. When the

body functions efficiently, the amounts of electrolytes excreted daily is in balance with the intake. Some amounts of electrolytes are lost through air exhaled from the lungs and through perspiration from the skin, but mainly they are excreted by the kidneys. If electrolytes are in short supply, the kidneys can reabsorb them as needed.

Potassium. Potassium, the main cation in the intracellular fluid, activates enzymes, processes and stores carbohydrates, and helps transmit nerve impulses to the heart and skeletal muscles. Poor nutrition, especially too little intake of fruits and vegetables, may result in potassium insufficiency. Also, persons on very low calorie diets or diuretics, as well as sufferers of anorexia nervosa, or chronic alcoholics may have low potassium levels. Potassium is lost through excessive perspiration, repeated enemas, severe burns and other traumas, uncontrolled diabetes, diseases of the intestinal tract and operations to correct them. Less common causes of potassium depletion are from the use of outdated tetracycline, and overindulgence in licorice.

Excessive potassium may result from using salt substitutes or from kidney failure. Signs of excessive potassium include diarrhea, irritability, muscle cramps, weakness, and pain.

Magnesium. Magnesium, another cation in the intracellular fluid, is involved in muscle contractions, nerve transmissions, and stimulation of enzymes involved in metabolizing fats, proteins, and carbohydrates. Magnesium deficiency may result from poor nutrition. Often, when magnesium levels are low, potassium and calcium levels are low, too. Use of diuretics, chronic alcoholism, diabetes, pancreatitis, and kidney damage may be related to magnesium deficiency.

Excessive magnesium commonly is due to impaired kidney function, and worsened by the use of magnesium-containing laxatives or antacids. Excessive magnesium can weaken reflexes, paralyze muscles, and depress respiration.

Sodium. Sodium, the main cation in the intracellular fluid, maintains proper fluid balance. Often, too little sodium is associated with dehydration caused by excessive sweating, diarrhea, or use of diuretics. Symptoms range from fatigue and muscle weakness to convulsions.

Use of salt tablets or sports drinks to replenish lost sodium is controversial. Many health professionals and athletic advisors believe that intake of adequate amounts of plain water and nutritious foods will replenish fluids and lost electrolytes. However, thirst is a poor indicator of fluids needed and proponents of sports drinks contend that such products, with flavorings and sweeteners, encourage people to drink more. The water proponents reply that water can be flavored and sweetened with fruit juice and achieve the same result. In addition, those who exercise lightly can replenish fluids adequately with water that is readily available and cost-free.

Excessive sodium results from too little water intake, especially in hot weather or if kidney function is impaired. Poor food choices, with many highly salted foods, results in excessive sodium and too little potassium. Symptoms of excessive sodium include thirst, dry and sticky mucous membranes, flushed skin, elevated body temperature, and lack of tears.

Calcium. Calcium, another cation in the extracellular fluid, is necessary for normal nerve impulse transmission, muscle contraction, and blood clotting. Although most of the calcium in the body is in a nonionized state in bones and teeth, a small amount is ionized. The ionized form may be decreased by certain diseases of the pancreas, kidney, and digestive tract, and surgical removal of parathyroid tissue. Signs of calcium loss include tingling of the fingertips, numbness, and over-reactive reflexes.

Although many Americans have insufficient calcium

REPLACING LOST FLUIDS

Experts suggest that athletes drink 13 to 20 oz of water before exercising, and 6 to 8 oz every fifteen minutes during exercising. This system is better than waiting to drink after exercising because it takes several hours to replace the lost water. Meanwhile, performance will decrease. Practice this system during training so that the body becomes accustomed to the fluid intake. Drink cold water (45°F to 55°F). Cool water is emptied rapidly from the stomach and therefore is absorbed and used quickly by the body.

intake, excessive amounts may also result from faulty diets, too much vitamin D, prolonged inactivity such as bed rest, overactive parathyroid gland, or kidney disease. Excessive calcium may result in loss of appetite, nausea, weight loss, kidney stones, and deep body pain.

Chloride, the main anion of extracellular fluid, usually paired with sodium, is needed for muscle contraction, balancing fluid level inside and outside of cells, and acid-base balance of extracellular fluids. Adequate chloride is essential to prevent bicarbonate, another important anion, from imbalancing the acid-base ratio.

Severe cases of electrolyte loss may require replacement fluids, including hospital-administered intravenous replacement fluids. However, most people can maintain electrolyte balance by eating nutritious foods, and drinking adequate amounts of water, especially in hot weather or when engaged in strenuous exercise.

SPECIALTY DRINKS

Commercial drinks used to be mainly carbonated sodas, cola beverages, or fruit drinks. The beverage market has expanded greatly, and presently offers a vast array. Some drinks fill unique niches.

Sports Drinks. One specialty is sports drinks. The American market for sports drinks is estimated to be more than $2 billion annually. When first introduced, the drinks were intended to replenish electrolytes lost from strenuous exercise. Now, these isotonic drinks are formulated to target muscle recovery. This requires restoration of body fluids, replenishment of muscle glycogen, minimizing muscle damage, strengthening the immune system, and rebuilding muscle protein.

For rehydration, isotonic drinks continue to achieve osmotic balance. The drinks usually contain a blend of sugars (such as high-fructose corn syrup, dextrose, or sucrose) with salt and calcium phosphate salts. More recently, glycerine or glycerol (a sugar alcohol which is less sweet than sucrose) has been added to some drinks to encourage water retention in muscle fibers, both during and after exercise.

The store of muscle glycogen, a carbohydrate derived from glucose (dextrose) is lost after exercise, and needs to be replenished. The process requires energy, glucose, and insulin (to get the sugars into the body's cells). The principal energy fuel in the body is adenosine triphosphate (ATP), which is built from a sugar molecule, D-ribose, to which are attached three phosphate groups. ATP is needed to fuel muscle activity, and to convert glucose into stored glycogen. Usually, it takes time to replenish ATP stores after exercise. This time can be shortened dramatically by bypassing the normal biochemical pathways that restore ATP by "pump priming" the body directly with ATP's precursor, D-ribose, which can provide a basic building block of ATP. Usually, D-ribose is synthesized slowly from glucose.

Creatine phosphate, another molecule, also can donate phosphates to ATP rebuilding. Both D-ribose and creatine phosphate can be used to formulate sports drinks that help replenish muscle glycogen.

Stressful muscle activity can result in small muscle tissue tears, along with inflammation and soreness. Stressed tissues release free oxygen radicals that induce further tissue damage. Antioxidants in muscle-recovery drinks can block or quench free radicals before they damage tissue. Some antioxidants, notably vitamin C, are water-soluble and can be added readily to muscle-recovery drinks. However, vitamin E is usually fat-soluble. A water-soluble form of vitamin E may be used as an antioxidant in drinks intended for muscle recovery. Green tea extracts, too, may be added for their antioxidant qualities.

Different protein sources are available for use in sports drinks intended to rebuild muscles. The most popular ones are whey and egg proteins, and soy protein isolates. Also, specific amino acids may be used. For example, L-arginine stimulates insulin production, which helps the cells absorb carbohydrates for energy. A metabolite of leucine (another amino acid) retards muscle breakdown that occurs during exercise, and helps muscles repair and recover.

Other substances may be added to sports drinks to relieve muscle pain and stiffness. Methylsulfonylmethane (MSM), a naturally occurring organic sulfur compound found in plant and animal tissues, known to alleviate pain and inflammation, appears to have multiple analgesic effects. It reduces muscle spasms and increases dilation of blood vessels, which enhances blood flow to inflamed tissues. Also, MSM seems to ease the pain of stressed joints, cartilage, and tendons that may result from strenuous physical activity.

Probiotic Drinks. Formerly, the main probiotic beverage was kefir, a fermented dairy-based product somewhat like yogurt, but in the form of a drink. Currently, probiotic beverages are being popularized by emphasizing their health benefits. Like yogurt, such drinks contain live and active cultures that help maintain or restore a favorable balance of bacteria in the intestinal tract.

Probiotics support the immune system in various ways. They lessen some problems associated with antibiotic use. Although an antibiotic may clear the targeted health problem, in the process it may destroy billions of beneficial bacteria that normally thrive in the digestive tract. This can lead to diarrhea or a secondary yeast infection. Probiotics, such as yogurt or the newer dairy-based probiotic drinks, can decrease the diarrheal effect and help restore the beneficial flora. Others who might benefit from the bowel-regulating effect of probiotic beverages include individuals with inflammatory bowel disease (IBD), those with travelers' diarrhea, and children infected with rotovirus.

Functional Drinks. Currently, the marketplace is flooded with drinks that promise to boost energy, cut fat, enhance memory, or deliver numerous other benefits. Such "functional" drinks may contain a dizzying array of ingredients, including spirulina, chorella, echinacea, astragalus, wheat grass, ginkgo, kava kava, St. John's wort, ginseng, guarana, green tea, yohimbe, gotu kola, and valerian root.

Consumers need to be informed. Are the combination of ingredients rational? Do they really bestow a specific health benefit? If so, how many drinks are needed daily or weekly to achieve a beneficial effect? What are the effects and how is the dose determined? Botanical extracts can be active biologically, but if the mechanism of their action is unknown, it is difficult to determine a dose that is both safe and effective.

Some functional drink processors may add an infinitesimal amount of a botanical merely to list its presence on the label of the product. No proof is offered that the low amount is effective. Critics dub this practice as one of dispensing fairy dust.

Certain functional drinks are not appropriate for the general public. What may be safe for an adult may not necessarily be safe for young children. For individuals on medications, certain botanicals in functional drinks may interact with the drugs. A drink with saw palmetto, intended for prostate problems, is inappropriate for women and children. Also, a drink with kava kava, a sedative, should not be consumed by truck drivers or persons operating machinery.

FOOD BARS: FOOD, CANDY, OR MEDICINE?

Various recent lifestyle and nutrition trends have combined to make food bars popular. Their sales are booming. Energy/sports bars accounted for more than $3 billion in sales in 1999. They are produced by more than seventy manufacturers, many of which are prominent food and beverage companies.

The food bars are popular because they are portable for people on the go. They replace lunch for people working at their desks. They provide late afternoon pick-me-ups to tide people over until their evening meals. The bars are regarded as a quick meal or meal replacement. They even substitute for breakfast.

For some people, food bars may be more acceptable than dietary supplement "pill popping." Certainly, they taste better, with their candy-like qualities of form, sweetness, chewiness, and chocolate enrobement. Yet some people who would eschew candy bars are not guilt-ridden in consuming food bars. The latter are regarded as healthy.

Indeed, the popularity of food bars has been built on the reinvention of the candy bar, with its new, frequently health-oriented, image. Reduced-fat candy bars are offered with five calories of fat per gram, instead of the usual nine calories. Reduced-sugar granola bars are made with one-third less sugar and one-third less fat. Of course, some of these bars are thinly disguised candies, consisting of nearly 50 percent sugar.

> The popularity of food bars has been built on the reinvention of the candy bar, with its new, frequently health-oriented, image.

Other trends contribute to the popularity of food bars. There has been a growth in the selfcare market, with easy access to health treatments. Some types of food bars target these concerns. The aging Baby Boomers are financially secure and health-directed. But, they are experiencing high stress, low energy, digestive disorders, obesity, heart disease, and increased risks of breast and prostate cancers. To meet these various conditions, specialized food bars are formulated to address concerns about cholesterol, diabetes, memory loss, weight loss/gain, lactose intolerance, muscle soreness, fatigue, oxidative stress resulting from exercise, "fat burning," and stronger bones. The lines have become blurred between food bars and foods, food bars and medicines, food bars and dietary supplements, and food bars and nutraceuticals.

Development of Energy/Sports Bars. Originally, energy/sports bars were formulated as performance-enhancing foods for marathoners, to eat at a critical period near the end of a race. The bars were perceived as health snacks that could provide energy for that last spurt.

Gradually, the bars were promoted and sold in health gyms and health food stores, intended for use in programs for weight training, body and mass building, and muscle recovery. Ultimately, sales were extended to sports enthusiasts, including runners, swimmers, cyclists, tennis players, and "weekend warriors," as well as mainstream America. The bars became available in numerous outlets for the general public. According to the Natural Marketing Institute, by 1999, conventional supermarkets became the main outlet for energy/sports bars.

The early energy/sports bars were formulated to be high in carbohydrates and low in fats, to conform to the concept of "carbohydrate loading" for athletes. Now, most of the bars contain higher levels of fat for greater palatability. Some contain about one-fourth of the saturated fats recommended for daily intake.

Early formulations were water-soluble, and the bars froze outdoors during cold-weather sports. People had to tuck the bars inside of clothing so that their body heat could keep the bars soft and edible. Now reformulated, the bars withstand temperature variations.

Energy bars are available with different ratios of nutrients, depending on various dietary fashions. Some have high carbohydrates/low fat ratios, intended for athletes. Others contain more than 20 grams of protein/2 grams of carbohydrates. Some are high protein/high fat/low carbohydrates, to meet the recommendations of the Atkins' dietary regime, or 40 percent carbohydrates, 30 percent protein, and 30 percent fat for the Sears' dietary regime.

Some bars are based on the glycemic index, with a ratio of 50 percent carbohydrates, 25 percent protein, and 25 percent fat. This ratio promises weight loss, fat-storage loss, lean-muscle gain, increased endurance, fat-burning recovery, and mental clarity. Purportedly, the glycemic index lowers the risk of diabetes and heart disease, manages weight, enhances performance, increases metabolism, maximizes hormonal function, and extends longevity.

What's in the Bars? Many of the energy bars are promoted for their protein content. Some bars contain more protein than is found in a fast-food outlet's quarter-pounder hamburger. Many high-protein bars are promoted with hyperbole, such as "for peak performance," "supercharge you with sustained energy," "push yourself to your personal best," or "power packed, high propulsion."

The protein in the bars often consists of whey (a dairy byproduct), soy protein isolates, or soy protein concentrates. Some contain soy protein and isoflavones (plant chemicals). These constituents are favorable selling points, especially since the Food and Drug Administration (FDA) approved health claims for soy protein.

Adequate protein is not a problem for most people. However, an overload of protein places an undue burden on the kidneys.

The so-called "quick energy" supplied by the bars may be provided by the sweeteners, complex carbohydrates, or even from stimulants, such as guarana, ginseng, or caffeine.

"No added sugar" is a claim on many of the bars. They may not contain table sugar (sucrose), yet still be loaded with sugars. Some of the sugars used included grain syrups from oats, rice, or barley; lactose, fructose, crystalline fructose, glucose, dextrose, or high-fructose corn syrup; grape juice or other fruit juices or concentrates; dehydrated cane juice; agave nectar, sorbitol, maltitol, honey, or molasses. Sugar is sugar, and the bars are sweet, chewy, and dense, like candy bars. The flavors of the bars reflect their candy-like quality, including coconut creme, double chocolate, chocolate peanut butter, and mint chocolate chips.

Some nutritionists and other health professionals express the same concerns about energy/sports bars as they had when low-fat cookies were introduced. Consumers may be so focused on the health claims of the bars that they lose track of how much they eat. An example was supplied by Kristine Clark, Director of Sports Nutrition at Penn State. One of her swimmers, who was fifteen pounds overweight, habitually consumed two energy bars before swimming practice, and consumed an additional bar after swimming practice. Then, she ate a full breakfast.

Antioxidants, vitamins, minerals, and amino acids may be added to the bars. Such additions supplement those already present in basic foods, or added in the form of dietary supplements. Both foods and supplements may be more cost-effective sources than the bars.

Many herbs are now added to energy bars. They include astragalus (to increase energy enhancement of the body's immune system, to fight diabetes, heart disease, and high blood pressure), schizandra (to stimulate the immune system, balance body functions, optimize energy, and reduce stress), rhodiola rosea (to increase resistance to infection and promote healing), green tea (for its polyphenols), and spirulina (for sustained energy).

Creatine may be added to bars. Creatine is the substance found in muscle tissue, and supplies energy for muscle contractions, boosting endurance, building muscles, increasing lean muscle mass, and for gaining strength during workouts.

Food Bars Fill Specific Niches. Diabetics are being targeted, especially with the bars that are based on the glycemic index. With a potential market of 16 million diabetic Americans, other types of products are marketed for this group, too. One pharmaceutical company offers "nibbles" to help control glucose blood levels of diabetics. The nibbles are to be eaten before bedtime to help prevent low-blood-sugar episodes during the night. Yet the need can be filled simply and less expensively by appropriate food.

Children are targeted for food bars. Some of the bars allegedly modify metabolic responses. These bars are geared to address behavioral problems such as attention deficit disorder (ADD), and attention deficit hyperactivity disorder (ADHD). But this approach is an oversimplified nonsolution to a complex problem. Even if these bars would be effective, there is the question of amount. How much is too much, or too little?

The candy-like appeal of the food bars is extended to the candy-like quality of some pharmaceuticals and nutraceuticals intended for children. For example, oral rehydration medication is available as frozen popsicles. Lollipops contain vitamins, pyruvate or chromium picolinate, along with active botanicals such as St. John's wort, ginkgo biloba, kava kava, passion flower, and echinacea. Snack foods enjoyed by children, such as corn chips, may contain kava kava for relaxation, cat's claw to increase longevity, and St. John's wort to combat depression. Gummy bears may have added chicory root for dietary fiber, as well as vitamins, antioxidants, and herbals.

Women are targeted for food bars, presumably to meet their special needs. The bars supply some of the minerals and vitamins that are low in the diets of many American women: calcium, iron, folic acid, and vitamin B_{12}, (cyanocobalamin). Some energy bars target women on weight-loss programs. Such bars have high carbohydrates/low fat ratios, and may contain ingredients such as soy and folic acid. Yet all these nutrients are readily supplied, at lower cost, with basic foods and dietary supplements.

As an extension of the successful food bars targeted to women, candy-like soft calcium chews (in chocolate, mocha, and caramel flavors) have been introduced for "active nutrition." The chews have added thiamine (vitamin B_{1}) calcium, and zinc, and such products are classified as a dietary supplement. The chews are described as "purseable" and "designed to delight the taste buds of women" in "convenient everyday form." Two or three chews daily provide an adult woman with the recommended calcium levels, plus minerals, and antioxidants, as well as vitamins D and K to improve absorption and reduce the risk of hip fractures. As with the food bars, the chews offer nutrients readily supplied, at lower cost, with basic foods and dietary supplements.

A recent entry into the candy-like supplement market is an herbal fudge-like food supplement described as a bite-size candy. The product is claimed to provide half the daily antioxidant requirements for adults, and 100 percent of the daily requirements for vitamins C and E.

Food, Candy, or Medicine? Some food bars are difficult to classify. Are they foods, candy bars, medicine, dietary supplements, or medical foods? An example is one ingredient, L-arginine, an amino acid found in many basic foods. Now, it is added to some food bars. Research shows that L-arginine improves the inner linings of blood vessels, and boosts the production of nitric oxide. The food bars with added L-arginine supposedly maintain a healthy heart and manage cardiovascular diseases. Two of the food bars with added L-arginine are reported to be equivalent to 12 to 18 dietary-supplement pills of this amino acid. The bars also contain other nutrients. Two bars, consumed regularly, are reported to improve circulation, increase pain-free exercise, and lower the total and LDL cholesterol levels. Are such bars foods or medical foods?

Medical foods are to be consumed under a doctor's supervision. They are formulated products that are intended to supplement oral intake as part of overall medical management of a condition or disease for which specific nutritional requirements are established by medical evaluation. Examples of medical foods are ones that manage cardiovascular diseases, kidney and liver diseases, compromised immune function, diabetes, burns, Crohn's disease, and short bowel syndrome. Some food bars are designed to provide specific nutrients depleted during dieting. Others are intended to complement major categories of common prescription drugs (example, heart medications) that deplete the body of nutrients such as potassium or magnesium. The overlap between medical foods and specialized food bars is apparent. Categorization is difficult.

Prebiotic food bars are difficult to classify. Commonly, such bars contain fructooligossacharides (FOS), a complex carbohydrate that stimulates growth of good bacteria, and inulin, a natural dietary fiber present in common fruits and vegetables. They are sold with claims that they stimulate the growth of bifidobacteria, ensure gut health, inhibit harmful bacteria, boost immunity, improve mineral absorption, lower triglycerides/cholesterol levels, prevent constipation, decrease stool weight, detoxify, are low in calories, and are suitable for diabetics. Similar results can be obtained, at far lower costs, with fermented dairy products (for example, yogurt or kefir), or with prebiotic dietary supplements.

Food bars with colostrum are also difficult to classify. Colostrum is a premilk fluid in mammary milk produced after the birth of offspring. It contains antibodies as well as growth immune factors that help ensure the health and vitality of the newborn. Colostrum from cows is used in food bars, with claims that the substance can support the human immune system, health in the gastrointestinal tract, and overall good health.

How does one classify a food bar to which substances are added, allegedly to improve memory and learning concentration? Some food bars (as well as chewing gums) have phosphatidylserine (PS) added to them. PS is present in the brain and important for neurotransmissions and synaptic communications.

Chewing gums, along with food bars, have candy-like qualities. How does one classify chewing gums that contain mushroom extracts to help deodorize or suppress odors generated in the digestive system? Such products are claimed to reduce functional burdens on the kidneys/liver, retard the progression of kidney failure, and suppress the formation of free radicals and allergens associated with disease and aging.

Milk-based chewing gums allegedly remineralize and strengthen teeth. Some dental gums promise to reduce plaque build-up by 35 percent provided that two pieces are chewed for twenty minutes after eating.

The difficulty in classifying such products is reflected by a marketing decision. In most mass marketing retail stores, food bars and similar products are now sold in *both* candy *and* health product sections of stores.

Chapter 5

Sugar: Desired but Undesirable

WHAT'S WRONG WITH SUGAR?

Why is sugar so bad when it gives a quick pick-me-up? Energy supplied by refined carbohydrate such as sugar causes the blood sugar in the body to rise quickly. But it falls nearly as fast. Refined carbohydrates, such as sugar, are rapidly digested, and produce a temporary oversupply of sugar in the blood. In turn, the liver and pancreas are stimulated to withdraw this excess, in order to keep the blood sugar level at an equilibrium. This is achieved by converting the excess energy into starch in the liver and storing it in the cells as glycogen, which eventually is converted into fat. The blood sugar level drops after the excess energy is withdrawn, and with this drop, the person feels hunger, fatigue, and a craving for more energy food. It is a vicious cycle.

If no food is eaten, the blood sugar remains at an undesirably low level until it is restored to a normal level, by reconversion of the stored glycogen into blood sugar. But, experiencing hunger, the person may eat before the glycogen is reconverted. Any excess of unused or unconverted glucose is converted into body fat.

High and low swings in the blood sugar level are undesirable. Complex carbohydrates (from potatoes, for example) are digested more slowly, and do not result in such fluctuations. The high and low swings, resulting from the quick energy supplied by refined carbohydrate such as sugar, are extremely damaging to the liver, the pancreas and the total functioning of the body. Over a period of time, the pattern of high and low swings in the blood sugar level can be devastating to the human organism, and result in health effects such as rapid aging, bodily deterioration, and a lowered resistance to sickness and disease.

Complex carbohydrates found in starchy vegetables, legumes, and whole grains contain many nutrients, bound up in cellulose fiber, that take longer to digest and enter the bloodstream. Complex carbohydrates, consumed along with proteins and fats, will sustain the glucose level in the bloodstream at a high, even level, and will not result in hunger, fatigue, or a craving for more energy food. The sugar in fruit, though rapidly digested, is combined with fiber and nutrients.

CONFUSING CONSUMERS ABOUT SUGAR INTAKE

How much sugar does the average American consume? It would appear that this simple question could be answered straightforwardly. But the official response misrepresents facts, misleads the public, and has significant health implications.

According to a joint statement by L. Jackson Brown, D.D.S., chief epidemiologist at the National Institute of Dental Research (NIDR) at the National Institutes of Health, and two economists from the University of Connecticut, Americans have been able to reduce their dental bills due to a decline in the per capita consumption of refined sugar—a drop of 33 percent during the 1980s. This is good news, because it is generally acknowledged that the amount of refined sugar eaten is related to the development of tooth decay—the greater the consumption, the more the decay.

Unfortunately, the news is untrue.

There hasn't been a drop in sugar consumption; on the contrary, consumption has been rising steadily, year by year.

This is of great concern to researchers and health professionals, who regard high sugar consumption as a serious health risk. Any improved dental health should be attributed to factors other than sugar consumption.

What accounts for this discrepancy? Semantics. By formulating an inexplicable and arbitrary definition, the Food and Drug Administration (FDA) has decreed that "refined sugar" solely denotes sucrose (table sugar derived from cane or beet), but excludes other caloric sugars—also refined—such as high fructose corn syrup (HFCS), glucose, and dextrose, as well as some minor caloric sugars such as honey and edible syrups—all designated as "sweeteners."

This limited definition of "refined sugar" is unscientific, because all caloric sugars are detrimental to teeth. With apologies to writer Gertrude Stein, not only a rose is a rose, but sugar is sugar. Although economists may not be expected to recognize this fact, surely NIDR researchers should acknowledge the potentially damaging effects of all caloric sugars. Additionally, emerging evidence from research at the U.S. Department of Agriculture (USDA) and elsewhere points to potentially harmful effects of high sugar consumption—the importance of which may be overlooked given the false reporting.

A More Accurate Picture. What are the facts? It is true that refined sugar (sucrose) consumption as defined by the FDA has been declining steadily from 83.6 pounds per person each year in 1980 to 64.6 pounds per person in 1994. However, this decline shouldn't be trumpeted, because it's misleading.

The figures for sucrose consumption are inextricably linked to those of corn sweeteners, mainly HFCS. The decline in sucrose consumption occurred as corn sweetener consumption simultaneously increased; corn sweeteners have been used as a partial or total sucrose replacer.

For a more accurate picture, it is necessary to look at the

figures for sucrose and corn sweeteners for the same years. In 1980, the corn sweetener consumption rate was 39.6 pounds per person; by 1994, it had risen to 83.2 pounds—more than double. The total of these two major sweeteners increased from 123.2 pounds in 1980 to 147.8 pounds in 1994, about a 20 percent increase.

When all caloric sweeteners are added—including sucrose, HFCS, glucose, dextrose, honey, and edible syrups—the grand total for 1980 was 124.4 pounds per person; for 1994, 149.2 pounds. Since then, sugar consumption continued to mount. By 2002, annual consumption per person reached 152.4 pounds. These figures are supplied by the USDA's *Sugar & Sweeteners* quarterly, contributed by its Economic Research Service (ERS).

The figures go higher when low-caloric sweeteners such as aspartame (NutraSweet, Equal) are included. The ERS, in a separate 1991 tabulation, cited total annual sugar and sweetener consumption as 164.9 pounds (more recent figures weren't available). It included aspartame: equivalency of 17 pounds of sugar sweetness annually per capita. (Aspartame's sweetening capacity is 200 times that of sucrose.) It also included saccharin (Sweet 'N Low), which is noncaloric, but omitted acesulfame K (Sweet One, Sunett), another low-caloric sweetener. All of the USDA's tables omitted consumption of the sugar alcohols, such as sorbitol and mannitol, which contain as many calories as sucrose. Despite these flaws, it is safe to assume that the current total is at least as high as the 2002 ERS numbers—probably higher, because sweetener consumption continues to escalate yearly in the United States.

In addition to the contradictory figures of the NIDR and the USDA regarding total sugar consumption, other groups also misrepresent and grossly underestimate actual caloric sugar consumption. In a leaflet called "Sweet Talk: Facts about Sweeteners," the American Dietetic Association (ADA) reported that "the average American consumes almost 43 pounds of caloric sweeteners each year, mostly from corn syrup and table sugar."

How did the ADA arrive at this number? Apparently it was based on information supplied by The Sugar Association, Inc., a trade group. In a "Consumer Fact Sheet," the association stated that "the USDA reports disappearance, not consumption, figures for sweeteners. The USDA estimates that in 1993, about 65 pounds of sugar (cane or beet); 79 pounds of corn sweeteners; and 1 pound of other sweeteners (honey, maple syrup) per capita were delivered into the food supply. That adds up to a total nutritive sweetener usage of about 145 pounds per capita."

So far, fine. But then, by a deft disappearing act, the total consumption was drastically reduced by over 100 pounds: "As disappearance data, these numbers do not account for waste, sugars used up in fermentation as in bread baking, or use in pet foods. Recently, the FDA estimated that the amount of added sweeteners (sugar + corn sweeteners + other) Americans actually consume is considerably less than disappearance—about 43 pounds per person, or about 11 percent of total calories."

How the FDA derived its estimates is not provided. By contrast, the USDA's own data—the source for consumption statistics—show Americans consuming 19 percent of their calories from added sweeteners. So the most authoritative data available add up to a significantly larger 80 pounds per person, per year. By all indications, this is increasing.

A Question of Health. Despite such conflicting data, dietitians, and the USDA's home extension service personnel repeat the FDA's questionable sugar consumption figures. The distorted data are picked up and repeated by food writers and widely read by the public.

At the same time, nutritional research findings suggest that the dangerous health effects from high consumption of sugar extend far beyond the oral cavity. Increasing consumption of high fructose corn sweeteners is of particular concern.

If per capita food supply estimates accurately reflect actual consumption, the USDA's journal *Food Review* reported, "each American, on average, now consumes significantly more added fructose than in 1980."

"This apparent increase," the report continued, "gives rise to concern among nutritionists because evidence has implicated diets high in fructose with increased blood lipid levels (lipids is the technical term for fats, waxes, and fatty compounds). A task force of scientists convened by the Food and Drug Administration found in 1986 no conclusive evidence that a high sugar intake is a risk factor for heart disease, whether by raising blood cholesterol, triglycerides (a fat in the blood), or blood pressure, 'in the general population.' However, some researchers suggest that a small number of 'carbohydrate-sensitive' individuals—such as those with insulin or triglyceride levels that are high to start with—may be particularly sensitive to sugar (especially fructose) and respond with raised cholesterol and triglyceride levels."

Sugar Intake, Heart Disease, and Diabetes. "I'm definitely concerned that sugar consumption at current levels is increasing risk of heart disease and diabetes in a small but significant percentage of the population," said Dr. Sheldon Reiser in 1991. Reiser had headed research on the effects of sugars and other carbohydrates on human metabolism at the USDA's Carbohydrate Nutrition Laboratory (CNL) at Beltsville, Maryland. Findings by Reiser and his colleagues affirmed that high sugar consumption poses health risks.

Some 15 percent of Americans are prone genetically to elevated fat levels (triglycerides) circulating in their blood.

Reiser and his colleagues showed that sugar raises triglycerides even higher in these people. Later, the researchers found that people with high triglyceride levels generally have elevated insulin levels, too. These are key risk factors, respectively, for heart disease and diabetes. As early as the 1960s, research showed fructose to be lipogenic (fat formative) in all people. The liver removes all of the absorbed sugar from the blood and converts it into triglycerides, which then are secreted back into the blood.

High triglyceride levels are recognized as a risk factor for heart disease, mainly because they usually accompany low levels of beneficial high-density lipoprotein (HDL) cholesterol. Persons with low HDL levels may not be able to remove cholesterol from their arteries promptly and may be at high risk for heart disease.

In subsequent studies, Reiser reported that sugar at levels and in diets reflecting what is consumed in the United States has usually produced significant increases in blood triglycerides in people with elevated triglycerides, insulin, or both. Studies conducted elsewhere showed similar findings.

Reiser and his colleagues found that in cases when increased triglyceride levels were not significant, the diets contained extra fiber or a higher ratio of polyunsaturated to saturated fat than most Americans eat. These food components seemed to counteract the harmful effects of fructose. Also, fructose did not appear to affect young women as it did men and postmenopausal women. However, it could interact with oral contraceptives and elevate insulin levels in women on "the pill." Fructose significantly increased triglycerides in men with normal levels, although the higher levels were still within a normal range.

At high levels, fructose promoted another recognized heart risk factor—high uric acid level—both in normal men and in those sensitive to fructose.

Studies at CNL, led by Judith Hallfrisch, showed that high fructose consumption caused people with both normal and high insulin levels to secrete more insulin during a glucose tolerance test. Those with high insulin showed the greatest increase. Subsequent studies by others confirmed these findings.

"High insulin is believed to be one of the earliest signs of noninsulin-dependent, or type II diabetes," noted Reiser. "Fructose has been suggested as a sugar that can be safely consumed by people with impaired glucose tolerance because the body does not use insulin to metabolize fructose. It's true that when consumed alone, fructose does not significantly increase either insulin or glucose levels in the blood. But fructose is almost always consumed along with glucose." For example, both HFCS and table sugar are about half glucose.

Studies indicated that somehow fructose reduces the affinity of insulin for its receptor—the first step for glucose to enter a cell and be metabolized. As a result, the body needs to pump out more insulin, in order to handle the same amount of glucose.

Reiser expressed concern about the increase of triglyceride and insulin levels as people age. "Fewer than 15 percent of young people are fructose sensitive, but more than 15 percent of older people are." Does the trait develop only in those with faulty genes? Or, do the years of eating high sugar levels push others into this danger zone, too? At present, there is no answer.

Otho Michaelis, a CNL research biologist, believes that sugar "could contribute to the time of onset and severity" of type 2 diabetes, "in its expression in people with a particular genetic background." Michaelis had searched for an experimental rat model that would resemble the 15 percent of the human population found to be sugar sensitive, and who would develop diabetes. Michaelis found three strains of genetically obese models suitable to study high blood pressure and diabetes, diabetes only, and gross obesity. By using the different strains, the influence of each factor influencing diabetic development could be studied. Rats genetically prone to diabetes developed the disease regardless of whether or not they were fed sugar. But, a high-sugar diet magnified blood glucose, insulin, and other hormones that regulate glucose, as well as triglycerides and cholesterol. Also, the high-sugar diet accelerated the structural damage to kidneys and, possibly, to other organs.

Another noted effect of high-fructose intake was that this sugar exacerbated copper deficiency in male animals. According to Meira Fields, also with CNL, numerous studies showed that young male rats developed severe anemia, enlarged hearts and livers, and died prematurely from copper-deficient diets when sugar (but not starch) was the main carbohydrate source.

Pigs have cardiovascular and digestive systems very similar to humans. Studies similar to those with rats were conducted with pigs on a low- copper/high -fructose diet by CNL researchers. When fructose comprised 20 percent of the total calories in the diet (only twice the level in the average human diet in the United States), the pigs developed pronounced anemia, liver damage, and severely enlarged hearts.

According to Fields, fructose (and other substances metabolized similarly, such as alcohol) "creates a unique environment in which copper deficiency can cause damage." Fields and her colleagues found that damage to the heart and to other organs depends on a change in the way animals handle another mineral: iron. Although all copper-deficient rats accumulate iron in their livers, those eating high-fructose levels cannot utilize the iron, which leads to anemia.

Much of the stored iron appears to be in a form that generates free radicals and results in liver damage.

Dr. Richard Anderson, who has researched high fructose corn syrup (HFCS) for twenty years, demonstrated that a loss in chromium is worsened if fructose is eaten along with another simple sugar, such as glucose, a component of table sugar. Low chromium levels, combined with high fructose intake, can lead to increased cholesterol and triglyceride levels in the blood.

"If you go into the general population and take people with slightly elevated blood sugar and give them chromium supplements, you'll see a drop in blood sugar in 80 to 90 percent of the people," Anderson reported. But, he believes that elevated blood sugar levels could be lowered simply if people reduced their intake of sweeteners such as table sugar and corn syrup.

Dr. David Milne at the USDA's Human Nutrition Research Center also has studied the effects of low-copper/high-HFCS diet on heart disease risks. At present, Milne is researching the effects of a high-HFCS diet low in magnesium—another mineral important for heart health. Copper and magnesium interact in the body. Milne suggests that a high-fructose/low magnesium diet could have similar adverse health effects as those of a high-fructose/low copper diet.

Sugar Intake and Cancer. Two studies from Europe produced new findings of the health effects of high sugar intake. One study of cancer of the biliary tract (including the gallbladder and bile ducts) was conducted at the National Institute of Public Health and Environmental Protection in The Netherlands. The most consistent finding of cancer risk was associated with high sugar intake. The effect was independent of other caloric sources, such as fat. Also, high sugar intake may predispose individuals to gallstones—which may be associated with biliary tract cancer. This finding had not been reported previously.

Another study was conducted in northern Italy, where researchers collected data between 1985 to 1992 on various dietary factors with nearly 1,000 colon cancer patients and more than 600 rectal cancer patients. The heavy sugar users had increased risks for both colon and rectal cancer, with the risk increasing in proportion to the amount of sugar consumed.

The study suggested that high sugar consumption may be a significant risk factor for colorectal cancers. If confirmed, the finding is significant as a public health issue. In magnitude, the relative risks in this study were comparable to those previously reported for such dietary factors as fats and red meats.

Danger of Current Recommendations. Reiser has noted that current recommendations to reduce fat intake by increasing carbohydrate intake may result in boosting sugar intake even higher. The current recommendation is to increase carbohydrates from the present 47 percent, up to somewhere between 55 and 60 percent. Although this increase should come from whole grains, fruits, and vegetables, Reiser is skeptical that Americans will make these prudent choices. Instead, people aiming simply to avoid "fatty" foods, often turn to "low fat" formulations, which are frequently high in sugar. People may think that one carbohydrate is just as good as another, as long as it is not fat. A *Newsweek* cover story highlights this phenomenon. The USDA acknowledges it: "Despite considerable progress toward a lower fat, higher carbohydrate diet in the past decade, per capita use of caloric sweeteners has reached an all-time high and average fiber intake remains very low."

High sugar intake may be an unrecognized risk factor in numerous health problems. Misrepresentations of actual sugar consumption obscure the issue and underestimate the role of sugar in health problems.

SOME PROBLEMATIC SUGARS

Some sugars, present in certain foods, are not well tolerated by all. Individuals born with certain genetic disorders of carbohydrate metabolism may lack specific enzymes needed to digest these sugars. An example is lactase, an enzyme needed to digest lactose, the milk sugar. In recent years, lactose intolerance (also termed lactose malabsorption) has been better recognized. Many strategies have been devised to cope with this problem. (See the article "Lactose Intolerance" on page 73.)

Galactose, a sugar component of lactose, also may create intolerance problems for those who lack the enzyme needed for its digestion. Galactosemia is a genetic disorder of carbohydrate metabolism. At present, galactose intolerance is at a similar stage as lactose intolerance was several decades ago: largely unrecognized and unexplored.

Galactose Intolerance. Galactose, the major component of the main carbohydrate in both human and cow's milk, must be avoided by galactosemics. Galactose intolerance is far less common than lactose intolerance. However, when experienced, it is far more severe. If not treated promptly after birth with a totally dairy-free diet, the galactosemic infant fails to thrive. The child may have stunted growth, cataract development, liver disorders, or even death.

Galactosemia affects one in every 30,000 to 60,000 infants. The acute symptoms occur a few days after birth in an apparently healthy infant. The baby may begin to vomit, lose weight, and become lethargic. Usually, the symptoms subside when dairy foods are replaced by a nondairy formula.

Because the galactosemic infant responds favorably to the same diet as the lactose-intolerant infant, galactosemia may be unsuspected at an early stage, and wrongly attributed to lactose intolerance. However, these two genetic diseases are distinctly different, which may become apparent during the next stage of the child's growth. The lactose-intolerant individual may continue to thrive when fruits, vegetables, and cereals are added to the diet. But the galactosemic may begin to show poor growth, mental retardation, and speech difficulties.

Recent galactose research may help explain this puzzle. A joint study, conducted by the Agricultural Research Service (ARS) of the U.S. Department of Agriculture (USDA) and Ross Laboratories, revealed that, in addition to dairy foods, many common fruits and vegetables, and possibly some grains, contain galactose.

As follow-up, baby food products from leading manufacturers were tested. Various amounts of galactose were identified in twelve fruit and vegetable products intended for infant feeding. High levels were present in applesauce, banana, and squash. The researchers examined 45 commonly consumed fresh fruits and vegetables. They identified high galactose levels in tomato, watermelon, papaya, and persimmon; and moderately high levels in banana, apple, date, kiwi, pumpkin, bell pepper, and Brussels sprouts. Unfortunately, the foods identified as galactose-free are those not likely to be used in baby food products: artichoke, mushroom, olive, and peanut. At present, there is a lack of information as to whether or not galactose is present in cereal commonly fed to infants, from grains such as rice, oats, or barley.

Based on this new information, fifteen galactosemic children, ranging from infants to teenagers, are being studied. Parents are keeping food diaries for the children. The ARS will make laboratory analyses of the foods to determine galactose intake levels. The goal is to learn whether galactose intake levels, present in nondairy foods, are sufficiently high that they need to be avoided by galactosemics.

Fructose Intolerance. Fructose, another natural sugar present in many foods, is problematic for some. Most people can convert fructose to glucose and burn it for energy. Fructose-intolerant individuals cannot make this conversion. They are unable to absorb fructose into the bloodstream. Instead, the fructose remains in the bowel, where bacterial fermentation produces carbon dioxide, hydrogen, methane, water, alcohol, and lactic acid. Both the alcohol and lactic acid can irritate the bowel lining. The gas, bloating, and abdominal distention, if chronic, can lead to hiatal hernia, or a blow-out of the thin weak-walled part of the colon.

Fructose intolerance may be a previously unrecognized factor associated with gluten intolerance. Also, it may be a missing piece in the puzzle of irritable bowel syndrome. Symptoms of fructose intolerance are surprisingly similar to those of lactose intolerance. A diet of benefit to some sufferers of ulcerative colitis and irritable bowel syndrome includes avoidance of fructose, as well as three other poorly absorbed sugars: lactose, sorbitol, and mannitol.

Not everyone with irritable bowel syndrome is fructose intolerant. Some may be intolerant only if the bowel already is inflamed or irritated from infections, drugs, lactose, sorbitol, and mannitol. Others may tolerate small amounts of fructose, but suffer serious effects if large amounts are consumed.

Fructose is found in fruits and honey. However, corn that is treated enzymatically can be converted to fructose. Corn-derived sweeteners and syrups have become increasingly important in the American food supply as high fructose corn syrup (HFCS). They either partially or totally replace sucrose in many foods and beverages. Heavy consumption of HFCS may induce or aggravate copper deficiency, which is thought to be a leading cause of ischemic heart disease (an obstruction of blood flow to the heart, usually as a result of atherosclerosis).

In animal studies, 30 to 60 percent mortality was induced

in copper-deficient rats merely by replacing dietary starch with fructose or sucrose. Both fructose and sucrose (which consists of linked sucrose and glucose molecules) aggravate symptoms of marginal and severe copper deficiency.

Dr. Sheldon Reiser and associates at the USDA (see "Sugar Intake, Heart Disease, and Diabetes" on page 175.) investigated the effects of fructose consumption on the copper status of twenty-four men who were fed alternately a diet comprised of 20 percent fructose and 20 percent starch. After the first few weeks, the study had to be terminated. Of the 20 percent fructose diet, four of the twenty-four men developed cardiac problems, ranging from severe tachycardia (abnormally rapid heart beat) to mild heart attack.

It is thought that the average American diet, consisting of many refined foods, is marginally copper deficient. This deficiency is worsened by heavy consumption of HFCS.

SUGAR ALTERNATIVES FOR WEIGHT CONTROL

Many people drink diet sodas containing the nonnutritive sweetener saccharin (Sweet 'N Low) or the low-calorie sweetener aspartame (NutraSweet, Equal), assuming that these sugar alternatives are useful for weight control. Is this assumption correct?

Results of various tests with nonnutritive and low-calorie sugar alternatives indicate that these substances are ineffective for weight control.

Saccharin. In 1974, on behalf of the National Institute of Medicine, Dr. Kenneth Melmon reported that "the data on the efficacy of saccharin or its salts for the treatment of patients with obesity, dental caries, coronary artery disease or even diabetes have not so far produced a clear picture to us of the usefulness of the drug."

Nevertheless, in 1977, when it appeared that saccharin might be banned as a carcinogen, the Food and Drug Administration (FDA) announced plans to reclassify the sweetener as a drug so physicians could prescribe its use for weight control, as well as diabetes and other health disorders for which weight control is important. (The reclassification was never implemented, as moratoria have been used, repeatedly, to stay the banning action. Ultimately, it was deregulated.)

After the proposed saccharin ban, Dr. Harold Rifkin, a diabetician associated with the American Diabetes Association in New York, reported that saccharin offered no health benefits for diabetics. Nor did saccharin offer any benefits for dieters, according to Norine Condon, a dietitian with the American Dietetics Association in Chicago.

In fact, animal studies demonstrate that saccharin, because of its ability to reduce blood sugar, is an appetite stimulant.

Cyclamates. Similarly, cyclamates—a group of nonnutritive sweeteners banned in 1969 as potential copromoters of cancer—lacked value in weight-control programs. Early in 1969, in the Netherlands, it was demonstrated in rat experiments that cyclamates actually stimulated appetite, and led to weight increase. The researchers concluded: "If this is true for man, then weight reduction will be more difficult if the diet contains cyclamates."

Instead of keeping weight down, cyclamates appeared to increase the craving for real sweets.

Aspartame. Recently, aspartame was investigated at Leeds University. Nearly 100 males and females, aged eighteen to twenty-two years, were given solutions of equal sweetness, containing either 188 calories of sugar (glucose) or three calories of aspartame. For an hour after drinking the solution, responses of pleasure, fullness and hunger were recorded every ten minutes. Both glucose and aspartame induced the pleasure response, but the effects of aspartame were only about half as strong. Glucose produced an increase in fullness, while aspartame had the opposite effect.

Also, aspartame did not suppress the appetite after the drink, as did glucose. In fact, in the second half of the test hour, the participants' appetites actually increased over the beginning level. Results showed that aspartame left the participants hungrier than those in the control group who had drunk plain water. It was concluded that aspartame may have appetite-stimulating properties.

Do Artificial Sweeteners Send the Body Mixed Messages? The American Cancer Society examined weight changes for one year in a homogeneous group of women aged fifty to sixty-nine years as part of a nation-wide study of more than a million people. More than 17,000 participants had never used artificial sweeteners (AS), while more than 61,000 had used them for at least ten years.

During the study year, the rate of weight gain was significantly greater among the AS users than nonusers within each weight group.

. . . the tongue perceives artificial sweeteners as food, but the rest of the body does not, and still craves more of both food and sweetness.

The percentage of AS users who gained ten pounds or more during the study year was significantly greater, regardless of their beginning weight. Dietary records showed no marked difference in the kinds of foods eaten by AS users and nonusers. No data were available about quantities of foods served.

It has been suggested that the body of an individual using these sugar substitutes may be receiving mixed messages—the tongue perceives artificial sweeteners as food, but the rest of the body does not, and still craves more of both food and sweetness. Confusion of psychological and biological information might even lead to less control over appetite, and result in disordered eating patterns.

For some, such as diabetics who depart from their customarily prescribed low-carbohydrate diet and become dependent on artificially sweetened foods, grave health consequences can result. Researchers at the Frances Stern Food Clinic in Boston had conducted studies with 100 diabetic women to learn whether artificial sweeteners could help them stay on a carbohydrate-restricted diet. The conclusion was that "there is little basis for implying that adherence or nonadherence to a carbohydrate-restricted diet is related to the use of a noncaloric [or nonnutritive] sweetener."

PLANT-DERIVED SWEETENERS

Sugarcane and corn, in the form of table sugar and syrup, provide most of our present caloric sweeteners. To a lesser extent, beet sugar is manufactured. But, in other parts of the world different plants supply sweeteners—some many times sweeter than our own.

Sweeteners Grown Abroad. Several are found in Africa. A red berry, from a plant in West Africa, was named the serendipity berry (*Dioscoroephyllum cuminsii* Diels) and has a sweet component—called monellin—that is about 2,500 times sweeter than those from sugarcane, corn, or beets.

Another African fruit containing an intensive sweetener is katemfe (*Thaumatoccus danielli*), termed the miraculous fruit of the Sudan. The plant grows from Sierra Leone to the Congo in West Africa, as well as Sudan and Uganda. The fruit contains three large black seeds surrounded by a colorless, mucilaginous substance. The two principal ingredients have been identified as proteins and are 1,600 times sweeter than table sugar.

The miraculous berry (*Synsepalum dulcificum*) is also found in a West African plant. The fruit is not especially sweet, but causes sour or highly acidic foods to taste very sweet. The taste distortion can last several hours. The sweet taste lingers in the mouth, and the sweetness is imparted to anything subsequently consumed. Anyone who has eaten a globe artichoke has experienced a similar taste distortion.

Stevia (*Stevia rebaudiana* Bertoni), indigenous to the northern sections of South America (Brazil and Uruguay) and Paraguay in Central America, is up to 300 times sweeter than sugar. The leaves of the plant retain their sweetness indefinitely, and have been called the "honey leaf." For centuries, they have been used, not only as a sweetening agent, but therapeutically, as a digestive aid, to support pancreatic function, and for wound healing due to the herb's ability to inhibit bacterial growth.

In recent times, stevia has been grown and used widely in Asian countries. It is exported mainly from China.

In 1991, the Food and Drug Administration (FDA) blocked stevia's importation, and regarded the herb as an unapproved food additive. Considering the investment that U.S. manufacturers have made in artificial sweeteners such as aspartame, they are unlikely to invest money for FDA approval for a nonpatentable substance like stevia.

Food and beverage companies, as well as the American Herbal Products Association, petitioned the FDA for "Generally Regarded as Safe" (GRAS) status, and submitted safety tests based on extensive Japanese scientific data, as well as the herb's long history of safe usage. The FDA denied the petition. Further petitions were submitted in subsequent years, and repeatedly denied.

After passage of the Dietary Supplement Health and Education Act (DSHEA) in 1994, the FDA classified stevia as a dietary supplement. Stevia products are sold in various forms as liquid extracts, in powders, capsules, and tablets. Maltodextrins are added as fillers to reduce the intense sweetness of stevia. Classified as a dietary supplement, no mention of it as a sweetening agent is permitted on the labels of such products. Nor is stevia permitted to be used as a sweetening agent in food or beverage products in the United States, although stevia is used for this purpose in many other countries. Ironically, in the United States, it is possible to purchase stevia capsules as a dietary product at levels reaching 1,000 milligrams (one gram), and to consume as many capsules as desired, without any official restriction concerning its safety. At the same time, stevia's use at an exceedingly low level to sweeten food and beverage products is forbidden, and regarded by the FDA as potentially unsafe.

Licorice (*Glycyrrhiza glabra*) is a sweetener generally known to Americans as a flavoring. Food processors have found that licorice intensifies other flavors and mellows a general harshness of synthetic flavors, and some food and beverage processors increasingly are using licorice compounds as sweeteners. In reviewing the safety of licorice, the FDA affirmed that licorice compounds were safe when used as flavoring agents, but the FDA has proposed to limit its use in foods as a sweetener. High consumption of foods containing licorice might interfere with drugs and decrease the efficacy of some used for heart conditions and blood pressure.

The active ingredient in licorice, glycyrrhizic acid, is related, chemically and structurally, to two adrenal gland hormones and can produce steroidal effects, exert estrogenic activity, and other biological actions. Other adverse health effects from high consumption of licorice include high blood pressure, paralysis of extremities, shortness of breath, swelling, weight gain, headache, and muscular weakness.

Sweeteners Grown Locally. At least three plants commonly grown in the United States contain sweeteners. Leaves of the herb, sweet cicely—sometimes called the candy plant (*Myrrhis odorata*)—have been used as a sweetener and flavor enhancer in conserves and with tart dishes. The dried leaves of the big-leaved hydrangea (*Hydrangea macrophylla* var. *Thunbergii*), and the rhizomes of the common fern (*Polypodium vulgare* L.) also contain sweeteners.

Increased consumer interest in a variety of sweeteners, especially sweeteners that won't damage teeth, may lead to the commercial use of these plant sources for alternative sweeteners. Unlike present sweeteners that are made from carbohydrates, those derived from protein might not damage teeth. However, when heated, they undergo irreversible breakdown and lose their sweetness. This characteristic is a drawback for food and beverage processors.

Although many of these sweeteners have been used traditionally in other areas of the world, they still need to undergo extensive safety testing before approval for food use in the United States. Just because substances are derived from plants and are therefore "natural" does not automatically assure safety. Also, just because substances have long been in use does not automatically assure safety, either.

Chapter 6

Fats and Oils: What You Should Know

WHAT'S WRONG WITH 'FAT-FREE' OLESTRA?

When the Food and Drug Administration (FDA) considered fortification of foods with folic acid, the agency's then Commissioner, Dr. David A. Kessler, issued a policy statement: "Whenever you fortify the entire American food supply with a pharmacologically active ingredient, you need to be sure you get it right and get it right the first time." This policy needs to be applied to other substances considered for approval. Did Kessler get it right the first time with the fat substitute, Olestra (sucrose polyester)?

Olestra Is Pharmacologically Active. Although the public has been led to believe that Olestra is not absorbed, this notion is inaccurate. Dr. George Pauli, from the FDA's Office of Premarket Approval, reported that Olestra is not absorbed in any *appreciable* amount. Long-term rat studies suggest that some Olestra is absorbed, as reflected by changes found in the animals' livers and spleens.

Procter & Gamble (P&G), Olestra's manufacturer, reported that the overall sensitivity of the tests was only about 2 to 3 percent of the administered dose. Later studies with rats, guinea pigs, and mini-pigs showed absorption ranging from 0.2 to 1.5 percent. The absorption problem, even at a low rate, may be critical for humans with impaired gastrointestinal tracts, as reflected in the tests with guinea pigs. One group was fed a substance known to cause intestinal damage. After three weeks, these animals with impaired gastrointestinal systems were fed Olestra and developed lesions in their tracts similar to those observed in acute and chronic human gastrointestinal diseases, such as ulcerative colitis and Crohn's disease. In feeding tests with mini-pigs—animals whose gastrointestinal tracts are anatomically and physiologically similar to those of humans—the animals absorbed 1.1 percent of the Olestra.

The FDA expressed concern about one aspect of the pharmacological activity of Olestra. In the colon, Olestra "has the potential to adversely affect the normal metabolic activity of the intestinal microflora. . . . Therefore, it is important to know whether consumption of Olestra affects microflora populations or alters fermentation processes in normal microflora metabolism" in the body. The FDA noted that "there is a hypothetical possibility that an organism capable of metabolizing Olestra at a low level could arise among the intestinal microflora."

Others expressed concerns about P&G's own test results in rat studies with Olestra that showed pituitary tumors in males and females; leukemias and premature deaths in males; abnormal and possibly precancerous liver changes in females; and deformed and stillborn offspring.

Inadequacies of the Testing Program. Among several objections to Olestra's approval, Dr. Henry Blackburn, an epidemiologist at the University of Minnesota who served as a member of the FDA's Food Advisory Committee (FAC), criticized the "unacceptably low power" of the human studies in the testing program. Blackburn was concerned that Olestra was approved for introduction into the food supply "without an agreed upon criterion for pre- and post-market testing to determine long-term effects."

Other critics charged that Olestra data lacked information about the health effects on potentially vulnerable segments of the population. No studies were conducted with healthy people over forty-four years of age, or those with poor nutritional status.

The studies with children were judged inadequate by Drs. A.R. Colon and J.S. Palma, pediatric gastroenterologists at Georgetown University Medical Center. They noted that the dose used in P&G's study with children, consisting of 7 grams (g) a day "is not realistic." They recommended realistic doses of 14 to 32 g a day, with longer studies of six to twelve weeks.

Dr. Patricia Rodier, senior scientist in obstetrics at the University of Rochester, a member of the Food Advisory Committee, said that the studies and database were deficient in information about the effects on the developing fetus when preformed vitamin A was added to Olestra.

Food Additive or Drug? In product development, Olestra has been invented and reinvented. In the 1960s, P&G considered but rejected Olestra as a potential nutritional supplement for premature infants. In 1971, P&G patented Olestra, and in 1975, sought approval for Olestra as an investigational new drug for cholesterol reduction. In 1988, P&G withdrew this application, because the company found that Olestra was not as effective as other available drugs for this purpose. At that juncture, P&G was reluctant to lose its expenditures in money and effort, and decided to salvage Olestra by reinventing it once more, as a fat substitute with foods.

P&G petitioned for Olestra approval as a calorie-free additive that would replace up to 35 percent of the fat in shortenings and cooking oils for home use, and up to 70 percent of the fat used in commercial deep-frying or snack foods. It became clear that there would be obstacles to gaining approval for widespread use. So, in 1990, P&G amended its petition, to limit Olestra's use as a fat replacer for savory snacks. The reasoning was that Olestra approval for a limited application might be achieved more easily, and would facilitate subsequent approvals, in incremental steps, for widespread applications. This technique had already been successful with another controversial food substitute, aspartame, which initially was approved for limited uses, and later, step by step, approved for numerous additional applications.

Some critics, including Blackburn, believe that the FDA should not have classified Olestra as a food additive, but rather as a drug, like the cholesterol reducer cholestyramine (Questran, LoCholest).

Olestra may not only act as a drug, but also may interfere with the effects of other drugs. Some physicians and researchers have voiced concerns, especially with Olestra's potential interference with blood-thinning anticoagulants such as warfarin (Coumadin).

Dr. Sheldon Margen, professor emeritus of public health nutrition at the University of California at Berkeley asked:

Mandatory Labeling Statement

The FDA required that the following labeling statement be placed on all products made with Olestra:

"This product contains Olestra. Olestra may cause abdominal cramping and loose stools. Olestra inhibits the absorption of some vitamins and other nutrients. Vitamins A, D, E, and K have been added."

As a condition of approval by the FDA, Procter & Gamble was required to conduct studies to monitor consumption of Olestra as well as to assess its long-term effects. The FDA would review these studies at a public meeting of the Food Advisory Committee after thirty months.

"Should FDA approve mineral oil or petroleum as a fat substitute?" and pointed out that such approval would be "absurd and dangerous." However, Margen noted that the physical properties of Olestra, "are virtually identical" to mineral oil. Years ago, the FDA had allowed mineral oil in the food supply. Like Olestra, it had no food value but pulled fat-soluble vitamins out of the body. By 1941, experiments showed mineral oil to be dangerous and the FDA proposed to ban it as a food ingredient. The proposal was challenged, and after a five-year legal battle, the courts exonerated the FDA by declaring that mineral oil could not be used as an ingredient in any food product. (Mineral oil still has limited uses, at very low levels, as a processing aid.) Will the case of Olestra become a *déjà vu* of mineral oil?

Olestra for Weight Reduction? If Olestra had been classified as a drug rather than as a food additive, not only would its safety have needed to be demonstrated, but also its effectiveness. Because Olestra is used with "fat-free" or "low-fat" food products, individuals on weight-reduction diets may be attracted to this feature. How effective is Olestra for weight reduction?

Dr. W. Mark Lafranconi, an Olestra researcher at P&G, reported that Olestra consumption had no effect on body weight or weight gain in mice. However, there was a 5 to 10 percent increase in their food consumption, attributed to the lower caloric density of the Olestra-containing diet. This finding is similar to those with sugar substitutes such as saccharin and aspartame. Neither the fat substitute nor sugar substitutes are useful for weight reduction.

Dr. Meir Stampfer, professor of epidemiology at Harvard University's School of Public Health, noted that "the single best dietary predictor of weight gain is saccharin use. It is a marker for the kind of diet that leads to just the kind of behavior that says, 'I'll drink this diet drink and then I can have a doughnut."' The same mentality may be applied to Olestra.

Dr. Walter Willett, chairman of the nutrition department at Harvard University's School of Public Health, confirmed the statement of his colleague, Stampfer. Willett reported "we have lots of data that over the last ten to fifteen years, fat intake has gone down as percentages of calories and weight have gone up dramatically in this country." Willett added that this demonstrates "that Olestra is definitely not the solution to the problem of overweight."

Overlooking Some Nutrient Losses. There is general consensus that fat-soluble vitamins A, D, E, and K dissolve readily in Olestra as this substance moves through the digestive tract, and these valuable vitamins are carried out of the body before they can be absorbed into the bloodstream through the intestine. Kessler's response was to require supplementation of Olestra-containing foods with these four vitamins to compensate for their losses. This response is an oversimplified solution to a complex problem.

Even supporters of Olestra's approval, such as Dr. Wayne Callaway, a specialist in endocrinology, metabolism, and clinical nutrition at George Washington University, noted that "supplementing Olestra with selected vitamins will not solve all of Olestra's nutrient-depleting problems."

By P&G's own estimates, Olestra can reduce daily carotenoid absorption by as much as 10 percent. Critics fear that, over time, such reduction gradually could deplete the body of important carotenoids.

Dr. Lilian Cheung, at the Center for Health Communications at Harvard University's School of Public Health, noted the "devastating" effect on blood carotenoids that will "jeopardize the impact of the hundreds of millions of dollars spent in cancer research and prevention each year." "Why," Cheung asked, "even continue the National Cancer

Institute's successful Five-a-Day for Better Health national campaign [to consume fruits and vegetables] when much of its benefits will be negated by Olestra?" Cheung predicted: "By the time Olestra has existed long enough to allow us to ascertain its adverse effects on cancer, heart disease, stroke, macular degeneration, and cataracts, it will be very hard to remove it." Also, as she predicted, after Olestra approval in the United States, approval followed in other countries. "We will be subjecting much of the world's population to a large-scale human experiment on the public health impact of a product that we already know has palpable adverse effects."

Others have pointed out that Kessler's dismissal of the problem of carotenoid depletion is inconsistent with the released *Dietary Guidelines for Americans*. This publication, issued by the Department of Health and Human Services, in conjunction with the U.S. Department of Agriculture (USDA), emphasizes the importance of adequate intake of carotenoids in the diet. Yet, as Willett pointed out, "the individuals who are most likely to consume substantial amounts of snacks containing Olestra are the same persons who are likely to consume small amounts of fruits and vegetables in their diets."

According to Stampfer, there is "highly suggestive data" associating adequate carotenoid intake with decreased risks of lung cancer, coronary heart disease, and stroke. As an epidemiologist, Stampfer took into consideration the health effects of Olestra from carotenoid depletion. He calculated that if the American population ate three 1.0-ounce Olestra-containing snacks per week, it would result in 400 additional annual cases of macular degeneration; 2,000 to 3,000 more cases of prostate cancer; 10,000 to 30,000 more cases of heart disease; and 2,000 more cases of lung cancer.

Olestra depletes foods of other nutrients, which were

Kessler Turns a Deaf Ear to Numerous Critics

Before arriving at a final decision, the head of the Food and Drug Administration (FDA), David Kessler, was obligated to consider the opinions of experts as well as to evaluate the scientific data. How well did he listen?

- Five out of the twenty committee members chosen to serve on FDA'S Food Advisory Committee expressed strong reservations about Olestra's unproven safety. By any measure, 25 percent opposition in safety matters represents a strong minority opinion that deserves attention.

- A petition opposing Olestra's approval was sent to Kessler, signed by 275 physicians, more than forty scientists, and organizations such as the American Public Health Association, the American Academy of Ophthalmology, and the National Association for the Visually Handicapped.

- A letter written to Kessler in November 1995 by seven physicians with prominent affiliations urged that Olestra not be approved. "We believe the potential benefits that could result from use of this product are far outweighed by the potential risks to the public health." The letter was signed by David Carpenter, dean of the School of Public Health, State University of New York at Albany; Mark Donowitz, director of Meyerhoff Digestive Disease Center, Johns Hopkins University; D. Mark Hegsted, professor of nutrition emeritus, Harvard Medical School; M. Peter Lance, chief of gastroenterology, State University of New York at Buffalo; Roy Maliakkal, assistant professor of internal medicine at the University of Mississippi; Hooshang Meshkinpour, acting chief of the division of gastroenterology, Medical Center, University of California at Irvine;

and Orlando Nives, dean of the graduate school of Public Health of Puerto Rico.

• A letter to Kessler from Dr. Fernando Trevino, executive director of the American Public Health Association (APHA) charged that P&G "has not adequately addressed long-term public health questions." APHA recommended that Olestra should not be approved.

• The National Association for the Visually Handicapped recommended that Olestra not be approved because it depletes carotenoids and increases the risks of macular degeneration, optic neuropathy, and other visual impairments. "P&G has not proposed to add back every carotenoid and other phytochemicals that Olestra affects."

• Dr. Herbert Needleman, professor of psychiatry and pediatrics, School of Medicine, University of Pittsburgh, commented that the marginal utility it [Olestra] offers can be completely and safely met by dietary education and control. . . . It would be a clear folly to introduce this product into the diet of children."

• Dr. Henry Blackburn, epidemiologist at the Univeristy of Minnesota, who served on FDA's Food Advisory Committee, wrote to Kessler that he was "unable to arrive at a reasonable certainty of no harm" from Olestra. A number of nagging questions remained unanswered; a lack of long-term trials with adequate numbers of humans; an insufficient follow-up on cancer findings in a mouse study; and a failure to test patients on blood-thinning drugs and on those with bleeding disorders.

• Dr. Arlo Kahn, associate professor, College of Medicine, University of Arkansas, questioned "how thoroughly the FDA has evaluated the potential impact of this additive on the health care delivery system." Kahn warned that health care dollars will be "wasted" on office visits and gastrointestinal diagnostic procedures that may result from Olestra's use.

• Dr. Lilian Cheung, mentioned earlier, wrote to Kessler in December 1995 that "from a public health perspective, the 'Olestra' scenario is worse than the 'cigarette' scenario—individuals, including children, who choose to smoke make a conscious choice to do so. However, individuals may not be aware that they are eating foods containing Olestra, as the use of Olestra is likely to be widespread."

In addition to the dissenting letters directed to Dr. Kessler from health organizations, physicians, researchers, and scientists, more than 700 written comments were filed at the FDA's Dockets Management Branch. The vast majority urged that Olestra not be approved. Nearly 300 were sent by health professionals. Among the rest were form letters urged by consumer groups, and some resulting from press coverage of the FDA's Food Advisory Committee meetings.

overlooked by Kessler. Among them may be valuable phytochemicals. Jed Fahey, a faculty research associate at Brassica Chemoprotection Laboratory at Johns Hopkins School of Medicine, wrote to Kessler to report that he was "distressed" by data showing that Olestra reduces many fat-soluble vitamins. "There are a great number of other fat-soluble phytochemicals, some of which we are investigating . . . for their anti-cancer potential." Fahey reported that many of these have not yet been isolated in pure form, and therefore are unavailable for testing. "The inclusion of Olestra in commonly consumed American foods has a high probability of affecting the wholesale reduction of a multiplicity of beneficial compounds from the diet of a great many Americans," and "based on overwhelming epidemiological evidence there is a high probability that the use of this product would have a negative health impact."

Was Olestra Approval Based on Science or Politics? On January 24, 1996, the FDA approved the use of Olestra in savory snacks. As noted in *Bloomberg Business News*, the date of Olestra's approval came in the nick of time for P&G to get a two-year extension on its patent, which had been scheduled to expire in late January 1996.

Many critics have condemned the composition of the reviewers chosen by the FDA, charging that some members had industry affiliations and/or biases, or previously had been paid testers or consultants to P&G. Individuals listed with academic affiliations were not necessarily independent of industry funding for their work.

Blackburn, in a letter to Kessler in November 1995, had stated frankly that "as one of the newest members of the Food Advisory Committee" he felt "a bit uncomfortable that the FDA staff could review only the literature and industry-provided test data rather than carry out its own studies." Blackburn continued: "The appearance of conflict that one perceives with the appearance of collusion by the committee and staff with industry is a shock for a new member familiar mainly with NIH [National Institutes of Health] review process." He added: "Beyond 'the appearance of intimacy' between industry and the FDA staff, under the conditions of absent legislation or funding for independent testing of foods and additives by the FDA, would it not be useful for all to know that a particular petitioner from industry had at least met all basic FDA testing requirements for short- and long-term safety in humans?"

The viewpoint of the FDA staff and advisory committee members was described by Blackburn as having "an orientation and mind-set which is entirely 'bench and clinical' rather than'public health and epidemiological'." Blackburn suggested that the FDA's orientation and mind-set "might be broadened by clear criteria for human testing of safety, as well as by renewed attention to the composition of the advisory committee to include a stronger proportion of disinterested public health experts."

Z-TRIM: A ZERO-CALORIC FAT

Z-Trim ("Z" signifying zero calories) is a noncaloric fat replacer. It is a bland mixture of insoluble fibers made from agricultural byproducts such as oat, soybean, pea, or rice hulls, as well as from corn or wheat bran.

This fat replacer has been developed by Dr. George E. Inglett and associates at the Biopolymer Research Unit of the National Center for Agricultural Utilization Research, U.S. Department of Agriculture (USDA), in Peoria, Illinois. Earlier, Inglett and his associates had developed a carbohydrate-based fat replacer "Oatrim" which is used commercially as a partial fat replacer in numerous food products.

Inglett and his associates spent three years in perfecting a technique to produce Z-Trim satisfactorily. The process crushes the hulls or brans in a mill that breaks apart the plant cells, and then treats the mixture with an alkali solution. Next, it is centrifuged to remove the alkali and other water-soluble components. Once again, the mixture is milled and centrifuged to refine it further. The final product is a fine, white, tasteless cellulose powder. It can absorb a great amount of water—up to twenty-four times its weight—and becomes a gel. Depending on the ratio of powder to water, the gel can vary from being a pourable liquid to a soft solid. The gel's consistency can be modified, depending on which hulls or brans are used to make the powder.

Most fat substitutes replace fat with carbohydrates.

However, the addition of sweeteners usually adds back as many calories as are replaced. Z-Trim is different. According to Inglett, Z-Trim could cut as many as 700 calories from a daily 3,500-calorie diet.

Potential Health Benefits. For a long time, microcrystalline cellulose has been used as a fat replacer. But its coarse texture makes it hard to digest. Unlike microcrystalline cellulose, Z-Trim is so fine that it does not irritate the gastrointestinal tract. Unlike the synthetic fat substitute, Olestra (sucrose polyester), Z-Trim does not cause gastrointestinal distress. Nor does it prevent fat-soluble vitamins and carotenoids in foods from being absorbed and utilized in the body, as does Olestra.

Richard Greene, a biochemist at the Peoria center, reported that Z-Trim could have health benefits because one would "replace fats and be removing calories, and eating more fiber."

Inglett expressed regrets that dietary fibers have been "refined out of our diets." Both insoluble and soluble ones offer health benefits, yet both types are in short supply in the typical American diet. The insoluble fibers help prevent constipation, speed digestion through the intestinal tract, and tone its function. The soluble fibers help lower serum cholesterol, handle glucose metabolism, and may help prevent colon cancer. Z-Trim is made from insoluble fibers; Oatrim, from soluble ones.

Most fat substitutes replace fat with carbohydrates. However, the addition of sweeteners usually adds back as many calories as are replaced.

Unlike Olestra, Z-Trim cannot withstand frying. Under such high heat, Z-Trim would collapse. However, Z-Trim is suitable for gentler heat, such as in baking. It can replace some of the fat and carbohydrates in formulations for chocolate, baked goods, cheeses, and ground beef. In studies at the Peoria center, it was found that Z-Trim could replace up to half the fat and carbohydrate in baked goods. Taste panelists judged the Z-Trim-containing brownies with only 15.5 percent fat to be as good as those made with 25 percent fat in a traditional recipe. Z-Trim, added to lean ground beef, cut its fat content by 15 percent. The hamburgers were judged to be tender and juicy. Other satisfactory results were obtained by combining Oatrim and Z-Trim to make a chocolate-covered snack bar, and a low-fat cheese spread.

Although Z-Trim could be used as a total fat replacer (and even as a partial flour replacer), Inglett suggested that some fat be used to enhance the flavor of products and to prevent them from drying out.

Potential Drawbacks. Are there any drawbacks with Z-Trim? Concern was expressed by a food technologist, Thomas H. Parliment, regarding the microbial stability of foods containing such water-containing fat substitutes. Parliment noted that "microbes are able to grow, and you can get mold."Like Oatrim, Z-Trim was developed under a research agreement with a commercial company. Mountain Lake Manufacturing of Mountain Lake, Minnesota made the agreement and will have the first marketing rights, after official approval. Inglett reported that the finished product, Z-Trim, will not be inexpensive. Although the starting materials are low-cost agricultural byproducts, the production technique is sophisticated, and the process is energy intensive.

Another concern is the potential allergenicity of grain— and legume-based fat substitutes. Some of the byproducts used are from grains and legumes that are not tolerated by some individuals. Yet the derivation of the substances in the fat replacer will not be noted on the labels of finished food products. This lack of information may limit the choices of those with food allergies in selecting products.

CONJUGATED LINOLEIC ACID: A NUTRIENT LOW IN THE MODERN DIET

Conjugated linoleic acid (CLA) is not exactly a familiar phrase, but it is a powerful substance with several benefits. CLA is a naturally occurring fatty acid that is found in many foods of animal origin. It was identified only about fourteen years ago in hamburger. Foods highest in CLA are beef, lamb, full-fat milk, butter, goat cheese, some cream, and full-fat yogurt. Other foods that contain some CLA are poultry, pork, and fish. The acid is produced by bacteria in the animal's rumen (a part of the digestive tract).

Formerly, CLA was abundant in the American diet. However, changes in agricultural practice have reduced its availability drastically. The current craze for low- and no-fat foods, and veganism (an extreme form of vegetarianism in which all animal products are shunned) have lowered CLA intake even further.

Benefits of CLA. Although CLA's parent nutrient, linoleic acid, at high intake may promote cancer development, CLA has been found to slow the progress of some types of cancer and heart disease. Despite being a fat component, CLA appears to help reduce body fat and increase lean muscle mass. High amounts of CLA also may help fight cachexia, a wasting disease that compromises the survival of many ill individuals such as persons with cancer or malaria.

CLA is one food component being examined in the complex relationship between diet and cancer. It has been found capable of inhibiting the growth of chemically induced skin and stomach cancers in mice, as well as cancer in the mammary glands of rats. Similar results have been noted in studies with other animal species. The lowest active dose of CLA in animals was within the range of what humans can obtain from eating foods from animal sources.

The amount of CLA present in foods from animal sources depends on the quality of the feed they consume. An animal scientist, Dr. Tilak Dhiman, and his colleagues at Utah State University, found that the CLA content of cow's milk was as much as five times higher when cows grazed on green pastures (predominantly ryegrass) than when they ate a mixture of "conserved forage" (such as hay from alfalfa and corn silage).

The researchers found that feeding higher amounts of conserved forage increased the CLA content in milk, but the level still was not as high as that found in milk from cows that grazed on green pastures. Dhiman suggested that something might be present in green grass that enhances the growth of particular bacteria in the animal's rumen that is responsible for CLA production. Or, perhaps cows grazing on pastures outdoors have different microbes in their rumens than cows fed silage indoor in barns. Dhiman said, "Today, we are producing milk more efficiently, but we need to couple this efficiency with milk quality."

"We have a tendency to get a little information and think that all fat is bad," observed Dhiman. "We must distinguish between types of fats." Dhiman and his colleagues are exploring ways to increase the CLA content in milk, cheese, and meat.

Elsewhere, scientists at the USDA's Dairy Forage Research Center in Madison, Wisconsin, found that livestock eating feed supplemented with CLA formed more lean tissue and less fat. Dairy cattle produced more milk. The highest CLA levels in the milk were obtained when the animals fed solely on pasture grass. This had been the earlier tradition in agricultural practice.

Increasing CLA Intake through Diet. CLA appears to be very stable. Different cooking methods (baking, broiling, frying, or microwaving) or processing do not produce any major changes in CLA.

The identification of CLA and studies about its benefits call to question any scientific basis for official recommendations to select no-fat and low-fat food products. It has already been demonstrated that many of these products are not low in calories, due to increased use of sugars. The CLA issue adds another dimension. Although CLA is found in milk, this beneficial fatty acid is a component of the fat grams. If the fat grams are reduced, the CLA benefit is lessened.

The International Dairy Foods Association estimates that, by 1996, American milk consumption dropped to about twenty-four gallons per person annually, compared with thirty-one gallons in 1970. Along with this decline, sales of nonfat and reduced-fat milk products doubled since 1970, and whole milk consumption dropped to less than half its 1970 level.

In the billion-dollar yearly business that has accompanied the drive for leaner bodies in America, health supplements containing CLA (synthesized from sunflower oil) are being promoted to replace its reduction in the present food supply. Dhiman observed that, nearly every month, new brands of CLA capsules are introduced in the marketplace. He plans to study this form of CLA by feeding the supplements to laboratory mice, and note any changes in their muscle and body fat compositions. Studies, already conducted elsewhere, found that rats, mice, and chickens fed CLA-rich diets had reduced body fat and increased lean body mass. Other studies are tracking long-term changes in humans who supplement their diets with CLA.

Meanwhile, consumers should question the wisdom of using low- and no-fat food products. By reducing or eliminating dairy and meat fats from the diet, beneficial CLA is lowered drastically. Those who are interested to increase CLA intake through diet can do so. The general CLA content of commonly available foods, in milligrams (mg) per gram (g) of fat, are: lamb, 5.5 mg; milk, 4.5 mg; beef, 4 mg; turkey, 2.5 mg; chicken, 0.9 mg; pork, 0.6 mg; and fish, 0.3 mg.

MISLEADING FOOD LABELING FOR FATS

The fat listings on the "Nutrition Facts" panel on food labels are oversimplified, inaccurate, and inadequate for consumers to make informed choices. Currently, fatty acids are grouped according to chemical structure. It would be more accurate to group them by their physiologic or metabolic effects. Individual fatty acids differ both in their composition and their effects on our bodies. Yet, on labels, all saturated fats are grouped together, as if they were all equal. They are not.

Stearic Fatty Acids. Stearic acid does not have the same effects of raising serum total cholesterol and harmful low-density lipoproteins (LDLs) as do other saturated fatty acids. Stearic acid has a neutral effect on serum cholesterol levels. In fact, it even may lower serum cholesterol concentrations when it is substituted for other saturated fatty acids. Also, stearic acid does not appear to increase blood clotting as do other saturated fatty acids. Blood clotting can be a factor in the development of heart disease.

Stearic acid contributes about 27 percent of the total saturated fatty acids in foods. It is found mostly in meats (beef, pork, and chicken breasts), fat-containing dairy products (butter), and products such as milk chocolate.

Information about stearic acid's unique effects on cholesterol raises a question about the validity of grouping it with other saturated fatty acids on food labels. It would be more accurate to list stearic acid separately. Also, the distinct characteristics of stearic acid deserve to be considered in any dietary recommendations.

Despite the evidence that stearic acid should be distinguished from the other saturated fatty acids, the FDA has postponed any policy of labeling individual fatty acids. Its sister agency, the U.S. Department of Agriculture (USDA), which regulates meat and poultry, permits an optional labeling of stearic acid.

***Trans*-Fatty Acids.** *Trans*-fatty acids form by hydrogenating vegetable oils. During hydrogenation, the naturally occurring *cis* form is converted to an abnormal *trans* form, which the human body handles differently. Current food labeling for fats is misleading for *trans*-fatty acids. According to Tim Byers, M.D., M.P.H. at the School of Medicine, University of Colorado: "Many of the 'hidden fats' in processed foods such as pastries and savory snacks are *trans*-fatty acids. Ironically, though, the question is not whether we should include *trans* fats on the food label. They are already there, hidden within the levels reported for polyunsaturates and monounsaturates, two classes of fats that are widely accepted as being healthful in terms of one's cholesterol profile." To include *trans* fats in this classification is inaccurate. Consistent and persuasive evidence shows that the *trans*-fatty acids have effects on serum cholesterol similar to that of most saturated fats.

"While we wait for complete knowledge about the health effects of eating partially hydrogenated vegetable oils, perhaps the best option is to change food labels so that fats listed as saturated reflect the content of saturated and *trans*-fatty acids combined," suggests Matthew Longnecker, a researcher at the National Institute of Environmental Health Sciences, a division of the National Institutes of Health. According to Longnecker, "Lumping *trans* and saturated fats together may be incorrect chemically, but physiologically, *trans*-fatty acids behave like saturated fats. Such lumping may unduly emphasize the effects of *trans*-fatty acids, but, from the public health perspective, it is more honest and safe than the present approach." Longnecker adds, "If manufac-

How to Determine *Trans*-Fatty Acid Levels in Foods

By sleuthing, you can learn whether these undesirable fatty acids are in a food product. Your first clue is the phrase "partially hydrogenated" or "partially hardened" in the ingredient listing. The next step is to add up the grams of saturated, polyunsaturated, and monounsaturated fats that are listed. You will find that the number is smaller than the "total fats" listed. The difference in the two sets of numbers consists of the *trans*-fatty acids.

turers are required to change the way they calculate the amount of fats listed as saturated fatty acids in the product—so that *trans*-fatty acids are included—their incentive to decrease the [*trans* fat] content will mount."

Byers agrees, noting: "The good news is that reducing our intake of *trans* fats may not be particularly difficult. The food industry has demonstrated a remarkable ability to respond rapidly to consumer demands. Disclosing the levels of *trans* fats in foods, reducing levels to a minimum . . . and avoiding the mistake of replacing *trans* fats with saturated fats in baked goods and in cooking fats could have meaningful effects on the public's health."

Omega-3 and Omega-6 Fatty Acids. Omega-3 fatty acids are concentrated in seafoods and in the green leaves of plants. The early traditional diet of humans was predominantly from fin and shellfish, meat, fruit, and vegetables (including starchy roots and tubers), which contributed ample amounts of omega-3s.

Omega-6 fatty acids are concentrated in dairy food and cultivated grains, which were introduced into the human diet only as recently as about 10,000 years ago, when agriculture became stable. The predominance of omega-6 fatty acids in the present diet has developed only in recent times, due to radical transformation of the diet. As a result, the ratio of omega-3 to omega-6 intake has become severely imbalanced. During early human history, it is thought that the ratio was about one to one. Presently, the diet in the industrialized world contains approximately fourteen to twenty times more omega-6s than omega-3s.

In many respects, our fat metabolism is quite adaptive. Our bodies can manufacture fats from sugars and starches. We can make short-, medium-, and long-chained fats, depending on the number of carbon atoms linked together to form fatty acid molecules. We can desaturate fats, and turn them into monounsaturates and polyunsaturates. However, our bodies *cannot* manufacture primary omega-3 or omega-6 fatty acids. These fatty acids must be obtained from food sources. Hence, they are termed "essential." After we consume them, they undergo chain lengthening and desaturation, and then go into the membranes of all of our cells. These fatty acids are the only fats that can become eicosanoids—the major fat regulators at the cellular level of most of our bodily functions.

Despite the importance of omega-3 and omega-6 fatty acids, present food labels give no indication of their presence or amounts in food products.

Numerous studies have associated the imbalance created by low amounts of omega-3s with health problems, including cardiovascular diseases, cancer, obesity, insulin resistance, diabetes, asthma, arthritis, lupus, depression, schizophrenia, attention deficit disorders, postpartum depression, and Alzheimer's disease. Recent findings about omega-3 and omega-6s have brought into question the "prudent diet" of low-fat and low-cholesterol-containing foods as a preventive measure against cardiovascular diseases. When the deficient omega-3 fatty acids have been supplied in the diet, high cholesterol and other fats in the blood have declined.

Despite the importance of omega-3 and omega-6 fatty acids, present food labels give no indication of their presence or amounts in food products. As the public becomes better educated about these essential fatty acids, and their roles in health, interest may grow to have them listed in the fat information.

The shortcomings of present fat labeling are obvious, in view of the knowledge about the different effects of individual fatty acids on metabolism and health. Fat labeling should be revised. Improved and accurate label information is a useful tool for consumers in order to make informed choices.

Chapter 7

Dispelling Some Popular Health Myths

SHOULD EVERYONE CUT BACK ON SODIUM?

In 1994, the U.S. Department of Agriculture (USDA) proposed to limit sodium in school feeding programs. The Salt Institute, a trade organization, promptly protested. The group contended that removal of high-sodium foods, such as milk and other dairy products, inevitably denies children other important nutrients such as calcium and potassium, present in such foods.

This challenge deserves scrutiny. The USDA's proposal, which forms public policy, is based solidly on scientific evidence. Correct? Incorrect!

Contrary to popular perception, *universal* sodium restriction is unnecessary, and possibly undesirable. A common notion is that sodium induces hypertension (high blood pressure) and that lowering sodium intake will prevent hypertension. Unfortunately, this notion has no scientific basis. Instead, many recent medical studies have brought into question the effectiveness and even the safety of universal sodium restriction.

There is a relationship between sodium and blood pressure, which is important for about 10 percent of the population, which is sodium-sensitive. For this group, sodium restriction is an important feature, along with other measures, for treatment. However, for about 90 percent of the population, there is no convincing scientific basis for the idea that sodium restriction will prevent hypertension.

Treatment Differs from Prevention. In earlier times, medically supervised sodium restriction therapy was common with hypertensives. For the general public, however, the Food and Nutrition Board of the National Academy of Sciences warned in 1954 that "harmful results may follow the restriction of sodium intake . . . when the diet is severely restricted in sodium for long periods . . . reduction of intake of essential nutrients, especially vitamins, may occur . . . [in studies] calcium, riboflavin (vitamin B_2), and protein were the principal nutrients in short supply. These dietary deficiencies were occasioned chiefly by the omission of milk. . . . Metabolic studies on patients with hypertension treated with sodium-restricted diets have revealed a number of changes . . . these changes are potentially dangerous, perhaps leading to . . . reduced renal (kidney) function."

Contrary to popular perception, universal sodium restriction is unnecessary, and possibly undesirable.

At that time, there was a medical consensus regarding the treatment of hypertension. In terms of prevention, one doctor warned the public against self-imposed sodium restriction that "affords no benefit to the normal individual. . . self restriction will not prevent disease . . ."

Another doctor noted that "thousands of misguided enthusiasts have eaten unpalatable food on a mistaken assumption that . . . high blood pressure would be prevented. The facts are simple. There is no evidence that excessive salt intake produces high blood pressure in humans."

Treatment focuses on an individual's medical problems, with all the unique characteristics that shape the person. *Prevention* focuses on entire populations and improvement of their average conditions. The medical and public health models differ. Physicians dealing with a patient follow the rule of "do no harm," whereas public health doctors hope to "do some good."

The Sodium Hypothesis. In the late 1950s, the difference between treatment and prevention of high blood pressure became blurred. Lewis K. Dahl, M.D. promoted the hypothesis that there was a direct correlation between sodium intake of populations and hypertensive incidence.

Dahl's sodium hypothesis was viewed by critics as being "packaged as a panacea." A few strategically placed advocates popularized the hypothesis. Over time, and with endless repetition, the hypothesis gradually became viewed as gospel.

There were skeptics. In a 1979 report, the National Institutes of Health Hypertension Task Force noted that the brevity of the section on prevention "is indicative of the lack of knowledge concerning basic mechanisms of hypertension. Research must supply new knowledge before confident statements concerning prevention can by made."

John H. Larach, M.D., a prominent hypertension researcher, commented in 1983 on the popular, anti-sodium policy, "Now, what can I possibly have against these well-intended efforts? Nothing except the fact that they are not supported by scientific evidence. They are based on assumptions that are either entirely false or entirely unproven."

In 1984, a group of thirteen scientists wrote on the subject in *The Lancet:* "The usual scientific standards for weighing evidence and for giving advice, which are now well established in drug development and prescribing, seemed to have been forgotten in an evangelical crusade to present a simplistic view of the evidence which will prove attractive to the media."

Larach, joined by Michael H. Alderman, M.D., assessed the impact of sodium intake on cardiovascular health among healthy people over the course of eight years. In 1991 they reported their finding. People on low-sodium diets had dramatically higher numbers of heart attacks.

Another skeptic of the sodium hypothesis was David A. McCarron, M.D. at the Oregon Health Sciences University. He argued that governmental concern about high-sodium diets was misplaced. Not an *excess* of nutrients such as sodium is the problem, but rather a *deficiency* of nutrients, especially calcium, is responsible for hypertension.

McCarron's "calcium hypothesis" reflected a renewed scientific interest in the interaction of electrolytes—electronically charged particles that play an important role in regulating body processes—mainly the interrelationships of sodium with calcium and potassium. (See "electrolytes" on page 154.) Numerous articles in medical journals noted that calcium and potassium deficiencies were implicated in sodium's blood pressure effects. Some studies found them to be even more important than sodium.

Unanticipated Risks. Researchers began to question, too, the lack of proven safety for universal sodium restriction. Studies began to identify unanticipated risks of low-sodium diets, resulting in elevated blood pressure in some individuals, and increases in serum creatinine (a waste product from a substance found in muscles, blood, and urine). Also, there was a rise in undesirable low-density lipoprotein (LDL) cholesterol, uric acid, and significantly higher fasting insulin levels. All of these features are disease risk factors.

In addition, low-sodium diets might lead to a reduced capacity to absorb other nutrients and a lowered resistance to problems such as diarrhea, hyperthermia (greatly increased body temperature), and bleeding. Low-sodium diets also seem to be related to sleep disturbances.

The sodium hypothesis proponents recognized that their scientific basis was being challenged. They devised a massive global study in an attempt to answer the skeptics' objections.

INTERSALT was funded by national blood pressure research groups, the National Heart, Lung, and Blood Institute, and the World Health Organization (WHO), in an attempt to provide a scientific basis for the sodium hypothesis.

By 1986, INTERSALT researchers had examined numerous population studies purported to link sodium and hypertension. The studies encompassed more than 10,000 individuals, at fifty-two centers, in thirty-two countries. Most of the studies, when evaluated, were found to be flawed, and were discarded. The number of quality studies was reduced to thirteen, of which ten failed to demonstrate any sodium-hypertension association. The results of the evaluation were summarized succinctly in the *British Medical Journal:* "Salt has only small importance in hypertension."

Thomas J. Moore, a medical writer, wrote that the INTERSALT results were "as clean an outright refutation as can be found in science, yet the findings of the INTERSALT study passed virtually unnoticed in the media and scientific journals in the United States."

William Ira Bennett, M.D., editor of the *Harvard Medical School Health Letter,* explained that the deafening silence by officials was because they had invested their credibility in promoting the sodium hypothesis. Bennett wrote that "little was said about the INTERSALT study because it was a kind of humiliation when you have a nutrition recommendation that you have to abandon."

Despite the lack of any confirmation of the sodium hypothesis from the INTERSALT study, federal officials continue to retain the recommendation that everyone should reduce dietary sodium. The 1988 Surgeon General's Report admitted that whether universal sodium restriction would lower population blood pressure or not, had never been tested.

Recognizing that the public policy was at odds with scientific findings, the National Heart, Lung, and Blood Institute convened a Salt and High Blood Pressure Workshop in 1989. The experts could reach no consensus.

The leaders of the INTERSALT project tightly controlled the release of analyses of the database for publication. They used meta-analysis, a technique of compiling all previous studies to gain the statistical power of large numbers of observations. However, the poor quality of many of the early studies, as already noted, was ignored, and the meta-analysis, by sheer numbers, was used to confirm the sodium hypothesis. Yet, publication of numerous new and well-designed studies reported in medical journals continued to undermine confidence in the sodium hypothesis.

The advice for hypertensives to decrease sodium intake remains sound. However, the same advice for the general public lacks a scientific basis. There is no proof, to date, that excess sodium actually causes hypertension, or that decreasing sodium intake will prevent hypertension from developing.

Support of the sodium hypothesis is based on population studies, which ignore the confounding variables that may determine sodium's role in hypertension. Precisely how sodium influences blood pressure is not yet firmly established.

Many Contributing Factors. There are many determinants of hypertension. Sodium appears to be only a minor player in a highly complex field. There are environmental factors of geography, location, temperature, and poisoning from heavy metals, such as lead and cadmium.

For example, cadmium, a toxic metal, is an important contributing cause of hypertension. With age, cadmium accumulates in the body, especially in the kidneys, from contamination by this heavy metal in the environment. Cadmium in foods results mainly from food processing and refining; in drinking water, from areas of "soft" water lacking in minerals such as calcium and magnesium, as well as from water piping; and in air, from industrial pollutants. Cadmium's role in hypertension development can be stopped if the body's zinc supply is adequate. Unfortunately, many Americans are low in zinc.

There are lifestyle factors of obesity, lack of exercise, mental stress, smoking, alcohol, coffee, and tea. Hypertension is far more common among overweight adults than among those with normal weight. Studies have shown that weight loss can reduce blood pressure significantly in obese adults. Heavy drinking is known to increase hypertensive risks. Even moderate drinking may be a risk factor, according to the findings of Jacqueline Witteman and colleagues at Harvard University. They found that women who consume two mixed alcoholic drinks daily may be 40 percent more likely than others to develop hypertension. Milk drinkers may lower this risk, possibly due to the calcium and other protective nutrients in the milk.

> . . . a lack of adequate calcium may be as important a factor in hypertension as is excessive sodium and . . . sodium-sensitive individuals may benefit the most by increasing calcium intake.

There are factors of genetics, race, gender, hormones, and age. A hormone has been identified and studied that is believed to be related to hypertension development. A sodium-pump inhibiting hormone appears to slow the activity of a protein that moves sodium out of the cells, according to Mordecai P. Blaustein, M.D. and John M. Hamlyn, Ph.D. at the Maryland School of Medicine.

There are nutritional effects of certain dietary components, and potable water quality. Studies that examine only sodium or any other single dietary component as a factor in inducing hypertension give too limited a view. Many components may be interrelated. Also, not all sodium compounds affect blood pressure as does sodium chloride (table salt). Nor do we eat sodium, per se, but rather as sodium compounds in foods.

Nutritional Factors. Hypertension is associated with certain nutritional deficiencies, especially with low intake of specific minerals, vitamins, proteins, fatty acids, carbohydrates, and calories. Excessive sodium intake is related to some of these nutrients.

The standard weight-reduction diets actually may *exacerbate* conditions that lead to hypertension by further reducing nutrients that are essential to maintain normal blood pressure.

As previously noted, Dr. McCarron and his colleagues suggest that nutritional deficiencies, not excesses, distinguish hypertensive and overweight Americans. In studies, individuals on low-sodium diets with low intake of dairy products were at two to three times greater hypertensive risk than those with high intake of dairy products. McCarron concluded that the standard weight-reduction diets actually may *exacerbate* conditions that lead to hypertension by further reducing nutrients that are essential to maintain normal blood pressure. By recommending sodium reduction, McCarron said, "we're setting up the dietetic community for failure."

Many Americans do not get enough calcium. McCarron believes that a lack of adequate calcium may be as important a factor in hypertension as is excessive sodium and that sodium-sensitive individuals may benefit the most by increasing calcium intake.

The ratio of potassium to sodium intake is important. Basic foods have favorable high potassium/low sodium ratios. Examples are fresh fruits and vegetables. This ratio becomes inverted in processed foods, whereby the potassium is reduced or even depleted, and sodium rises, sometimes dramatically. Examples are canned string beans and potato chips. In industrialized countries, the average diet contains a large excess of sodium—far beyond the physiologic needs of this essential mineral—and too little potassium to meet its physiologic needs. Processed foods account for up to 80 percent of the daily sodium intake in the American diet. (See the article "Modern Food Processing: Nutritional Shortchanges" on page 10.)

Studies have suggested that the chloride component in sodium chloride (table salt) might also be a factor. In rat studies, blood pressure increased far more following ingestion of sodium chloride than with other sodium-containing compounds. Chloride might enhance sodium's effects on blood pressure.

Although table salt may increase blood pressure in hypertensives, many other sodium-containing compounds may not. In a study conducted by Dr. Theodore W. Kurtz and his colleagues at the General Clinical Research Center, University of California, men with high blood pressure were given table salt supplements for a week. As anticipated, their blood pressure rose sharply. But, when they received the same amount of sodium in other sodium-containing compounds, such as sodium citrate (a common additive in many foods and beverages) their blood pressure remained constant.

A clearer designation would be "sodium chloride-dependent hypertension" rather than "sodium-dependent hypertension."

Many Americans have diets low in magnesium. Burton M. Altura, M.D. at State University of New York (SUNY), Downtown Medical Center in Brooklyn, NY, reported that low magnesium levels may be related to hypertension. A group of normal rats, fed a magnesium-deficient diet for twelve weeks, developed hypertension. The interior of the fine branches of their veins and arteries had constricted in size, which caused the blood pressure to rise. The lower their intake of magnesium, the smaller their blood vessels became, and the more their blood pressure rose.

In human studies conducted in The Netherlands, ninety-one middle-aged and elderly women with untreated mild to moderate hypertension were given magnesium supplements at levels difficult to achieve solely by dietary changes. After six months, they showed beneficial blood pressure reduction.

Some segments of the American population may be severely magnesium depleted, including chronic alcoholics, and individuals taking diuretics—widely used prescription drugs. The diuretics, used by hypertensives to expel sodium, also expel magnesium. A Swedish study found patients given a magnesium supplement along with the diuretic avoided this problem.

Tin may be a factor, not yet well recognized, in hypertension. The animal model used most frequently to study hypertension is a spontaneously hypertensive rat (SHR). In tests, a tin compound (stannous chloride) was found to keep blood pressure normal in the young SHR during a fourteen-week study, but had no similar beneficial effect on SHR adults. Selenium deficiency has been found to accelerate the development of hypertension in SHR.

In epidemiological studies, as well as in animal experiments, an adequate intake of high-quality protein food has been shown to be beneficial for sodium excretion, improvement of arterial walls, and lowering of blood pressure.

The type of fat in the diet may be related to hypertension. In a review of nondrug therapies for hypertension, reduction of saturated fat intake was recommended in the *American Journal of Hypertension* (February 1989). This dietary change causes a modest lowering of blood pressure, as well as counteracting the cholesterol-raising effect of some commonly used antihypertensive drugs. Vegetarians and others whose fat intake consist mainly of polyunsaturated fats have lower blood pressure levels than those whose fat intake consists mainly of saturated fats.

The American diet is low in omega-3 fatty acids, found in fish and fish oil supplements. Increased fish consumption may reduce the risk of pregnancy-induced hypertension. Results have been inconsistent with many studies using a high-fish diet or fish-oil supplements to reduce high blood pressure. However, data from studies of more than 1,300 subjects, analyzed by scientists under the auspices of the National Institute of Environmental Health Science of the National Institutes of Health, suggested overwhelmingly that fish oil lowered blood pressure moderately in the majority of hypertensive subjects. Generally, larger amounts of fish oil produced greater declines in blood pressure than did smaller amounts. Very low supplemental dosages had virtually no effect. Nor did it produce changes in the blood pressure level of healthy subjects. The effects of fish oils, however, might be harmful for hypertensives with impaired kidney function or poor blood clotting ability.

Sugar is a food component that, at high intake, is known to enhance the increase of blood pressure caused by salt in sodium-sensitive rats. In a study involving monkeys, larger amounts of sugar as well as salt in the diet induced high blood pressure. The animals fed a diet containing 3 percent salt and 38 percent sugar developed higher blood pressure than those on a high salt, but sugarless, diet. Both groups developed higher blood pressure than animals fed their normal monkey chow. The study demonstrated that a diet high in both sugar and salt—much like a typical American diet—also could raise the cholesterol level in the animals' blood.

Deficiencies of certain nutrients and food components may be additional factors in hypertension. These constituents include some vitamins (A, niacin, and C); bioflavonoids; certain amino acids (tyrosine and tryptophan); and inadequate intake of water and dietary fibers. Food allergy, especially gluten sensitivity to certain grains (wheat, rye, oat, and barley) has been suggested by Lloyd Rosenvold, M.D., formerly of Loma Linda University Medical School, as an unrecognized factor in some cases of hypertension. There may be other nutritional factors, as yet unrecognized, that play a role in hypertension.

CAN YOU TRUST CHOLESTEROL TESTS?

Americans have been urged to have their cholesterol tested, and in past years nearly two-thirds of adults have complied. At social gatherings, an individual's cholesterol figure may be mentioned as nonchalantly as one's golf score. What do cholesterol tests tell? How accurate are they?

It is highly unlikely that a single measurement of cholesterol is accurate. Cholesterol values should be viewed in terms of a range rather than as absolute fixed numbers. Furthermore, a test that merely measures total cholesterol offers too little information to make it meaningful. It is necessary to learn the measures for different components of total cholesterol.

Cholesterol is transported in blood plasma through lipoproteins. The three major lipoproteins are *low-density lipoproteins* (LDLs), which contain 60 to 70 percent of the total serum cholesterol; *high-density lipoproteins* (HDLs), which contain 20 to 30 percent of the total serum cholesterol; and *very low-density lipoproteins* (VLDLs), which contain 10 to 15 percent of the total serum cholesterol. The VLDLs are precursors of LDLs. *Triglycerides,* too, are an important class of blood lipids, or fats, and usually are measured in conjunction with cholesterol values. Recently, attention has been given to *apolipoprotein* groups, which are subcomponents of these different types of cholesterol, because they may be better predictors of certain risks associated with coronary heart disease, such as degenerative arterial wall changes.

HDL cholesterol, regarded as beneficial, is the smallest in size of all the lipoproteins, and is difficult to measure accurately. Using current criteria for acceptable laboratory testing, leeway is given in the accuracy of HDL measurement. A figure is acceptable even if it is as much as 30 percent higher or lower than the standard measure.

LDL cholesterol, regarded as unfavorable, appears to be the main component that causes plaque formation on arterial walls. Yet to date, no error standard for LDL cholesterol measurement has been established. Direct LDL cholesterol measurement can be done with expensive, time-consuming tests, but generally they are unavailable in most cholesterol test settings. Instead, LDL cholesterol is calculated from other laboratory measurements by reliance on measurements of total cholesterol, HDL, and total triglycerides. As a result, if any of these measurements are inaccurate or imprecise, the measurement error for LDL will be compounded.

Triglyceride levels usually are measured along with lipoproteins. At present, calibration of one testing technique using enzymes is not linked to any validated standard. Another technique, which uses an acid, is considered the best means for accurate measurement, but a figure is acceptable even if it is 25 percent higher or lower than the standard measure.

Several methods measure different apolipoprotein components, but they have not yet been standardized and cannot be done in most laboratories. To date, no comparative reference base has been established by means of any comprehensive, statistically sound study.

Factors of Variation in Measurements. Even if a single cholesterol measurement were accurate and precise, the value would not reflect the individual's cholesterol variation from day to day. Total cholesterol, as well as HDL cholesterol levels, vary over time and are influenced by many factors.

Some fluctuations and variations of an individual's total HDL and LDL cholesterol are normal. Some people experience dramatic week-to-week fluctuations, while others experience virtually no change during the same period of time. Overall, biological variation of total cholesterol is reported to average more than 6 percent; HDL, more than 7 percent; LDL, more than 9 percent; and triglycerides, more than 22 percent. Because of these fluctuations and variations, individuals whose test levels measure close to a classification between "border-line risk" and "high risk" should have several testings performed over a period of time. Because present measurements for HDL and LDL are imprecise, such repeated testings are critical, especially before a diagnosis is made.

Biological variations are so wide that some individuals move into, or out of, one of the risk categories, and some even move two categories, from "desirable" to "high risk" levels of cholesterol.

LDL and total cholesterol levels of any individual may vary by season. Both average higher in winter than in summer. The HDL cholesterol level has not been found to vary seasonally.

Gender is another factor in biological variation. Total cholesterol concentrations may average 20 percent lower during the luteal phase of the menstrual cycle. This is the time period immediately following ovulation.

As a person ages, the total cholesterol level tends to increase.

Every individual has biological cycles that produce variability. As a result, cholesterol levels can vary considerably between measurements. Normal cholesterol level fluctuations are estimated to account for about 65 percent of the variation in individuals for both total and HDL cholesterol, and about 95 percent of variation for triglycerides.

Lifestyle factors appear to have varying effects on the cholesterol levels of different people. In some, it may have a large effect on total and LDL cholesterol levels. In part, this may be related to the estimates that only one-third of an individual's cholesterol level is linked to diet. The body produces the remaining two-thirds by manufacturing cholesterol in the liver. When the individual takes in a low amount of dietary cholesterol, the body compensates by manufacturing more.

Often, blood cholesterol samples are drawn after the individual has fasted, especially if a lipid measurement is to be made. Otherwise, after eating a typical fat-containing

CHOLESTEROL IS ESSENTIAL

Despite popular misconception, cholesterol is essential in the body. It is necessary for many processes, affects the production of steroid hormones and bile acids, and serves as a structural component of cellular membranes.

Cholesterol is a fatlike substance (lipid) manufactured by the body, and also obtained, in lesser amounts, from foods. In addition, certain saturated fats raise the blood cholesterol level more than any other nutrient component in the diet. Thus, an elevated cholesterol level may be the result of a diet heavy in certain saturated fats as well as cholesterol. Also, it is possible that the liver is manufacturing high levels of cholesterol and triglyceride, or that cholesterol is being removed too slowly from the body.

meal, the individual's lipid level will change, and the effect will last for about nine hours. Typically, triglyceride and VLDL cholesterol levels will increase, whereas the LDL cholesterol level decreases significantly.

Dietary cholesterol is incompletely and variably absorbed by different individuals, ranging from as little as 18 percent absorption, up to as much as 75 percent. Those with the greatest absorption appear to have the highest LDL cholesterol levels.

Individuals respond differently to changes in dietary fats. For the same increase in dietary cholesterol, the cholesterol levels of most persons will increase, but some will remain essentially unchanged, and a few will increase dramatically.

Vigorous exercise just before testing will cause a significant rise in HDL levels. Thus, patients should avoid strenuous exercise for 24 hours before having a blood specimen drawn so as not to distort the measurement.

Moderate alcohol intake appears to increase HDL cholesterol, and greater alcohol consumption lowers LDL cholesterol and raises triglycerides. Any unusual alcoholic intake before drawing a blood specimen also may skew cholesterol measurement.

Obese individuals who repeatedly gain or lose weight, when tested for cholesterol, may show significant variation in lipoprotein levels. It is recommended that an individual's weight be stabilized, and that the person follow his customary diet for at least two weeks before having a blood specimen drawn for a cholesterol test.

Clinical Factors. Pregnancy is associated with changes in lipid levels in the second and third trimesters, when total and LDL cholesterol, triglycerides, and certain apolipoprotein levels increase significantly. Because of these changes, cholesterol testing is not recommended until three months after the woman has given birth, or three months after she has stopped breast-feeding.

An individual's cholesterol measurement may also be affected by acute infections or metabolic diseases. An underactive thyroid can raise total and LDL cholesterol levels. Diabetics may have high total and LDL cholesterol, as well as elevated triglycerides. Higher levels of insulin are associated with unfavorable levels of total and LDL cholesterol, triglycerides, and some apolipoprotein.

Other diseases, including Tay-Sachs (a rare, fatal, hereditary disorder in children), rheumatoid arthritis, and infections can alter lipid levels. (A heart attack may be accompanied by decreased total and LDL cholesterol levels.)

Drug Factors. Medications such as diuretics, some betablockers, and sex steroids can change lipid levels. Oral contraceptives, high in progestin, can increase serum total and LDL cholesterol, and decrease HDL cholesterol levels, while contraceptives with high amounts of estrogen have the opposite effects. Similar changes are found in postmenopausal women on estrogen supplements.

Testing Procedures. Conditions under which a blood sample is taken are critical for obtaining accurate measurements. Capillary blood taken from a finger-stick sample can differ markedly from blood taken from a vein, even when analyzed by the same device. One large research study found that capillary blood total cholesterol was approximately 7 percent higher than venous blood samples, when both were measured with the same analyzer. Such disparities may account for "contradictory results" from different tests of the same individual, if capillary blood is drawn for some tests, and venous blood for others.

The procedures used for taking the specimen and preparing it for analysis can affect lipid level measurements. Knowledge and experience of the laboratory technician are important. For example, the length of time a person is sitting or standing before having blood drawn has been shown to influence cholesterol test results. The individual should be seated for at least fifteen minutes before a venous sample is taken. If used, a tourniquet should be applied only for less than one minute before the specimen is taken for a lipid analysis.

Proper storage of the blood sample is important to avoid changes in the composition and to ensure accurate measurement results. Use of a standard collection policy by a trained laboratory technician can help minimize variability and inaccuracy.

How Accurate Are Cholesterol Measurements? Even if all the variable factors in cholesterol measurements are taken into account, there is still another hurdle: how accurate and precise are the measuring devices?

Cholesterol tests are conducted in a variety of settings, ranging from hospitals and physicians' offices to mass screenings at health fairs. In addition, some home test kits are available.

The biological variabilities plus the inaccuracies or imprecisions of the testing devices combine to make cholesterol measurements, at best, tentative information. . . . They do not necessarily reflect the health status of an individual.

Cholesterol testing devices consist of three types: large stationary analyzers that are capable of performing multiple tests daily on many analyses for hundreds of specimens. They are found in large independent laboratories, hospital laboratories, and in major testing organizations that serve the medical community. Cholesterol tests with processed blood tend to act differently from fresh serum samples on many instrument reagent systems used in large stationary

Cholesterol Ratings

The National Cholesterol Education Program classified American adults without evidence of existing coronary heart disease into three levels based on total cholesterol levels:

- Desirable: below 200 milligrams per deciliter (mg/dL)
- Borderline High: 200–239 mg/dL
- High: at or above 240 mg/dL

An HDL cholesterol level of less than 35 mg/dL is considered "low" and as a contributing risk factor of coronary heart disease.

LDL cholesterol levels are classified as:

- Desirable: less than 130 mg/dL
- Borderline High: 130–159 mg/dL
- High Risk: at or above 160 mg/dL

analyzers. In studies, total cholesterol tests done on fresh serum samples in a select group of clinical settings met the established accuracy standard, whereas processed control materials resulted in greater inaccuracy.

Desktop analyzers are small, portable or semiportable devices used to measure cholesterol, either in a physician's office or in a nontraditional setting. A recent study concluded that "in general, desk-top analyzers give fairly accurate measurements on average, but tend to be somewhat more variable than laboratory-based methods in individual samples." In tests, even under optimal operating conditions, some desktop analyzers were found to be inaccurate and imprecise for total, HDL, and LDL cholesterol measurements. Several studies showed misclassification rates ranged from 17 percent to nearly 50 percent. The General Accounting Office (GAO), which reported on the accuracy of cholesterol measurement, advised consumers to be "aware of the potential uncertainty associated with test results" produced by desktop analyzers.

As for home test kits, which measure total cholesterol, GAO cautioned: "While these may prove to be useful, questions about their precision and accuracy should not be overlooked." Also, the issue has been raised as to whether the user may interpret cholesterol measurements incorrectly, or initiate a self-prescribed treatment without proper medical feedback and monitoring.

Cholesterol testing may be helpful, along with other tests, in indicating one's health status. However, its limited usefulness should be understood. The biological variabilities plus the inaccuracies or imprecisions of the testing devices combine to make measurements, at best, tentative information. Also, the classifications of "desirable," "borderline high risk," and "high risk" assigned to different cholesterol levels have been set arbitrarily, based on broad population studies. They do not necessarily reflect the health status of an individual.

ARE NATURAL AND SYNTHETIC VITAMINS IDENTICAL?

"The evidence that has accumulated over many years since we've identified nutrients makes it very obvious that a nutrient is a nutrient is a nutrient, or a vitamin is a vitamin is a vitamin," Ogden C. Johnson, Ph.D., Director of the Office of Nutrition and Consumer Sciences, Food and Drug Administration (FDA), once remarked in a published interview.

Repeatedly, FDA officials, many members of the drug trade, and some nutritionists who have apparently missed some important findings in reading the literature of their profession, all keep assuring consumers that vitamins and other dietary supplements are identical, regardless of whether they are derived from natural or synthetic sources. How reliable is this information for individuals who purchase supplements?

If "identical" refers only to the chemical compositions, the statement is true with some limitations. A molecule of crystalline ascorbic acid, synthesized in the laboratory, may be "chemically" identical to a molecule of ascorbic acid derived from a natural source such as citrus fruit. However, the analysis should not be limited to a simple determination of the chemical composition. By failing to explore the subject further, and by ignoring other characteristics, writers on the subject have misled the public. Indeed, distinct and important differences do exist, and consumers have a right to be aware of them before making choices in the marketplace.

Absorption and Utilization. A synthetic vitamin contains one pure substance, or at most, a few pure substances. It lacks other constituents that are present in a natural product and that possibly may be vital for its full effectiveness in restoring or maintaining health. For example, the synthetic form of vitamin C consists solely of the isolated pure substance, crystalline ascorbic acid. The natural form of vitamin C, derived from foods (such as citrus fruits, rose hips, acerola cherries, and black currants) in addition to its ascorbic acid content, also has other vitamins, minerals, trace minerals, enzymes, and coenzymes, as well as other important nutritional elements. These substances, in combination with the ascorbic acid, as well as with one another, may exert marked effects. Such interactions may determine the degree to which the ascorbic acid is absorbed and utilized. The medical literature contains numerous reports that suggest that, in many instances, natural vitamin C has been found to be more effective than synthetic ascorbic acid.

This fact has been recognized for at least as early as 1954, when it was reported that cases of scurvy failed to respond to doses of synthetic vitamin C. A cure was effected when the individuals suffering from scurvy were given a natural food substance containing vitamin C. For some reason, inexplicable at the time, the curative results that failed with the administration of synthetic vitamin C were achieved with the vitamin in its natural medium.

Artificial fruit drinks, with synthetic vitamin C added, are advertised as being nutritionally superior to real fruit juice. This claim is questionable. For example, in a 1971 study by R. E. Hughes and P. R. Jones, two groups of guinea pigs on a diet without vitamin C were given equivalent amounts of vitamin C (that is, L-ascorbic acid) from black currant juice concentrate, and from dried acerola juice. A third group received an equal amount of synthetic vitamin C in water. The overall growth rate was greatest with the group fed the black currant juice; intermediate with the acerola juice; and lowest with synthetic vitamin C.

The highly purified nature of synthetic vitamins makes them readily soluble, a feature that may be undesirable. Vitamins that are crude natural extractives, being less soluble, need to undergo digestive processes before being absorbed. Because of this characteristic, they may be deposited in the tissues and utilized more effectively.

Different Forms Show Different Biological Activity. Although molecule for molecule, synthetic and natural vitamins may appear to some government spokesmen and writers for the popular press to be chemically identical, distinct differences can be demonstrated with polarized light. The plane of a beam of polarized light is rotated by all natural substances either to the left (L-form) or to the right (D-form). (See "chirality" on page 118; also discussion on page 108.) Substances not occurring in nature may not cause rotation of the plane of polarization and these substances are said to be optically inactive (DL-form). What is the significance of these different forms of the same basic substance?

Commercially prepared natural vitamin E concentrates (derived from edible vegetable oils or from the byproducts of their refining) rotate the plane of polarization to the right, and hence they are D-form. D-alpha tocopherol (natural vitamin E) has been found to be considerably more active than DL-alpha tocopherol (synthetic vitamin E). Different forms of vitamin E show very different biological activity. All synthetic tocopherols, in one way or another, have been shown to produce different physiological effects. Some of the synthetic ones differ from D-alpha tocopherol in the manner in which they transfer across cell walls and accumulate in desirable concentrations where needed. To date, no completely nontoxic synthetic substitute for D-alpha tocopherol has been found.

Pantothenate, another nutrient, demonstrates distinct

Read Labels

Label reading is important for those who wish to know whether a vitamin product is from natural or synthetic sources. In addition to looking for the D- or L-forms, the following ingredients may be listed. Natural sources of:

- vitamin A—fish oils
- vitamin B—yeast, liver, and soybeans
- vitamin C—citrus, rose hips, acerola cherries, and currants
- vitamin D—fish oils
- vitamin E—mixed tocopherols, wheat germ oil, and d-alpha tocopherol—wheat germ oil, and sunflower, corn, or soybean oils

differences with various forms. The complete chemical structure of calcium pantothenate was determined when a method was devised to extract it from liver. All of the configurations of molecules were found to be D-form. When the pantothenates were made having only *slightly* different atomic arrangements, they were found to be ineffective. The L-form, for example, was termed "useless."

Natural food protein, as well as protein in the human body, contains only L-forms of amino acids. The body possesses L-enzymes to handle L-amino acids, but has none for other forms. Natural L-amino acids are absorbed immediately in the digestive system by means of the L-enzymes, but with D- or DL-forms, absorption is delayed. When processed foods are fortified with amino acids, the DL-forms are used. It is questionable whether the body can utilize DL-amino acids efficiently.

Another critical difference between natural and synthetic supplements has been supplied in testimony from allergists, who have noted that two substances, even though chemically identical, may affect individuals quite differently. A synthetically derived vitamin may cause a reaction in a chemically susceptible person, whereas a naturally derived vitamin may be well tolerated. The most frequently reported reactions to synthetic vitamins that have been observed clinically are especially those involving thiamine (B_1) and vitamin C (ascorbic acid).

It becomes clear that the public is grossly misled by official statements that "a nutrient is a nutrient is a nutrient" or that "a vitamin is a vitamin is a vitamin."

The subject of natural versus synthetic encompasses far more than a comparison of vitamins. As the trend continues toward a diet comprised of highly "fabricated" manufactured, factory modified and processed foods, infant feeding formulas, fortified breakfast foods, as well as agricultural practices based on similar assumptions regarding the safety of human "improvements" over nature, it is especially important to examine the subject carefully. It becomes clear that the public is grossly misled by official statements that "a nutrient is a nutrient is a nutrient" or that "a vitamin is a vitamin is a vitamin." Chemically? Perhaps. Biologically? It's definitely not so.

THE DOWNSIDE OF SOY

Despite the many alleged benefits of soy, which are being promoted enthusiastically, and the Food and Drug Administration's (FDAs) approval of a health claim for soy, there is also a downside to soy, which largely is being ignored. Soy contains many antinutrients. The downside of soy needs to be considered in any overall evaluation, official recommendation, and endorsement.

Antinutrients. Raw soybeans are anticoagulants and have antienzyme agents. Their anticoagulant activity is not reversed by vitamin K—the blood-clotting vitamin. Soy's anticoagulant properties are attributed to its antitryspin activity. Tryspin is a special enzyme that is needed to digest protein. It allows vitamin B_{12} (cyanocobalamin) to be assimilated. Soybeans also have antiproteolytic activity that increases the requirement for vitamin B_{12}. At the same time, soy's antitryspin activity may actually create a vitamin B_{12} deficiency.

Raw soybeans contain other antinutrients. Phytic acid, from phytates, present in soybean, binds up and prevents the absorption of minerals (especially zinc, calcium, and magnesium). Phytic acid is present in grains as well. As a result, vegetarians who depend on large amounts of soybeans and soybean products, as well as grains in their diets, are at even higher risk for deficiencies of these minerals.

Many studies confirm these findings. Phytates are present in plant foods, but do not exist in animal foods.

Another group of antinutrients in raw soybeans are hemagglutinins. These substances have the ability to agglutinate (clump together) the red blood cells in humans and in other animal species, and suppress growth significantly. These antinutrients are known also as "phytoagglutinins" or "lectins."

The downside of soy needs to be considered in any overall evaluation, official recommendation, and endorsement.

Although the level of many of these antinutrients present in raw soybeans can be reduced somewhat by proper heat treatment or by sprouting of the beans, the substances will still be present, at lower levels. The only satisfactory method known to deactivate these antinutrients is by means of traditional fermentation. This process involves a slow chemical change, triggered by bacteria, molds, and yeast. Fermentation deactivates the antinutrients present in raw soybeans, such as the enzyme inhibitors, trypsin inhibitor, phytic acid, hemagglutinins, and vitamin antagonists. Fermentation makes the nutrients in soybeans much more available and digestible.

Unfortunately, the fermentation process is used with only a few soybean products, and ones that are not especially familiar in the American cuisine, nor readily available. The main fermented soybean products are tempeh (a soybean-based entree), miso (a soybean paste used in soups and sauces), and natto (fermented whole soybeans). Tempeh and miso are available in some health/natural food stores in the United States. Tempeh is a food, but miso is only a flavoring. Natto, common in Japan, is unfamiliar and unavailable to most Americans. Natto is reported to have a strong odor, a sticky texture, and is not generally favored by novices.

Soybean products such as tofu and bean curd, familiar and available to Americans, are *not* fermented. Rather, they are processed by precipitation, a method that deactivates *some* but not all of the antienzyme agents, and deactivates only a *little* of the phytates.

Some Thyroid Effects. Soybeans, even processed ones, have antithyroid properties. Often, this characteristic is not noted, but consumers deserve to know more. The estrogenic isoflavones in soy—genistein and daidzein—are much touted for their alleged health benefits. What is unpublicized is that they happen to be antithyroid agents. Individuals who habitually consume soybean products may encounter long-range thyroid disturbances. Animal studies relate the isoflavones in soy to thyroid disorders, including goiter. Other studies have related soy consumption negatively not only to hypothyroidism, but also to low energy levels, poor mineral absorption, and infertility.

Even at exceedingly low levels, hormones can exert profound biological effects, either beneficial or detrimental. The estrogenic isoflavones in soy are being promoted enthusiastically as health promoters. Although estrogenic isoflavones appear to prevent breast cancer if supplied early, they may *promote* breast cancer at a later stage. Both human and animal studies suggest that soy may *increase* the risk of breast cancer.

Frequently, studies are cited of the low breast cancer rate of Asian women who consume soy. However, confounding dietary factors must be considered. Asian women who forsake their traditional diets and embrace the Western diet increase their risk of breast cancer. Soy cannot be singled out as the sole factor.

Several Downsides. How beneficial are soy products being offered to Americans? The antinutrients in modern soy products, including soy flour, can inhibit animal growth. In humans, they can cause intestinal problems, reduce protein digestion, and lead to chronic deficiencies in the uptake of amino acids.

Soy contains a high amount of omega-3 fatty acids, which turn rancid rapidly when the soybean is converted into soy flour. Full-fat soy flour is especially prone to such deterioration, and has a disagreeable taste that is difficult to mask. Rancid foods are toxic and should be avoided.

Textured soy protein (TVP), an inexpensive filler, became popular at one time as a hamburger extender. Presently, it is used extensively in processed foods, despite the fact that it contains antinutrients such as phytic acid, the trypsin inhibitor, and antithyroid agents.

Soy protein isolates are used in powder mixes intended as meal-replacement drinks. The isolates are produced by a high-temperature process that denatures the protein extensively. In its damaged form, the protein is rendered low in nutritional value. Soy protein (and other protein) isolates cause negative calcium balance in humans and animals, and can contribute to the development of osteoporosis. The soy protein isolates are still high in mineral-blocking phytates, thyroid-depressing phytoestrogens, and potent enzyme inhibitors. Also, the high heat used in processing the isolates has been reported to increase the likelihood of forming carcinogenic compounds.

Soy "milk" is used as a cows' milk replacer, and marketed for the general population. Also, it is used as a substitute for cows' milk in infant feeding formulas intended for babies who are allergic to cows' milk. Soy milk is *not* the equivalent of milk from humans or cows (or goats or sheep). Soy milk has several undesirable features that need to be considered whenever it is used as a substitute ingredient in infant-feeding formulas.

Soy can have adverse effects on the hormonal development of infants. Soy milk formula is devoid of cholesterol, a substance that is vital for the proper development of the brain and the central nervous system in infants. A study of infants fed soy formula showed a concentration of estrogenic compounds as much as 22,000 times higher than those in human breast milk or in milk-based formula. This finding caused speculation in the *New Zealand Medical Journal* that such an overload of estrogen in infants might result in precocious development of breasts and secondary sex characteristics in very young females. In addition, it raised worries that such an overload might result in male organs not developing normally at puberty.

Another factor to consider about use of soybeans as edible fats is that soybean oil is likely to be partially hydrogenated. This processing results in the formation of undesirable, unhealthy *trans* fatty acids in the oil, and in food products made with the oil. To date, the vital information about *trans* fatty acids is not included in the "Nutrition Facts" panel of food labels.

Frequently, the soybean has been touted as a "complete" protein from a plant-derived food. The soybean may have a better nutritional profile than other beans, but it is low in some essential amino acids, which makes it an unbalanced source of protein. Only when beans, including soybeans, are supplemented with some complete and balanced protein from an animal-derived food, can the combination be considered as a complete protein food.

Soy as a Major Food Allergen. Infants fed soy milk formulas in order to avoid cows' milk allergy may develop allergy to soy. Individuals of all ages have developed soy allergies, attributable to the proliferation of soy and soy constituents in many commercially formulated products. Since the FDA approved the health claim for soy, it is predicted that more than 1,000 new soy-containing products will be introduced. As soy is promoted more and more, and is available in more and more food and beverage products, the number of soy-allergic individuals keeps increasing. At present, soy is among the major food allergens in the American diet.

It is difficult to avoid soy and soy constituents unless one chooses basic foods and avoids processed ones. Even then, soy gets into the basic diet, indirectly, from the soy constituents in the feed of farm animals and of farmed fish (in aquaculture).

". . . no other dietary staple has so many antinutrient drawbacks as soy. Conversely, no other food has so many public relation firms and lobbyists working for it."

The soy health claim now permitted is based on 25 grams of soy protein daily, alleged to reduce the risk of heart disease. Such a daily overload of soy inevitably increases the risk for soy allergenicity. The FDA determined that diets with four daily servings of soy can reduce levels of low-density lipoproteins (LDLs). Four daily servings of soy protein not only promote the risk of more allergenic reactions, but replace high-quality protein foods that have no antinutrients with low-quality protein foods that have many antinutrients. In addition, the recommendation narrows the food base and negates the sound principle of choosing from as wide a variety of foods as possible. (See the article "Our Narrowing Food Base: A Perilous Trend" on page 18.)

The FDA approved the health claim for soy protein, in response to a petition by a leading soy producer. In view of the overall evidence, is the health claim justified? Previous health claims have been approved in response to commercial interests, and similarly based on highly selective evidence. One critic observed that "no other dietary staple has so many antinutrient drawbacks as soy. Conversely, no other food has so many public relation firms and lobbyists working for it."

IS NUTRITION POLICY BASED ON ACCURATE DATA?

The U.S. Department of Agriculture (USDA) is engaged in important basic research at its several human research service centers. The work uses information from different fields of science. Technological and analytical advances, computer science, and statistical data contribute to the research. Unfortunately, some statistical information derived from federal figures of food composition, and from federally sponsored food surveys, may be unreliable.

Inaccurate Food Composition. The USDA's Agricultural Handbook No. 8, which contains tables of the nutrient compositions of foods, has long been valued as the world's source of nutrient information. A wide spectrum of primary groups—including some twenty-two federal agencies, international organizations, and researchers—depend on data from the Handbook. It serves as a guide for a broad range of federal programs, including school lunches, recommended daily allowances (RDAs), feeding the military, and the nutrition-labeling program.

This icon of reliability came crashing down in 1993 with a critical report issued by the U.S. General Accounting Office (GAO). Among its findings, the GAO reported: "In some cases, data have been accepted into the data base with little or no supporting information on the testing and quality assurance procedures used to develop the data. For example, data on bacon cheeseburgers. . . . came primarily from brochures provided by fast-food chains; the brochures generally did not explain how the nutrient values were determined. Consequently, HNIS [USDA's Human Nutrition Information Service] cannot be assured that all the data in Handbook 8—used in so many nutritional decisions—are reliable."

The GAO found that about 85 percent of the information in the Handbook was obtained either from the food industry or from scientific literature, rather than from actual laboratory analyses at the USDA. The Agency budgets only $200,000 annually for nutrient analyses, and a single analysis can cost $2,000.

The GAO questioned the HNIS's data for accuracy, adequacy of analytical methods used to produce the data, and the sufficiency and adequacy of the documentation used for validation. Similar concerns had been raised in 1989 by a federal interagency working group, but none of the concerns raised nor the recommended changes had been addressed up to the time of the 1993 GAO report.

The tables in the Handbook have been used for years by dietitians and researchers to estimate nutrient intake, as well as by regulatory agencies to formulate federal food policies and programs. It had long been suspected that some of the values listed in the Handbook might be overestimations. Commonly, the nutrient composition figures for meat, milk, and other farm products have been based on well-raised animals on demonstration farms at land-grant colleges or universities, reflecting higher values than those commonly found on private farms in less ideal settings.

A valid database is critical for many current issues. For example, the method used to calculate the number of calories people actually obtain from foods, known as "metabolizable energy," was developed at the turn of the twentieth century. Because of the current emphasis on increasing dietary fibers and decreasing dietary fat, researchers have been critical of the continued use of an outdated method. In a ten-week human study, metabolized energy values were found to be lower than those in the Handbook, which overestimates high-fiber diets by 5 percent and high-fat diets by 8 percent.

The meat industry has charged that dietary fiber measurements in meat and poultry are not precise enough to allow fiber to be a compliance criterion for products made with these ingredients. This point is critical for accuracy on the nutritional labels.

The issue of whether or not to fortify foods with folic acid has become controversial. Among the opponents is Marion Nestle of the Department of Nutrition at New York University. Among her objections were faulty statistics. Although surveys suggest that average folate intakes are well

Agriculture Handbook: A Standard Reference

Basic food composition tables were first compiled and evaluated by the USDA's nutritional pioneer, W.O. Atwater. In 1886 the agency issued *The Chemical Composition of American Food Materials* (USDA Bulletin No. 28), the first in a long series of food composition tables. With each new bulletin, the work was expanded to include newly discovered vitamins, minerals, and other essential nutrients, and the roles they played.

Farsightedly, Atwater regarded Bulletin No. 28 as a work that would be "a standard reference until it shall be replaced by a larger and more complete compilation." Ultimately, Agriculture Handbook No. 8 superseded USDA Bulletin No. 28.

By 1976, Agricultural Handbook No. 8 was greatly expanded as a series of subdivided handbooks, issued singly over more than a decade. Subsequently, the Handbooks have been put in a database available online, and are constantly updated.

below recommended levels, Nestle contends that the standard has been based on faulty food composition data that underestimate actual folate intake. The method of calculating this nutrient has changed, but the USDA never adjusted its figures on the composition tables.

The USDA itself has cited inaccuracies known to exist in the Handbook. For example, the Handbook lists the figure of 5 grams (g) of fat in 3.5 ounces of soft tofu and 10 g of fat in the same amount of hard tofu. Independent tests reported only 3 g of fat in the former, and only 5 g of fat in the latter. Similarly, the Handbook lists 3.1 g of fiber in an orange, whereas the Produce Marketing Association, basing its figures on actual testing, reported 5.8 g.

At best, the composition of food tables can give only *averages,* and does not reflect the true values for an individual food. The nutritional value may vary considerably from one batch of food to the next, due to factors that include genetic stock, location, weather conditions, agricultural practices, soil composition, the degree of ripeness, and even the location in a plot of land or on a tree. Some examples serve to demonstrate:

- On average, avocados from California contain 15 percent more fat than those from Florida; navel oranges from California, 34 percent more vitamin C than those from Florida.
- Oysters from the Atlantic Ocean contain higher levels of some nutrients than those from the Pacific Ocean. On a per calorie basis, the former contain 10 percent more protein, 54 percent more calcium, 28 percent more phosphorus, 5 percent more iron, and 171 percent more niacin than the latter.
- The age of a vegetable or grain affects its nutrient content. As carrots mature, their vitamin A level increases appre-

ciably. Ripe red tomatoes contain 3.6 times as much vitamin A as green ones. Mature red sweet peppers have 7.5 times as much vitamin A as immature green ones.

- The season of the year affects the riboflavin (vitamin B_2) content of wheat, corn, and milk. The vitamin D content of butter from cows fed on summer grass is higher than from those fed on winter hay.

Despite these wide variations, the averages provide ample supplies of nutrients. However, averages may be inadequate for research that requires precise data.

Survey Shortcomings. One method used by the federal government to measure food intake has little to do with actual consumption. It is based upon the disappearance of food into the marketing system.

At best, the composition of food tables can give only *averages,* and does not reflect the true values for an individual food.

The USDA's Economic Research Service calculates each year the amount of food available in the United States for human consumption, based on records of commodity flows from production to end uses. The total available supply consists of production, beginning inventories, and imports. The availability of food for human use is figured as the residual component, after subtraction of other uses from the available total supply. Per capita consumption is calculated by dividing the total food disappearance by the total U.S. population.

Food disappearance is a proxy to estimate actual food consumption. The data provide an upper limit on the amount of food available for consumption.

However, estimates can overstate the actual intake because they include food that is discarded in processing, lost in spoilage, and thrown away in homes or fed to companion animals. Therefore, food disappearance data may serve as trend indicators of consumption patterns, rather than offer any precise measurement of absolute amounts of foods consumed. Even as long-range indicators, food disappearance data may be unreliable. Changes in product forms, marketing channels, and consumer behavior may alter the relative disparity between food disappearance and foods actually eaten. In recent years, dramatically different food patterns have developed.

Self-Reporting Shortcomings. Frequently, data are gathered in national surveys based on self-reported food intake or for other health features. Self-reported food records are used to judge the nutritional status of populations, to assess consumption patterns, and to develop health guidelines. If the survey findings are inaccurate, public policy can be faulty.

A survey by the National Center for Health Statistics found that overweight women underreported their weight by an average of seven and one-half pounds, and overweight men by an average of three pounds. Even an experienced registered dietitian underreported by five pounds.

Large-scale surveys of food consumption have used twenty-four-hour recall for total food energy intake, derived from total dietary fat and from saturated fat. The intake was found to be underreported by as much as 25 percent.

A study conducted by Dr. Walter Mertz, while serving as a scientist at the USDA, showed that Americans may be consuming far more calories than government surveys show. Mertz found that 81 percent of volunteers for a study underreported their caloric intake. The shortcomings of self-reporting could explain why average body weight in the U.S. population has increased while reported food intake has decreased.

The 1993 USDA Agricultural Yearbook, *Nutrition, Eat-*

ing for Good Health, noted that "People's perceptions about their diets don't always match reality." An example was cited: about 40 percent of households' main-meal planners responding to a survey about the USDA's Dietary Guidelines believed that their diets were "about right" for fat intake. Yet, only about one-quarter had fat intakes that actually met the guidelines' limitation of total fat to 30 percent or less of total calories. Similarly, about 50 percent of the meal planners believed their diets were "about right," yet fewer than one-quarter reported intakes that met the guidelines' limitation of saturated fat to less than 10 percent of calories.

In study after study, the inaccuracy of self-reported data has been demonstrated. Consistently, people omit or underreport amounts eaten of items perceived negatively, such as calories, fat, and sugar, and overreport items perceived positively, such as fiber intake and physical activity.

Similar shortcomings were noted by the Centers for Disease Control and Prevention (CDC) in a study of alcohol consumption among women of childbearing years. The CDC admitted that the findings were limited, partly because the estimates of frequent drinking were based on self-reported data "which usually underestimates actual alcohol use."

Other Shortcomings. Nationwide food surveys have been conducted about every ten years for the National Food Consumption Survey (NFCS), a program begun in 1936. Loss of data and inaccurate data break a half-century continuum. Such disasters can be serious setbacks for nutritional research as well as for policies and regulations.

The NFCS conducted from 1987 to 1988 was under contract with the USDA. The finished survey was reviewed by the GAO and found to be seriously flawed and probably useless for establishing important governmental policies. The survey was characterized as mishandled, with an ex-

Additional Flawed Surveys

• The epidemiologic evidence linking dietary fat and breast cancer may be flawed because it is based on the "food disappearance" calculation of the fat content of the food supply. The fat consumption of persons in the United States according to this method *overestimates actual intake by more than 50 percent.*

• In 1990, the FDA conducted a survey to investigate the safety of bottled water products. The survey cost $850,000 and, according to the GAO review, proved nothing because the survey was not designed as a probability-based statistical sampling. Results reflected only a limited number of both plant inspections (forty-nine) and bottled water test samples (112). Also, the GAO faulted the FDA testing for only nine of thirty-one federally regulated contaminants.

• An unsatisfactory USDA survey involved a supplemental food program for infants. Over the objections of the study's chief researcher, the conclusions were purposely changed to make it appear that, the program had failed to improve the beneficiaries' health.

• The GAO criticized the USDA's costly efforts to collect data on the amount of pesticide residues remaining on selected food crops when they reach consumers. The data were flawed by a lack of uniform requirements for commodity sampling methods, laboratory testing procedures, and quality assurance practices.

• Researchers with the USDA's Continuing Survey of Food Intakes of Individuals (CSFII), gathered from 1989 to 1991, three days' recall of data on nearly 12,000 people for foods prepared at home, purchased prepared, or eaten away from home. "CSFII remains an imperfect tool," according to David Haytowitz, of the USDA's Human Nutrition Information Service (HNIS). An example cited by Haytowitz: a person who reports having eaten lasagna fails to provide a list of ingredients in the dish. Instead, the HNIS computer program calls up standard recipes for lasagna and then calculates how much the portion eaten was comprised of pasta, tomato, and other ingredients in the dish. The HNIS also has data on fats such as oils, shortenings, and margarines used in food preparation. However, there is no distinction made among them or whether the fat is hydrogenated. All these flaws leads to imprecise information.

- Two official publications, *The Surgeon General's Report on Nutrition and Health* and the National Research Council's *Diet and Health,* include a graph that has been criticized by researchers as "highly inaccurate" for estimating obesity when weight and height are known. Health professionals have been cautioned against reliance on the graph.

- In 1992, the GAO reviewed the USDA's Pesticide Data Program and found the data were "not statistically reliable" and "of limited use in making upcoming decisions on pesticide safety in food products." The GAO noted that, historically, pesticide usage and residue data used by the EPA have been "incomplete, statistically unreliable, or not readily accessible."

ceedingly low response rate and no follow-ups. There were billing errors and a cost overrun of $1.4 million above the original contract of $6.2 million. The contractor also lost thirty-four laptop computers supplied by the USDA for the survey.

The GAO criticized the survey as poorly designed, with

eighty-nine pages of questions that would require several hours to answer on the first day of a three-day monitoring period. Each respondent received two dollars for cooperating, up to a maximum of twenty dollars per household. The response rate was so poor that the GAO suggested that the people who did respond might not even be representative of the total population. Only 34 percent responded, which fell far short of the goal of 74 percent and only about half the rate of the prior national survey in 1977–1978.

After the GAO report, the survey was reviewed by the Federation of American Societies for Experimental Biology (FASEB). This independent group recommended against using data from the survey or, if used, to include "a strongly worded cautionary statement concerning the nonresponse bias."

After completion of these two reviews, the USDA had to make a decision. The agency could reject the flawed NFCS from 1987 to 1988 and base its policy decisions on the prior NFCS conducted a decade earlier (1977–1978). However, within the scientific community, the validity of that earlier survey also had been questioned. The response rate had been only 62 percent, a very low rate compared with other surveys conducted at that time. Also, in the 1977 to 1978 survey, there had been no follow-ups of nonrespondents.

Another choice for the USDA was to base its policy decisions on the U.S. Department of Health and Human Service's Health and Nutrition Examination Survey (HANES), conducted from 1976 to 1980, also considered an outdated study. However, it had a response rate of 77 to 86 percent. In the judgment of many health professionals, data from the HANES studies were more reliable reflections of the U.S. food consumption patterns.

There are great disparities between NFCS (1977–1978)

and HANES (1976–1980). For example, in the former study, it was reported that women were consuming 41 percent of their calories from fat; in the latter study, 36 percent. With many discrepancies, national policies and guidelines can be formulated and launched that lack a solid scientific basis.

Despite the serious flaws, the USDA decided to base its plans for the school food programs, the Thrifty Food Plan, and the food stamp allotments on the 1987–1988 NFCS. The FDA also opted to use this survey for its programs. The Environmental Protection Agency (EPA) preferred to continue using the 1977–1978 survey. Despite its flaws and datedness, the EPA considered it more reliable than the newer survey. Thus, federal agencies are basing public health policies on different sets of data.

The implications of using flawed data are significant because they affect the well-being of the entire population. Public policy decisions of many federal agencies rely on food composition and consumption data. Hundreds of millions of dollars are spent annually to implement food nutrition-related activities such as nutrition monitoring, labeling, and related activities. The soundness of these programs depends on reliable data.

CHAOS IS HEALTHY

Some scientists consider that the three most important scientific breakthroughs of the twentieth century have been the theory of relativity, quantum physics, and—the most recent—theory of chaos. Since the 1970s, chaos has been found in patterns as disparate as human health, economics, cotton prices, stock market fluctuations, electronic transmission noises, electromagnetic fields, and river flooding.

Chaos does not mean disorder, as the word is commonly used. At first, chaos may appear as unpredictable randomness, but actually is a predictable order, but without periodic repetition. A chaotic system is determined completely by a very simple mathematical formula. Once the formula is known, the next number in the chaotic series, no matter how complex, can be predicted with complete confidence. A chaotic system is extremely sensitive to the initial condition. Very small changes lead to large differences. But behavior in chaotic systems has a definite form, and is bounded. It cannot go off randomly.

Practical Applications. Chaos has application in many health fields, including cardiology, neurology, immunology, psychiatry, and epidemiology. For example, chaos may provide a healthy flexibility to the heart, brain, liver, and other systems of the body. Loss of chaotic flexibility may result in many health problems. A healthy physiological system has some innate variability, and transition to a less complicated and more orderly state may signal an impaired system. This healthy variability is not mere random, uncontrolled fluctuation, but rather is a well-developed chaos.

In terms of cardiac health, a heartbeat may appear to be quite regular and periodic. In reality it varies from day to day, hour to hour, minute to minute, and even second to second. Analyses of these variations show that they are chaotic, complicated, and seemingly unpredictable. They result from the way the heart regulates its beatings, and they are not random fluctuations.

A comparison of electrocardiograms (EKGs) of normal, healthy individuals with those of heart disease patients shows more variability in the heartbeat of the former than the latter. The former are more chaotic. Extreme regularity of heartbeat may lead to certain types of heart failure.

Understanding chaos' role in cardiac fibrillation may bring about new therapeutic strategies. A chaos-analysis machine is reported to surpass a traditional electrocardiograph in diagnosing coronary artery disease. Chaos' role may lead to "smarter" pacemakers and defibrillators. With pacemakers, for example, rather than stimulating the heart at regular intervals as present pacemakers do, they might be designed to mimic one of the low-dimensional chaotic patterns that exist in healthy hearts. Smaller voltages might be used to stop fibrillation in defibrillators. Understanding chaos may bring new understandings about thrombotic occlusion of pulmonary arteries and vascular changes associated with pulmonary hypertension.

Similarly, chaos may play a vital role in the brain by providing a healthy variability that allows the organ to respond quickly to a variety of stimuli. A normal brain is much more chaotic than a brain undergoing a seizure, at which time the brain becomes very regular and periodic. Extreme regularity may lead to brain seizure.

Additional Applications. It is thought that chaos helps the brain to be in a state of readiness, keeping it alert to receive new stimuli. The brain's normal background neural activity is chaotic, and mental activity occurs as an imposition of patterns on this chaotic background. In a chaotic state, the brain can switch quickly into any other pattern.

The brain responds to stimuli from the senses, such as smell. In the olfactory system, the brain's chaotic background state allows it to be alert and ready to react to completely new as well as to familiar odors.

It is thought that chaos plays a role in other physiological systems too. For example, in some leukemic patients, the number of white cells that fight infection may fluctuate cyclically and represent a loss of chaos. In contrast, healthy people have chaotic fluctuations in their white blood cell levels.

Laboratory experiments on pituitary cells show that healthy cells respond to the chemical order of their natural regulators, but tumor cells do not. The tumor cells are locked into a fixed rhythm.

Chaos may have practical applications in epidemiology. For example, if chaos is a factor, it may describe the actual data from childhood epidemics. It may explain a recent recurrence of measles by examining the effects that different vaccination levels have on disease rates. Chaos may be useful in understanding why some diseases occur in outbreaks, whilst others are more regular.

Chaos in the body may be a means of avoiding strictly periodic behavior that is destructive. This feature can be compared to a group of soldiers breaking step before crossing a bridge, because a march in unison could resonate with the bridge and cause it to collapse. In muscle activation, as a health example, if any individual motor units were fixed periodically, they might tend to synchronize and produce undesirable tremors. Thus, an active desynchronization mechanism in sustained contractions can spread out the motor-unit timing to fill the time interval of the activity. Applying this concept, Parkinson's disease, characterized by uncontrollable muscle tremors, may be caused by a loss of variability in some systems. The aging process, too, may involve a loss of variability; the young body is more chaotic than the older one.

Some scientists claim that chaos is a key to health, a formula for feedback among all the many systems that function in the body.

Formerly, any information that failed to fit into any pattern of disease was regarded as "noise" and dismissed. Those interested in chaos applications to health claim that such data should not be discarded, but analyzed more deeply. Meaningful patterns can be much more complex and disguised than formerly appreciated.

Some scientists claim that chaos is a key to health, a formula for feedback among all the many systems that function in the body. They suggest that disease is the breakdown of chaos into more conventional order.

NITRIC OXIDE: A HEALTH-RELATED GAS

Formerly, nitric oxide (NO) was regarded as a noxious reactive byproduct of burning fossil fuel, and as an environmental pollutant in smog, an ozone destroyer, an acid rain precursor, and a suspected carcinogen. However, since the 1970s, various investigators, working independently of each other, discovered that this sometimes poisonous gas is crucial in human physiology, and affects the body's cardiovascular, digestive, central nervous, immune, and respiratory systems. The researchers were startled to find that they were studying different facets of the same molecule.

NO has joined a group of known messenger molecules with roles in the arteries, immune system, liver, pancreas, uterus, penis, peripheral nerves, lungs, and brain. NO is the smallest, lightest molecule, and is the first known gas to act as a biological messenger in humans and in other mammals. It is synthesized in creatures as diverse as the barnacle, fruit fly, horseshoe crab, chicken, and trout, as well as in the human. With merely one atom apiece of nitrogen and oxygen, NO is among a group of biological agents—hormones, enzymes, and nucleic acids—composed of thousands of atoms and complex structures. As a free radical, NO vanishes rapidly after functioning. Its lifespan is unknown.

NO is the smallest, lightest molecule, and is the first known gas to act as a biological messenger in humans and in other mammals.

Modulator of Blood Pressure. One of NO's important functions is to modulate blood pressure. NO is produced by the amino acid, L-arginine, in the endothelial cells that form the band of muscle that encircles blood vessels. NO dilates these vessels by signaling neighboring smooth muscle cells to relax. People with high blood pressure may produce insufficient NO in the blood vessel walls, or may destroy NO too rapidly. Lack of adequate relaxation may lead to chronically narrowed arteries, essential hypertension, atherosclerosis, and renal failure.

Understanding NO's role in blood pressure has led to useful drugs. Septic shock, a leading cause of death in U.S. hospitals' intensive-care units, is related to NO overload. Lives are saved with NO inhibitor drugs. Life-threatening low blood pressure may occur when the body responds to bacterial infection. NO inhibitors can raise the low blood pressure promptly out of the danger zone. NO inhibitors serve as adjunct therapy to maintain normal blood pressure when patients are treated for skin or kidney cancers.

Neurotransmitter-like Role. NO plays a crucial role in the central nervous system. It functions like other neurotransmitters, yet it does not look or act like them. Usually, when a neuron fires, it releases a neurotransmitter from a special storage facility into a gap (synapse). The receiving cell picks up the neurotransmitter and becomes activated. However, NO lacks any special storage facility and has no special release mechanism. NO seems merely to make a neurotransmitter when and where it is needed, and simply diffuses it from the producing cell.

Most neurotransmitters are composed of amino acids or a string of peptides which couple with precisely configured receptors on the cell surfaces. However, NO uses no receptor gates. It simply passes through membranes and targets enzymes deep within cells. NO carries its messages to all cells within reach.

NO may help brain cells store and retrieve information.

The cellular basis for learning and memory may rely on strengthening the connections between sending and receiving neurons.

Depending on how much NO is released, NO acts either as a messenger or killer. During a stroke, for example, NO's targeted neurons may kill neighboring cells by overstimulation with excessive neurotransmission releases that flood them. Also, in other degenerative brain conditions, such as Alzheimer's and Huntington's diseases, excessive NO may kill brain cells. NO inhibitor drugs may reduce such damage.

NO's neurotransmitter role extends to male sexual function. The brain sends messages to key pelvic nerves, and in response, they produce NO, which dilates blood vessels throughout the crucial areas of the penis. Blood rushes in for penile erection. If NO synthesis is blocked, the blood vessels fail to dilate. Understanding NO's role has been important in developing drugs that address male impotency.

Other Therapeutic Roles. NO operates in the body's immune defense system. A group of immune system cells, called macrophages, may engulf and destroy disease-causing microbes. Or, the macrophages may approach the microbes and release NO to kill them. NO attacks a wide range of infectious microorganisms. It combats *Salmonella typhimurium* by putting the bacterium in suspended animation to prevent replication. It destroys the tuberculosis bacterium. It guards against the ravages of malaria. The higher the NO concentration in the blood, the lower the parasitic malarial load, and the milder the illness. *Plasmodium falciparum,* known as cerebral malaria, is a deadly type that provokes release of NO.

NO is involved in digestion, by triggering the series of wavelike contractions and relaxations in peristalsis to move food through the stomach and intestines. In infants, lack of

NO is responsible for a grave digestive problem known as infantile hypertrophic pyloric stenosis.

In the respiratory system, NO is inactivated rapidly by hemoglobin in the blood, so that inhaled NO may be localized in the lungs. Inhaled NO diffuses to pulmonary vascular muscles to produce vasodilation. NO can reverse pulmonary hypertension, and has become a therapeutic option in patients with severe adult respiratory distress syndrome. NO inhalation is useful, too, in cases of high-altitude pulmonary edema by helping to distribute blood flow in the lungs. Inhaled NO is used, also, in critically ill infants with hypoxic respiratory failure, and is thought to be able to reverse the defect that causes sickle-cell anemia.

By the 1990s, NO was a rising star. Following a yearly tradition, in 1992, *Science* selected it as the "molecule of the year." A journal, *Nitric Oxide,* was founded to publish the plethora of scientific findings on this subject. By the close of the 1990s, a novel was published called *NO,* and "creams" are sold containing L-arginine, an essential amino acid that increases nitric oxide conversion. Such products are targeted to men "for erectile restoration and enhancement" and to women "for orgasm enhancement." Is NO destined to be the health fad of the twenty-first century?

Chapter 8

FOOD ADDITIVES AND YOUR HEALTH

U.S. CERTIFIED FOOD COLORS: A GUARANTEE OF SAFETY?

In the early nineteenth century, many food colors were hazardous to health. Pickles were colored, green with copper sulfate; cheeses with red lead and vermillion (red mercuric sulfide); spent tea leaves were colored with copper arsenite, lead chromate, and indigo so that the leaves would appear "fresh" for resale, and candies for children were colored brightly with lead chromate, red lead, and vermillion. These toxic compounds made many people ill and resulted in deaths.

By the mid-nineteenth century, synthetic industrial dyes were being applied to foods. No regulations existed regarding their purity or uses. Concern for public health led the U.S. Congress to pass the Food and Drug Act of 1906, which restricted use of synthetic colors to those that could be judged safe with foods. The legislation drastically reduced some eighty synthetic colors used with food to only seven. The legislation also established a voluntary certification system, and the synthetic colors became known as "certified colors." In 1907, eight additional certified colors were added to the list. By 1938, previously approved certified colors were re-evaluated for safety. Those approved were relisted; some permanently, and others only provisionally. In the intervening years, some have been "delisted," that is, banned.

The words "U.S. Certified Color" on a food label should be a reassuring phrase to consumers and should imply complete safety of any chemical used for dyeing foods. Unfortunately, the history of U.S. certified food dyes has been and continues to be a repeated story of careless and indifferent control by public agencies over the sale of harmful food ingredients. (See footnote on page 293 for the definition of certified food color.)

The chemical classes of dyes derived from coal tar—from which the U.S. certified food colors are made—are azo, triphenylmethane, and xanthene. Tests of examples of all three classes have shown potential for harm.

It has long been known that certain azo colorings can induce liver cancer in rats. The coloring is bound to the protein of the liver. The toxicity of the azo dyes depends on how they are metabolized within the body. Some merely pass through, and are excreted in an unchanged form. Others break down into innocuous products and are excreted. Some are reduced to supposedly harmless substances by living organisms normally found in the gastrointestinal tract. But at times azo dyes are absorbed into, and become bound to organs and tissues of the body. This action can do harm.

A number of azo colorings produce foreign particles in the blood (Heinz bodies). Some have produced sarcomas (malignant tumors) at the site of repeated injection of the dyes under the skin of experimental animals. There is some disagreement among experts as to whether the production of sarcomas by this technique necessarily indicates that the substance may be a cause of cancer when the dye is consumed in the normal way in foods and beverages.

On the basis of animal experiments, triphenylmethane coal tar colors are judged to be potential human carcinogens. Xanthene coal tar colors have demonstrated mutagenic qualities (a capacity to produce sudden, fundamental changes in the genes—elements of the germ plasm that transmit hereditary characteristics).

Although the coal tar food colors continued in widespread use, the lack of information regarding their metabolism, excretion, and toxicity was officially acknowledged. A report on food colors issued in the United Kingdom in 1954, warned that "we cannot accept the contention that, because coal tar colors have been used in foods for many years without giving rise to complaint of illness, they are, therefore, harmless substances. Such negative evidence in our view merely illustrates that in the amounts customarily used in foods the colors are not acutely toxic but gives no certain indication of any possible chronic (long-term, continuing) effects. Any chronic effects would be insidious and it would be difficult if not impossible to attribute them with certainty to the consumption of food containing coloring matter." (Acutely toxic means having a short and relatively severe poisoning effect, with pronounced symptoms.)

In fact, it became apparent that a large number of coal tar colors *were* toxic. In the 1950s the federal FDA initiated an animal testing program that required more testing and higher feeding levels than the earlier pharmacological studies. The agency redefined "harmless" to mean a substance incapable of producing harm in test animals in any quantity and under any conditions. As a result of these stricter standards, the FDA in 1956 delisted, for food use, FD&C Orange No. 1 and No. 2, as well as FD&C Red No. 32. In 1960, FD&C Yellow No. 1, No. 2, No. 3, No. 4, as well as FD&C Red No. 1 were delisted for food use.

It became apparent that a continued full implementation of this interpretation of no harm in test animals when fed in any quantity and under any conditions would lead to the delisting of practically all food dyes of coal tar origin. The Certified Color Industry Committee (comprised of manufacturers of over 90 percent of all certified colors produced in the United States) worked closely with the FDA to modify the testing standards and establish "safe" limits for the use of certified food colors. Jointly, the Committee and the FDA proposed legislation, which, when enacted, became the Color Additives Amendment of 1960 (Public Law 86-618).

The new legislation weakened consumer protection in respect to food color safety. The new regulations provided for less stringent interpretation of "harmlessness." Human safety would thereafter be determined by a safety factor established by means of a "no-adverse-effects level" in test animals. Furthermore, food colors were given "provisional" listings. Under this practice, the FDA has allowed food colors to be used in the manufacture of foods and to be consumed by the public while tests are still being conducted to determine whether or not they are safe, and so become appropriate for permanent listing, or exclusion from the approved list. Repeatedly, the FDA has granted liberal extensions of time. Some food colors have been in use under "provisional" listings for decades.

There is no assurance that the food dyes now permitted are any safer for use in and on consumer food products than those that have been delisted.

In 1969, the FDA issued permanent listings for three coal tar food dyes long in use; and for two additional ones, with certain limitations. The FDA also added a new one that had been recently developed. How safe are the U.S. certified colors now in use? The record is far from reassuring.

FD&C Blue No. 1. Also known as Brilliant Blue FCF, FD&C Blue No. 1 is a triphenylmethane dye. Injected in large doses into experimental rats, this color produced a significant incidence of malignant tumors. Officials in the United Kingdom considered this color to be one of "probable toxicity" and did not recommend its inclusion on the permitted list of food colors. The Joint FAO/WHO (Food and Agriculture Organization of the World Health Organization) Expert Committee on Food Additives placed this color in a category "for which the data available are not wholly sufficient to meet the requirements" of acceptability for use in food. In FDA studies, this color produced a high incidence of malignant tumors at the site of the injection. Two of the tumors metastasized (metastasis is spreading of the tumor, usually through the circulation, to produce tumors in other areas).

Though the mortality rate was high, a so-called "no-effect" level was established, and the color was listed provisionally. The FAO/WHO Committee reevaluated this color and shifted it to the category "found acceptable for use in food." In 1969, the FDA listed it as permanently acceptable. FD&C Blue No. 1 is used principally in beverages, including bottled soft drinks. Also, it is widely used in candies, confections, bakery goods, and dessert powders. Uses of less importance are in ice cream, sherbet, dairy products, pet food, cereals, sausages, maraschino cherries, snack foods, and inks used for marking meat in packing house operations.

FD&C Blue No. 2. Also known as indigotine or indigo carmine, FD&C Blue No. 2 is an indigo-related coal tar dye, and was among the seven coal tar dyes originally approved for use in foods. The United Kingdom considered this color "provisionally acceptable" and the FAO/WHO Committee reported a need "for further information concerning its safety-in-use." The committee requested further data from a two-year study in a nonrodent mammalian species. Short-term toxicity studies with pigs showed that indigotine resulted in blood changes. Some animals had slightly reduced levels of hemoglobin and red cell counts. One animal developed liver abscesses, the FDA engaged in two-year feeding studies with

FD&C Blue No. 2 in the diet of rats and dogs. No adverse effects were observed and a "no-effect" level was established, although the color did produce malignant tumors at the site of injection under the skin of experimental animals.

When rats were given single oral doses of this dye it was absorbed. Only 3 percent of the color was excreted in the urine after three days, with up to 80 percent of it in the feces during the same period of time. There was negligible excretion of the color in the bile. The researchers experienced difficulty in identifying the breakdown products of the dye in the feces. Then, the color was given intravenously to rats. Substantial amounts of the color, and relatively smaller amounts of two breakdown products were found excreted in the bile. Some of the two breakdown products were also excreted in the urine.

These data were both surprising and disturbing. Apart from the use of this color by the food industry, it has been used in hospital practice to determine kidney function. In the past, it had been assumed that all of the injected dye was excreted in an unchanged form by the kidneys. The animal study with rats, showing the presence of breakdown products from the dye in the bile as well as in the urine, demonstrated that its use could yield misleading results for a kidney-function test. (As was demonstrated with cyclamates, the synthetic sweeteners, it is vital to evaluate the toxicity of breakdown products as well as the toxicity of the original substance.)

FD&C Blue No. 2 is provisionally listed. Its principal use is in pet food, but also it is widely used in candies, confections, beverages, dessert powders, and bakery goods. There is some use of it in ice creams, sherbets, dairy products, and cereals.

FD&C Citrus Red No. 2. An azo coal tar dye (not to be confused with the "delisted" FD&C Red No. 2), FD&C Citrus Red No. 2 was fed to rats and mice at different levels for two years. Males of both species, fed at the higher level, showed growth retardation with corresponding reduction of food intake. Significant post-mortem findings were changes in the bladder: thickening of the wall, tissue hyperplasia (excessive formation of tissue—an abnormal increase in the number of normal cells in normal arrangements), one cancerous bladder tumor with four pigmented stones, and other bladder abnormalities.

In another experiment, FD&C Citrus Red No. 2 was added, in various amounts, to the diet of mice up to eighty weeks. At the three highest levels the dye caused increased morbidity and deaths. The feeding test was terminated. At a lower level of the dye, the mortality rate in both sexes increased, and there was an increased incidence of degenerative changes in the livers of female mice. Other groups of mice in the same experiment received repeated injections with FD&C Citrus Red No. 2 for eighty weeks. The females showed an increased incidence of malignant tumors, and these growths appeared earlier than those that appeared in the control group.

As early as 1965 the FAO/WHO Committee had classified this food dye as one that had been "found to be harmful and that should not be used in food."

On the basis of the accumulated evidence, as well as additional data, the FAO/WHO Committee issued a second and stronger statement in 1969. The committee warned that since FD&C Citrus Red No. 2 "has been shown to have carcinogenic activity and the toxicological data available were inadequate to allow the determination of a safe limit, the Committee therefore recommends that it should not be used as a food color."

Despite this recommendation of the international food protective organization, FD&C Citrus Red No. 2 is in current use in the United States with official government sanction. Food use of Citrus Red No. 2 is limited to the coloring of the skins of oranges that are not used or intended to be used for further processing; the level of dye is not to exceed two parts per million (ppm) of the weight of the fruit. Permitting the use of the dye is based on the assumptions that the orange skins will not be consumed and that none of the dye will migrate into the edible portion of the fruit. But orange skins are sometimes used in marmalades, as candied rinds, powdered rinds, and with roast duck or cocktails. Children frequently peel oranges with their teeth.

FD&C Green No. 3. Also known as Fast Green FCF, FD&C Green No. 3 is a triphenylmethane coal tar dye. It produced a significant incidence of sarcomas at the site of repeated injections under the skins of rats. Chronic toxicity studies conducted by the FDA in rats, dogs, and mice showed the color to be "without significant toxic effect" at the dosage levels fed, and a "no-effect" level was established. FD&C Green No. 3 is provisionally listed. Its principal uses are in beverages, candies, confections, and maraschino cherries. Also, it is widely used in dessert powders, bakery goods, ice creams, sherbets, dairy products, and in mint-flavored jelly.

Orange B. Orange B, an azo coal tar dye, is a comparatively new food color to those originally approved. Its food use is restricted to the coloring of casings or surfaces of frankfurters and sausages at a level of not more than 150 ppm. Orange B is closely related in chemical structure to FD&C Red No. 2, a dye discussed later in this article. Lifetime feeding studies were conducted with Orange B using three different species of animals. Tests failed to substantiate the safety of Orange B. Liver nodules formed in dogs whose diet contained 2 percent or more of the dye. The significance of this nodule formation is unknown. The FDA established a "no-effect" level.

FD&C Red No. 3. Also known as erythrosine, FD&C Red No. 3 is a xanthene coal tar dye. It was among the seven originally approved for use in foods and beverages. Although the FAO/WHO Committee found this color to be "acceptable for use in foods," the committee assigned to it a temporary acceptable intake level for humans, with two recommendations for further investigations. Studies were needed for information on the metabolism of erythrosine in several species and preferably in humans. Additional studies were needed for information on the mechanism responsible for the effect of this dye on levels of iodine bound to blood plasma.

The German Research Institute for Food Chemistry in Munich found that erythrosine had a slight but significant mutagenic (gene altering) effect on a common microorganism (*Escherichia coli*). The Institute tested other xanthene dyes and found that they had a similar mutagenic effect on bacteria. Some of the compounds displayed high activity. Erythrosine showed a very slight but statistically significant mutagenic effect on the bacteria. Subsequently, the basic substance, xanthene, was found to be mutagenic. Additional experiments showed that erythrosine had a significant mutagenic effect on certain strains of *E. coli.* These findings are significant. Frequently, when substances have mutagenic properties, they may also be carcinogenic.

FD&C Red No. 3 was provisionally listed until a "no-effect level" was established. In 1969, it became permanently listed by the FDA. Its principal uses are with candies, confections, bakery goods, dessert powders, sausages, and maraschino cherries. It is also widely used in cereals, beverages, pet foods, snack foods, ice creams, sherbets, and dairy products. Of lesser importance is its use in meat-marking inks and imitation jellies.

FD&C Red No. 4. FD&C Red No. 4, also known as ponceau SX, is an azo coal tar dye. Officials in the United Kingdom found evidence of "possible toxicity" for this dye and recommended its withdrawal. The FAO/WHO Committee categorized it as a color that was "found to be harmful and that should not be used in food." The FDA completed seven-year tests feeding FD&C Red No. 4 to dogs. The results showed conclusively that this food dye damaged the animals' bladders and adrenal glands.

Early in 1965, the FDA issued an order prohibiting further use of this dye in food. However, the trade association of the cherry industry as well as an organization representing maraschino cherries and glacé fruits sought and obtained an "extension" to be in effect while further experiments were being performed. When the extension period ended, the FDA announced that new tests had cleared FD&C Red No. 4, and a "no-effect level" was established. The new relaxed ruling permitted the continued use of this color with maraschino cherries at a level not to exceed 150 ppm by weight of the fruit. In addition, the color was given the classification Ext. D&C Red No. 24, with unrestricted use in externally applied drugs and cosmetics, and restricted use for drugs taken internally.

In addition to its use in coloring maraschino cherries, FD&C Red No. 4 formerly had been in widespread use to color the skins of frankfurters, gelatin desserts, in drugstore pills, and in liquid medicines.

FD&C Red No. 40. Also known as allura red AC, FD&C Red No. 40 is an azo coal tar dye. Its use in foods, developed to replace FD&C Red No. 4, was approved in the United States in April 1971. Data on this food dye have not been made available to the public. FDA has followed a policy of treating safety studies of company applications for agency approval of new additives as proprietary information ("trade secrets") to be protected from disclosure outside the government's own agencies.

FD&C Yellow No. 5. FD&C Yellow No. 5, also known as tartrazine, is a pyrazolone coal tar dye. It is one of the few coal tar dyes that has had universal acceptance in countries where the addition of dyes to foods has been officially permitted. Despite this fact, allergists have reported numerous cases of human sensitivity to tartrazine.

A "no-effect" level was established for FD&C Yellow No. 5, and in 1969 the FDA gave this food color a permanent listing. It is one of the most widely used dyes in foods. Its principal use is in pet food, and also extensively used in beverages, bakery goods, dessert powders, candies, confections, cereals, ice creams, sherbets, dairy products, snack foods, sausages, maraschino cherries, and imitation strawberry jelly. To some extent, the color is used in meat-marking inks.

FD&C Yellow No. 6. Also known as Sunset Yellow FCF, FD&C Yellow No. 6 is an azo coal tar dye. Although it is one of the dyes extensively studied for its effects on animals, information is lacking regarding the metabolism of FD&C Yellow No. 6 in humans. In a seven-year study, dogs fed this dye at the rate of 2 percent of their diet suffered eye defects, sometimes accompanied by blindness. In short-term toxicity studies conducted with miniature pigs and rats, as well as in acute toxicity studies with rats and mice, animals suffered from slight diarrhea, although no adverse effects were noted on their growth or food consumption. A "no-effect" level was established. FD&C Yellow No. 6 is one of the most widely used food colors. Its principal use is in beverages, including bottled soft drinks, but also it is used extensively in sausages, candies, confections, dessert powders, bakery goods, cereals, ice creams, sherbets, dairy products, pet foods, and snack foods. The dye is used to some extent in maraschino cherries.

Delisting of FD&C Red No. 2. The appalling record of human hazards from food dyes was demonstrated with the

FDA's delisting of FD&C Red No. 2. It was one of the seven originally approved, long in use, and one of the few azo coal tar dyes that had universal acceptance in countries that permitted food colors. Until its delisting, FD&C Red No. 2, known as amaranth, held first place as the food dye of greatest use in foods in the United States. Although its principal application has been in beverages, it had been widely used in candies, confections, pet foods, dessert powders, bakery goods, sausages, ice creams, sherbets, dairy products, and cereals. Of lesser importance, it was used in maraschino cherries, snack foods, and in meat-marking inks. In addition to its many food uses, FD&C Red No. 2 had been an ingredient in lipsticks and drugs. Use of this dye was not limited to items obviously shaded red. Frequently, FD&C Red No. 2 had been blended with other dyes, and present in unexpected items, even having been used to give an exact shading to white icing, to chocolate syrups, and ready-to-eat cereals. An FDA official was quoted as saying, "FD&C Red No. 2 is so ubiquitous that if every food with Red 2 self-destructed tomorrow, a lot of people would starve."

The FAO/WHO Committee had categorized amaranth as a color that was "found acceptable for use in food" and the committee had established an unconditional acceptable daily intake level for humans. However, allergists reported cases of human sensitivity to amaranth.

Comprehensive long-term tests on rats, mice, and dogs failed to reveal that FD&C Red No. 2 had any cancer-inciting properties. Repeated injection of this dye under the skin of rats demonstrated "no appreciable tissue reaction" and a "no-effect" level was established.

In 1968, however, Soviet researchers studied amaranth and reported finding carcinogenic properties of the color. In the investigators' first experiment, they fed amaranth to fifty rats for twenty-five months. When the initial daily dietary level of 4 percent of the color was not well tolerated, the amount fed was reduced to 2.5 percent for the next thirty weeks. Then, the dye was withheld for four weeks and reintroduced at a dietary level of 2 percent for the remainder of the experiment. After nineteen months, four tumors were found in four of the eighteen surviving animals. At the end of twenty-five months, eleven of the eighteen animals had developed tumors, while none of the surviving thirty-five control animals had developed tumors. The majority of the tumors were sarcomas of the peritoneum (membrane lining the walls of the abdominal cavity). The sarcomas infiltrated into the intestine. The first tumor to appear was in the thigh muscle. One of the abdominal tumors affected the spleen.

In the second Soviet experiment, daily doses of 10 milligrams of amaranth in solution were fed orally to mice, while weekly, one of two known potent skin-cancer inciters was applied to the skin, which produced papillomas (benign skin tumors). The papillomas appeared three to four weeks earlier, and in a greater number of mice, than in the control group treated with the skin-cancer inciters on their skin but not fed the amaranth solution. The benign tumors in the treated mice became malignant sooner, and in more animals than in the control group. The researchers recommended that amaranth food usage be discontinued.

Further tests by the Soviet scientists, reported in 1971, showed that amaranth diminished fertility in rats and caused some stillbirths.

As a result of the Soviet findings, the FDA took several actions. The agency ran its own tests, which confirmed the data regarding decreased rat litter size. The agency recommended reduced use of this dye, and ordered the food industry to provide, by October 31, 1971, lists of all products in which the color was used, as well as the levels of use. The

FDA ordered food manufacturers to conduct animal tests with all food dyes in order "to show whether the color additive produces any adverse effect on reproduction." In the past, such tests were not required, nor generally conducted. On the basis of present animal studies, there is no reliable method to estimate the potential harmfulness of a food dye on the human fetus. Therefore, wisdom would dictate that if animal tests reveal any signs of harming the animal fetus, an additive such as a food dye ought to be banned promptly. Doubts should always be resolved in favor of the consumer, because there is no dire necessity to use any food dye if there is doubt about its safety in long-time use.

The FDA conducted its own year-long tests with FD&C Red No. 2. Although the FDA's studies failed to confirm any carcinogenic properties of this food dye, the agency found that the dye induced malformed and macerated (discolored and softened) animal fetuses.

Despite these highly significant and disturbing findings, the FDA failed to take prompt, vigorous action. In September 1971, the agency merely announced plans to limit the future use of FD&C Red No. 2.

Editor's Note: Since publication of this article nearly three decades ago, all of the U.S. Certified Food Colors are still approved for use. However, numerous medical reports have attested to the adverse reactions experienced by many individuals to tartrazine (FD&C Yellow No. 5). The reports forced the FDA to take action, albeit limited. The presence of tartrazine in any food, drug, or cosmetic must be declared on the product's label.

FOOD FLAVORING ADDITIVES: HOW SAFE ARE THEY?

The French Academy of Medicine opposed officially all practices that lead to the introduction of foreign substances into foodstuffs, even those reputed to be harmless. Rejections included natural aromatic or analogous synthetic substances. The French government permits the use of only seven synthetic flavorings in foods, which makes France the only European country with highly restrictive legislation in this regard. By contrast, in the United States, well over a thousand flavorings and flavor adjuncts are used. Numerically, they form by far the largest single group of food additives, and pose, according to a prominent critic, "one of the areas of greatest toxicological uncertainty at present."

After enactment of the federal Food Additives Amendment of 1958, food additive manufacturers were made responsible for determining the safety of their products. In an effort to evaluate synthetic flavorings and adjuncts, the food additives committee of the Flavoring Extract Manufacturers Association of the United States (FEMA) collated data from an industry-wide questionnaire concerning the identity, composition, and uses of these substances. Data for more than a thousand substances were reviewed by an expert panel of toxicologists and pharmacologists, to determine which food flavor additives could be considered "Generally Recognized as Safe" (GRAS)—a vague and questionable category.

GRAS Status for Food Flavoring Additives Prior to 1958. Food flavorings and adjuncts used prior to 1958 could be granted GRAS status in one of two ways. The substance could be evaluated "by experience based on common use in food," or by scientific procedures. Common use or long-time use in food has been shown, repeatedly, to be an unreliable method to determine the safety of a number of major food additives. For nearly seventy-five years, coumarin, a food flavoring, was widely used. Long overdue tests showed that coumarin caused liver damage in rats and dogs. It then was banned for food use. Safrole, a flavoring substance long in use as the chief flavoring ingredient in root beer, finally was tested in long-term feeding experiments with rats and dogs. Safrole was found to be a potent inciter of liver cancer, and was banned from food use.

The review of scientific data by FEMA was inadequate to determine the safety of food flavoring additives in use prior to 1958. In many instances, then, as today, information was lacking, incomplete, or outdated. Tests had been conducted for short-term animal ingestion, not for long-term human ingestion. Nor did the data include areas of concern that we now recognize as vital: chronic toxicity (poisonous qualities that become evident after a long period of use); allergenicity (capacity to cause allergic reactions); carcinogenicity (capacity to cause or contribute to cancer); mutagenicity (tendency to cause genetic mutations, abnormal deviations in hereditary characteristics); teratogenicity (capacity to develop defects or malformations in offspring); and other subtle biological damage such as impairment of learning ability or behavioral problems inflicted on the body by ingested substances in foods or beverages. Even with what, in present perspective, appears as a totally inadequate yardstick for evaluation, FEMA admitted that some 100 to 200 food-flavoring additives would probably have to be dropped for lack of supporting safety data, or suspected toxicity.

Of some 1,400 food flavorings and adjuncts in use, 191 were covered by FDA "white lists" of official approval and 343 were granted "extension" status (tentatively continued in use). FEMA, on the basis of its review, decided that 662 of the additives could be considered GRAS. Additives on the GRAS list automatically enjoy certain privileges. They are exempt from the regulatory requirements that apply to chemicals legally classified as food additives; they are not subject to regulations concerning food additives as long as they remain on the GRAS list.* Food flavorings and flavor adjuncts that came into use after 1958 could be placed on the GRAS list only after scientific data were submitted and acceptable to the FDA.

FDA Safety Studies. Recognizing that toxicity data were woefully lacking regarding many food flavorings, the FDA conducted studies for acute oral toxicity in rats, guinea pigs, and mice with a large number of the additives. (*Acute* toxicity refers to harmful effects that occur within a short period of time, contrasted to *chronic*, which refers to lasting or lingering injuries to health.) Numerous adverse effects were observed, including rough fur and scrawny appearance, diarrhea, soft stools, bloody urine, intestinal irritation, hemorrhaging, anatomic or functional manifestations of disease conditions in the liver, lacrimation (tearing), salivation, gasping, respiratory failure, tremors, depression, ataxia, coma, and death.

Flavor additives include compounds with a wide variety of chemical structures and mixtures of variable compositions derived from synthetic sources as well as a much smaller number of "isolates" or plant extractives from natural products. Natural flavorings include spices, herbs, and essential oils. In later studies, the FDA tested certain food flavorings and related compounds for subacute and chronic toxicity in rats. Many of the substances caused retarded growth; increased mortality; damage to organs such as liver, kidneys, and heart; stomach ulceration; bone changes and

*The original GRAS list established by the Federal Food Additives Amendment in 1958, was drawn up by the FDA after polling some 900 experts of its own choice. Only 355 responded. Of these, only 194 concurred with the submitted list, or made no comments. In preparing the GRAS list, the FDA dismissed many critical remarks received from its own experts on the grounds that "common sense as well as scientific principles require us to accept the opinions of some and reject the opinions of others."

malignant tumors. The FDA's policy was not to publish its findings about the toxicity of additives. Reports of its studies with flavoring materials were unavailable in technical periodicals or in publications available from the Government Printing Office.

Many essential oils used as food flavorings have been on the GRAS list. However, in tests for chronic toxicity, some essential oils were shown to be mildly irritating to the mucous membrane of the mouth and the digestive tract. Their ingestion in large amounts irritated the kidney, bladder, and urethra. In the presence of a preexisting inflammatory condition of the urinary tract, small doses of ingested essential oil appeared to worsen the condition. Essential oils, applied to mouse skins, produced moderate to marked skin, hyperplasia (abnormal increase in the number of normal cells in normal arrangement in a tissue). In some cases, areas of necrosis (death of tissues) with ulceration, oozing or weeping of fluid, and crusting developed. Some essential oils were found to promote skin tumors. Benign warts and malignant skin tumors appeared in some animals, which had been pretreated with a known cancer-inciting substance, and then had repeated skin treatments with an essential oil.

Continued Paucity of Data. Presently, there is still a great lack of trustworthy toxicological data for many, perhaps most, food-flavoring additives used by food processors. These compounds are regarded as "proprietary information" (valuable trade secrets), and are treated by government agencies as privileged materials. Safety studies, even when they exist, as we have noted, are not published in professional journals as, of course, they ought to be. Nor have they been made available by the FDA for purposes of public review.

In 1970, some $150 million worth of flavoring additives were used with foods and beverages in the United States. These additives were the "top sellers" among all classes of food additives. The greatly increased demand for flavoring additives is related to the phenomenal rise in the use of "convenience foods," which often are so poor or characterless in flavor that they would not do well in repeat sales without having their flavor "stepped up" by the addition of various flavors.

Although the consumer should have the right to know the specific flavorings and flavoring adjuncts that have been used in foods and beverages, the presence of these substances is stated on labels only in such a nonrevealing term as "artificial flavor added," In view of what is already known, and what yet remains to be learned, the safety of many of the numerous flavors appears to be more than dubious. Because use of chemical flavor additives is principally with convenience foods, the use of such items should be limited, or, better still, eliminated from one's choice of foods.

SULFITES: PRESERVING FOODS AT A PRICE

Five to ten percent of the roughly nine million asthmatics in the United States might be sensitive to sulfites, the chemicals used to preserve the freshness and natural appearance of a variety of foods. Nonasthmatics are also affected. In fact, to date, 500 reports of illness and twelve deaths have been linked to sulfites, and the Food and Drug Administration (FDA) estimates that about half the people who consume sulfites are exceeding the recommended upper level.

Why has the problem of sulfite sensitivity developed in recent times? Societal changes are key factors. With the expanded manufacture and consumption of highly processed foods and beverages, higher levels of sulfites are present in our diet. Greater wine consumption, increased use of factory-prepared convenience foods both in homes and in restaurants, more dining out, and the increased popularity of salad bars are all contributing to the rise in sulfite use.

What Are Sulfites? Six sulfiting agents are permitted for use in the food supply: sulfur dioxide, sodium sulfite, sodium or potassium bisulfite, and sodium or potassium metabisulfite.

According to current FDA regulations, all six sulfiting agents may be used in any food except in the meats and other foods that are recognized as valuable sources of thiamine (vitamin B_1). As a result, twenty-two established categories of foods are likely to contain sulfites, and some seven million pounds of sulfites now enter the American food supply each year.

Sulfites are applied to foods as sprays or dips for various reasons. They are used as antibacterial, antioxidant, and antibrowning agents (to prevent wilting and discoloration in such foods as raw mushrooms, peeled potatoes, cut apples and lettuce during distribution, storage, or preparation). They act as a general preservative to conserve carotene and vitamin C in foods (although they destroy thiamine). They

SULFITES AND ASTHMA

When sulfiting agents are ingested, they release sulfur dioxide gas—a known asthma inducer—in the mouth, which is then inhaled. Asthmatic attacks induced by sulfites are characterized by numerous breathing problems, including shortness of breath, labored breathing, tightness in the chest, airway constriction, coughing, and wheezing. Other symptoms might include a rapid pulse, faintness, weakness, sudden generalized flushing, lightheadedness, cold clammy skin, hives, itching, severe abdominal distress, diarrhea, swelling of tongue, and difficulty in swallowing. Severe reactions could result in loss of consciousness, anaphylactic shock, cyanosis (blue discoloration of the skin caused by insufficient oxygen in the blood), coma, and death.

arrest fermentation in wine making. They control certain bacteria without inhibiting the desired yeast development. They soften the hard kernels of corn in the wet-milling process of cornstarch manufacture. They act as bleaching agents (for example, to make raisins lighter in color). They are pH-control and stabilizing agents, which help to maintain a desired acid/alkaline balance in certain foods. They serve as conditioning agents in bakery products to make the dough less adhesive. And, finally, they can sterilize food containers, and sanitize food-processing equipment.

By far, the greatest single amount of ingested sulfiting compounds comes from drinking wine. The practice is old. In ancient Rome, wines were treated with sulfur dioxide. Sulfites are used as antimicrobial and antioxidant agents in the growing of grapes. Many vineyard owners would like to find suitable alternatives. They have not only become con-

As little as 7.5 mg of sulfites taken orally can trigger a reaction in a person who is sensitive to these compounds. The average nonalcoholic American consumer probably consumes 2 to 3 mg of sulfites daily. Wine or beer drinkers might consume an additional 5 to 10 mg daily.

Some physicians who have treated sulfite-sensitive individuals have reported that vitamin B_{12} (cyanocobalamin) is a metabisulfite blocker. They recommend that sensitive individuals should ingest 1,000 to 2,000 micrograms (mcg) of vitamin B_{12} before eating any factory-prepared foods. Other physicians report that the inhalation of sodium cromoglycate blocks the provocation of asthma in people exposed to sulfur dioxide. However, sulfite-sensitive individuals should discuss these preventive measures with their physicians.

cerned about the adverse reactions suffered by sulfite-sensitive individuals, but they note the development of adverse flavors and color changes in certain grapes, notably muscadine, when sulfur dioxide is used.

Frequently, additional sulfites are used in bottling the wine. Sometimes the bottles are sanitized with sulfites and even the corks are likely to be treated. In home wine-making kits, sodium metabisulfite is provided for this purpose.

The World Health Organization (WHO) set 35 milligrams (mg) of sulfur dioxide per liter of wine as the upper limit for safety for daily adult absorption. Yet the sulfite level of twenty-two common table wines range from 56 to 250 mg per liter (l). In France, 225 mg/l of sulfites of red wine and 300 mg/l for white wine are established limits. At these levels, even a moderate daily consumption exposes drinkers to far higher levels than the WHO considers safe.

Along with numerous sulfite exposures from foods and beverages, people are also exposed to sulfites from drugs and from air pollution. Many medications taken orally, injected or inhaled, such as adrenergics and corticosteroids, contain sulfites as preservatives. Some intravenous medications as well as dental anesthetics contain sulfites. To determine if a medication contains sulfites, a sulfite-sensitive individual may need to contact the drug company directly.

Sulfite Sensitivity. The average American diet provides more of the sulfur-containing essential amino acids (cystine and methionine) than the body can use and retain. In the normal metabolism of the body, any excess sulfur in these amino acids is converted to sulfite, and then, with the help of an enzyme (sulfite oxidase), the sulfite is converted to harmless sulfate, and excreted in the urine. Presumably, the body metabolizes sulfites added to foods in the same way.

Individuals who have a congenital deficiency of sulfite oxidase are unable to convert sulfite to sulfate. In other cases, adverse sulfite reactions might be allergenic reactions. Sulfite sensitivity could also develop as people age: the vast majority of known cases of sulfite sensitivity are among people forty-five years of age or older.

Some researchers believe that adverse reactions to sulfites actually are toxic reactions. Others believe that sulfites can react with a body protein or a body cell membrane and trigger numerous inflammatory mechanisms. Whatever the immediate reactions might be, it is generally accepted that, in the end, sulfites destroy thiamine and that, at high levels, they lead to a deficiency of this important vitamin.

Animal experiments conducted prior to 1935—and responsible for the false assumption that sulfites were safe—were conducted without awareness of what was discussed above. Hence, findings from these early tests might be flawed and fail to show the true toxicity of sulfites. Also, it is known now that sulfites are subject to rapid change through oxidation, volatilization, evaporation and long storage. As a result, the actual levels of sulfites administered to the test animals might have been far lower than intended.

Despite these shortcomings, early tests with high levels of sulfites demonstrated toxicity in three different animal species. The first evidence was the appearance of occult, or barely detectable, blood in animal feces. Another effect, noted in rats, was the reduction of relative weight gain in the second generation of animals. In 1970, it was learned that sulfites act on nucleic acid components. (Nucleic acids are groups of complex compounds found in all living cells. Their components are purines, pyrimidines, carbohydrates, and phosphoric acid. Nucleic acids in the form of DNA and RNA control cellular function and heredity.) This observation raises questions about the possible genetic effects of sulfites. In fact, mutations have been produced in the bacteria *Escherichia coli* in laboratory experiments with sulfites. At

Where to Find Sulfites

The presence of sulfites is required by law to be declared on the ingredient listing of retail packaged foods. However, there are limitations. For example, 70 percent of all imported shrimp and 50 percent of domestic shrimp are treated with sulfites on boats, but these products do not bear any label statement about the treatment.

Labels on packaged mushrooms might also be incomplete as regards the presence of sulfiting agents. Some packers say "washing" mushrooms in a solution of sodium bisulfite is not "adding" the sulfiting agent; therefore, the treatment is not noted on the label. Or, the package might be marked "no preservative added when packaged," although the mushrooms might have been treated with sulfites before being packaged. And, if sulfites are used in the early stages of processing a food (for example, to treat cookie dough to make it less sticky, or in the manufacture of corn syrup and cornstarch), they are not required to be listed among the ingredients on the label. Thus, reading ingredient labels, although important, is not always enough when trying to identify foods treated with sulfites.

high concentrations of sodium bisulfite, mutations were produced in viruses, too.

Ban Denied. Even though sulfites have enjoyed the FDA's "Generally Recognized as Safe" (GRAS) status since 1958, the FDA had throughout the 1980s requested several sulfite safety evaluations and reevaluations from scientific groups both outside and inside the agency. But when it became apparent that the greatly expanded use of sulfites was raising total daily intake for the entire population (and therefore causing greater health problems for certain groups

> The following foods—found in retail stores, restaurants, vendings machines, and the fare served by caterers—are apt to be treated with sulfiting agents: breads, hot roll mixes, corn bread, muffin and pancake mixes, cookies; preserved meats such as uncooked sausage mixes and mincemeat; processed cheeses and cheese spreads; fresh and frozen shrimp and other shellfish, and dried cod; fresh salad mixes in packages and canned vegetables; dehydrated vegetables such as peas, green peppers, carrots and onions in dried soup mixes; frozen pizza and other frozen entrees; canned or dried sauces and gravies; sweet and sour sauces, jalapeno peppers, prepared dips such as avocado and guacamole, horseradish, cole slaw, pickles, relishes, and sauerkraut; dried fruits; gelatin, packaged desserts, molasses, syrups and toppings; dehydrated potatoes in all forms, and mixtures of white rice and wild rice; French fried potatoes and potato chips; salad dressings made with vinegar, bottled lemon juice, wine and apple cider vinegars; white grape juice, cider, fruit juices, fruit fillings and fruit pulps; and imitation fruit drinks, instant teas, soft drinks, wine, wine coolers, cordials, and beer.

of people), the FDA chose not to strip sulfites of their privileged GRAS status, nor to take any curbing actions.

At the time, the agency said it could not prove that sulfites caused any danger, a required condition for any ban. Also, the agency pleaded lack of manpower necessary to enforce notification of the presence of sulfites in foods. Instead, the agency recommended that state and local health authorities require restaurants and food wholesalers and retailers to inform customers about the presence of sulfites by providing "easily readable labels, signs, placard or menu statements." The recommendations, however, appeared unworkable because, with a few notable exceptions, there was no compliance.

The National Restaurant Association (NRA) opposed mandatory menu labeling on several counts. The NRA claimed that restaurants do not always have a constant supplier of foods, making it difficult to keep track of sulfite uses. Moreover, the NRA feared that labeling might dissuade people from dining out, cause some patrons to panic, and others to sue. In sum, the NRA suggested that the sulfite content of foods and beverages should be controlled at the sources. If the substances are harmful, the NRA contended, then it is the FDA's responsibility to ban them.

Nevertheless, according to the NRA, most restaurants discontinued the use of sulfites on the premises. NRA advised patrons that the restaurant foods not apt to be sulfite-treated are chicken, eggs, meat and cheese. However, if these foods appear in sauces, gravies, soups or stews, the other ingredients might contain sulfites.

Seeking Safe Alternatives. Food processors responded to the sulfite alarm by seeking safe alternatives to sulfites. Among these are water-soluble antioxidants and antibrowning agents, which contain items such as lemon juice, ascorbic acid, citric acid or erythorbic acid, in various combinations. The Produce Marketing Association (PMA) also took action by discouraging the use of sulfites on fresh produce. (Cases had been reported of personnel having adverse reactions after handling fresh produce treated with sulfites.)

Plant breeders are searching for safe alternatives to the sulfiting agents by attempting to develop apples that are relatively low in levels of enzymes and phenols, which are responsible for turning cut fruits and vegetables brown.

Chemists experimented by adding a small amount of honey to apple juice to prevent browning. A characteristic protein present in honey interacts with the browning products in apple juice and creates large molecules that precipitate out, which can be removed. This processing results in long-lasting clear juice, previously obtained with sulfiting agents.

In another approach, chemists infused dehydrated apples, cranberries, or cherries with sugar. The dried fruit exhibits more stability in color, flavor, and shelf life than when sulfiting agents were used.

The U.S. Department of Agriculture (USDA) earmarked some research money to seek alternatives to sulfites. Among promising substances are proteases, a group of naturally occurring enzymes such as ficin in fig, actinidose in kiwi fruit, and other enzymes present in papaya, pineapple, and other types of fruit. The proteases can keep cut fruits and potatoes from browning. These substances could serve as "processing aids" which would not make it necessary to declare them on food labels.

A Ban on Sulfites. The FDA acknowledged that the "acceptable daily intake" level of sulfites might be exceeded by some people. The agency admitted that information was lacking about the specific levels of sulfite residues in treated foods and beverages. The agency proposed that sulfites used in the early stages of processing should be labeled, especially if a detectable level remained in the final product, as it does, for example, in cornstarch.

In 1985, the FDA's expert panel on the risks of sulfiting agents in food decided that warning labels were insufficient and recommended a ban on sulfites. In the panel's final report, the panel concluded that for sulfite-sensitive individuals, "additional labeling requirements alone would not assure protection.... It would seem advisable to specify safe conditions for the use of sulfites in situations where levels shown to elicit adverse reactions in sulfite-sensitive individuals are likely to occur at the point of consumption."

CARRAGEENAN: RELATED TO HUMAN ULCERATIVE COLITIS?

Carrageenan, also known, as Irish moss, has had a long history of use as a food in western Europe and the United States. This seaweed, with jellying properties, when cooked with milk and seasonings, was turned into a popular custard, blancmange. Supplies of carrageenan were carried by the colonists to the New World, and continued to be imported until some choice sources were discovered along the coasts of New England and the Maritime Provinces of Canada. Harvesting carrageenan in those areas began as early as 1835.

Due to its mucilaginous quality, carrageenan also had extensive medicinal use. It was given for diarrhea, urinary disorders and chronic chest inflammations, including tuberculosis.

Assumed Innocent. As with many other food additives, carrageenan was assumed to be innocuous because of its plant origin, its long-time use, and its apparent record of safety. Toxicity studies were begun in 1959. High levels (25 percent) of carrageenan in the diet of mice and rats produced in a few animals liver lesions that suggested cirrhosis. Most of the animals showed retarded growth. Because carrageenan was known to depress peptic activity, investigators attributed the adverse effects to some dietary deficiency. There was no increase in mortality, nor any consistent cause of death. No colonic ulceration, nor scarring was observed.

Ten years later, another animal experiment with carrageenan produced results totally different from the earlier studies. The new findings were unexpected, and there were great discrepancies of results between the old and new study. Concentrations of only up to 5 percent degraded carrageenan in the animals' drinking water caused weight loss within two to three weeks in guinea pigs and rabbits, but not in rats or mice. However, all four species developed pinhead size ulcers in the caecum (a pouch at the beginning of the large intestine), colon, and rectum. These lesions resembled ones found in human ulcerative colitis. At later stages, other pathological changes developed in some animals. The findings were important in view of an increasing incidence of ulcerative colitis in humans.

The investigators extended the studies. One group of guinea pigs was given low levels (1 percent) of undegraded carrageenan in their drinking water; another group, was given higher levels (5 percent) of degraded carrageenan. Both groups developed ulcerative lesions, beginning in the caecum and spreading to the lower colon and rectum. Although such a distribution is not the typical pattern in human ulcerative colitis, the tissue damage in the animals, examined microscopically, appeared similar to that in humans. Other effects included blood and mucus in the feces, and retarded growth.

Then the researchers gave rabbits carrageenan in drinking water. A low level (1 percent) produced diarrhea and ulceration in all of the rabbits. Even at one-tenth the level (0.1 percent), ulceration was produced in half of the rabbits. Lesions were mainly in the caecum. Microscopic examination showed an infiltration of carrageenan into the cells, and the presence of abscesses and polyps.

These findings created a controversy that continues, up to the present. Additional studies have produced conflicting evidence. Some experiments have reaffirmed earlier findings of the antipeptic activity of carrageenan, but have failed to confirm ulceration.

Despite Importance, Doubts Are Raised. Carrageenan is of great importance to food processors, as well as to the cosmetic and pharmaceutical industries. This derivative of a seaweed is used in many kinds of consumer goods, includ-

A Versatile Food Additive

Carrageenan, one of the most versatile of food additives, is used as:

- a suspending agent to keep chocolate from settling in chocolate milk and chocolate-flavored milk drinks; to stabilize fruit juices, fruit nectars, and soft drinks
- a clarifier in beet juice, vinegar, wine, and beer; to stabilize and control beer foam
- an ice-crystal inhibitor in frozen desserts (ice cream, frozen custard, sherbet, and ice milk); to stabilize milk protein; to prevent whey separation
- a stabilizer to prevent oil-water separation, minimize surface hardening, and improve spreading properties in cream cheese, other soft cheeses (Neufchatel type), processed cheeses, cheese spreads, and cheese foods; to induce small curd formation in cottage cheese; to prevent contrasting streaks of colors or flavors from mixing in variegated ice creams, syrups, and purees
- an emulsifier and stabilizer in pressure-dispensed whipped cream, yogurt, evaporated milk, coffee whiteners, filled and imitation milk, whipped toppings (liquid and dry), and salad dressings
- a gelling agent in water-, milk-, and starch-based puddings
- a bodying agent to improve mouthfeel in soups, sauces, gravies, soft drinks, fruit drinks, syrups, and toppings; to thicken salad dressings, relishes, mustard, and catsup; to improve mouthfeel in low-calorie foods that lack sugar and oil; to replace all, or part, of the starch in low-calorie puddings and

pie fillings; to provide bulk for a feeling of satiety and to mask the aftertaste of artificial sweeteners in low-calorie foods

- a water binder, adhesive, and emulsifier to improve the appearance of processed meats; a gel in fillers and binders for sausages, caviar, and pet foods; to prevent textural breakdown in canned fish, poultry, soft meats (tongue) and canned solid, ground, and jellied meats
- an adjunct to antioxidants in edible coatings on frozen poultry and meat; with antibiotics, to improve uniformity of distribution on fish
- a flour conditioner that acts on the flour protein during baking to improve the dough strength, loaf volume, shape, and finished texture in a variety of baked goods
- a texturizer for cake batters; to reduce the fat absorption and improve the texture of yeast-raised doughnuts; to give a moist texture and even distribution of fruit in fruit cakes; an adjunct in other bakery ingredients (fruit and pie fillings, bakery jellies, toppings, icings, and citrus oil emulsions)
- a sugar-crystal inhibitor in certain confections (caramels, nougats, and taffies); to emulsify fat and keep it evenly distributed throughout some confections: also in jelly candies, candy bars, and marshmallows

ing toothpastes, hand lotions, deodorants, spermatocidal jellies and medications.

Because carrageenan is known to inhibit pepsin and other gastric enzymes in the human stomach, it has been used therapeutically to treat gastric ulcers. Proponents say that this therapy has been used with many patients who do not appear to have suffered ill effects. To reaffirm this argument, degraded carrageenan was fed experimentally to baboons at levels used therapeutically for humans. There was little absorption from the gastrointestinal tract.

Despite its use with gastric ulcers, carrageenan is known to have inflammatory effects. Injected under the skin, it readily produces an inflammation. This suggests that, in high concentrations, it has an irritant effect when it is in direct contact with tissues. Tests with experimental animals have confirmed this fact. Carrageenan injected in rats directly under the capsule of the liver led to the formation of liver fibrosis. The connective tissue formed with carrageenan was reabsorbed after the injected material disappeared. In other studies, carrageenan produced tumors. In guinea pigs, a single injection of carrageenan under the skin led to the formation of a certain type of tumor (collagen granuloma). In rats, malignant tumors (sarcomas) developed at the site where carrageenan was injected.

In the wake of the cyclamate ban in 1970, the Food and Drug Administration (FDA) requested a review by the National Academy of Sciences and National Research Council of many food additives about which doubts have been raised (including carrageenan). In examining carrageenan, there are differences in this substance from various sources and in different forms. For example, do nondegraded and degraded carrageenan produce the same reactions? Are there differences among the plant species? Does carrageenan act the same as its salts? Present processing procedures are radically different from traditional methods. Formerly, carrageenan was sunbleached, cleaned in seawater, and sun-dried. Presently, it is bleached with sulfur dioxide, cleaned with alkali, decolorized with charcoal, and precipitated with alcohol. Of dubious safety are other food additives that serve similar purposes as carrageenan, including related-seaweed derivatives (agar-agar, algins, and furcellerans) and synthetic substances (carboxymethyl cellulose).

What is definitely established is that ulcers can be induced by carrageenan under certain conditions in some animals. These animals apparently possess an ability to absorb this material in the intestinal tract. Whether this is similar in humans remains to be demonstrated. Meanwhile, consumers are being exposed to a possible hazard of unknown dimensions. Ulcerative colitis is a particularly unpleasant, serious, and sometimes fatal condition. The question has been raised, but remains unresolved: Is the current widespread use of carrageenan and related substances safe, or may it be contributing to human ulcerative colitis?

NATURAL FOOD COLORS: VEGETABLE, ANIMAL, MINERAL?

The old parlor game "Vegetable, Animal, Mineral?" can be applied to so-called "natural" food colors, because they can be derived from all three sources. Actually, the term "natural colors" for food has no legal basis, and is not permitted on food labels. Food colors are either "certified,"* signifying that the colors are synthetics, or "noncertified" for colors that are exempt from certification. The latter include colors from pigments derived from vegetables, animals, or minerals, as well as man-made counterparts of natural derivatives,

*The term "certified food color" has been misunderstood by many consumers. The term does not ensure safety of the substance, but rather denotes quality control. It guarantees that one batch of the color is similar to all other batches, in composition, consistency, and strength of the color. Certified colors are designated as FD&C (followed by a number). FD&C designates that the color may be used with foods, drugs, and cosmetics. Some are only D&C, which means that they cannot be used with foods.

termed "nature-identical." Both certified and noncertified food colors are subjected to standards of safety prior to approval for food use.

At a symposium hosted by the Institute of Food Technologists, titled "A Spectrum of Natural Colors for the Year 2000," the announcement given to food and beverage processors stated: "The current demand for 'all natural' products is real and the wave of the future, a need which will encourage the use of natural colors."

Increasingly, food and beverage processors are eager to use natural pigments to color their products. This trend is a response to consumer interest in "natural" foods, based on the assumption that such ingredients and food products are safer and more nutritious than their synthesized counterparts. According to Winston Bach, director of Ohio State University's Food Industry Center, concerns about some synthetic food dyes as carcinogens have heightened interest in researching colors from plant materials.

As a result, a wide range of food colors has become available to food and beverage processors, based on pigments in fruits, vegetables, and other plant materials. Additional ones are being investigated, both here and abroad.

A Meaningless Term. Despite the increased interest in and use of "natural" colors, the term is meaningless. Under Food and Drug Administration (FDA) regulations, no color added to a food product can be considered "natural" regardless of its source. Only the color found naturally in the food would be considered "natural." For example, the strawberry juice in the berry gives strawberry ice cream its pink hue. However, if red beet color is added to color strawberry ice cream, it would not be considered "naturally colored" because the beet juice is not a natural component of strawberries or of strawberry ice cream. Although food processors and consumers might consider the noncertified color of beet juice as "natural," products made with it cannot bear a claim "naturally colored" on the label. Instead, beet juice is listed specifically, among the ingredients on the label. The manufacturer has other options: "color added;" "artificial color added;" "colored with" (followed by the name of the noncertified color, which in this instance, would be beet juice); or name of noncertified color (beet juice) followed by the word "color." Actually, such specific information benefits consumers, and is more informative than if the vague term "natural color" were permitted, without revealing the source. Such specific information helps individuals who are sensitive to certain substances and need to avoid them.

Colors from Plants. Four types of pigments from plants serve as food colorants. Anthocyanins range from orange-red to red to blue; betacyanins, red; carotenoids, yellow to orange to red; and chlorophylls, green to olive green.

- *Anthocyanins.* Anthocyanins are pigments present in many fruits, including berries (such as strawberry, blackberry, raspberry, blueberry, cranberry, chokeberry, and elderberry), as well as in grape and apple. Anthocyanins are present in other plants, such as in red beech leaf, rose, and hibiscus.

One anthocyanin, enocianin, in a water solution or a dehydrated water-soluble powder, can be prepared from the skin of wine grapes. It is purplish red, and can be used as a colorant in beverages.

Another pigment is prepared from the lees (dregs) of pressed Concord grapes. This extract contains common components found in grape juice, but in different proportions. During the steeping process, sulfur dioxide is added, and most of the extracted sugars are fermented to alcohol. In concentrating the extract, nearly all of the alcohol is removed, but a small amount of sulfur dioxide may remain.

This residue can be a problem for some individuals, especially asthmatics, who react unfavorably to sulfur dioxide residues, even at extremely low levels. (See the article "Sulfites: Preserving Foods at a Price" on page 279.)

Despite the increased interest in and use of "natural" colors, the term is meaningless. Under FDA regulations, . . . only the color found naturally in the food would be considered "natural."

The FDA permits the use of grape-skin extract to color carbonated beverages and fruit drinks, flavored syrups, instant beverage base powders, alcoholic drinks, ice creams, fruit yogurts, jams, jellies, chewing gums, candies, confections, pharmaceuticals, and cosmetics.

The pigment in red cabbage, an anthocyanin, is pressed out of the vegetable and concentrated so that it can be used as a food coloring. Different varieties of red cabbage produce different hues. The pigment is used with processed meats, yogurts, and other acidic foods. Red cabbage may serve as a more satisfactory source in red color than others, such as beet or grape juice, which fade when heated or exposed to light.

The red cabbage pigment gives a bright pink to cherry red color to hard candies, even when they are exposed to heat as high as 220°F in their manufacture. The cabbage color retains its redness in beverages even after storage in clear bottles for more than a year. The red cabbage extract is deodorized so that it does not impart any unusual flavor or odor to the foods or beverages in which it is used.

Although anthocyanins have been used as colorants for thousands of years, few toxicologic data exist.

- *Betacyanins.* Betacyanins consist of a relatively small group of pigments, with red beets as the best known source. These pigments are found, as well, in cactus fruit, red chard, pokeberry (a poisonous plant), and in the colorful tropical flower, bougainvillea.

The betacyanins from beets can be extracted, and the concentrated colorant can equal the strength of synthetic red colors. The purification process can remove the strong beet flavor that might be undesirable in a final food product. When beet juice is purified to yield the pigment only, it is classified and regulated as a food additive.

- *Carotenoids.* Carotenoids are very common, both in plants and animals. It is estimated that nature produces a billion tons of carotenoids annually. They are present as yellow to orange to red pigments in the green leaf, red tomato, paprika, corn, butter, palm oil, and red salmon, as well as in the marigold petal and marine alga. Colors from carotenoids can fade easily, if exposed to oxygen and sunlight.

Beta-carotene from carrots is familiar with its orange-colored pigment. Beta-carotene is only one of many in this group of carotenoids. Some of them are synthesized, but classified along with the "natural" colorants in the list of noncertified food colors. Beta-carotene, yellow-orange in hue, was among the first carotenoids to be synthesized. Subsequently, apo-carotene and apo-carotenal (beta-apo 8′ carotenal), and canthaxanthin (with a red hue) were synthesized to serve as yellow-to-red coloring agents. They have a unique characteristic. Although they are synthetic, they possess vitamin A activity, which makes them useful for purposes of fortification and supplementation, as well as for coloring. They are less expensive to produce than their plant-derived counterparts.

Low levels of canthaxanthin as a food color is considered safe. However, safety questions were raised about high levels of its use, associated with crystal formation in the human retina. As a result, the FDA lowered the allowable daily intake (ADI) level.

Carrot oil, with an orange hue, is solvent-extracted and contains both alpha- and beta-carotene. Tomato contains lycopene, a red hue. Tagetes, from the petals of the marigold flower, is used as a colorant in poultry feed.

Paprika, the dried ground fruit of the red pepper (*Capsicum annuum*), yields red to orange to yellow hues, depending on where the peppers are grown. The oleoresin (a mixture of oil and resin) is extracted from the pod, and contains three main carotenoid pigments: capsanthin, capsorubin, and beta-carotene. However, as many as twenty or more additional pigments may be present, including zeaxanthin, which, in combination with beta-carotene, produces a strong yellow hue.

Paprika is used in meat products, cheeses, spice mixes, salad dressings, and toppings. It is a characteristic component of Middle European ethnic dishes. Paprika adds flavor as well as color to foods, and ranges from sweetness to being slightly pungent. In addition, paprika contributes vitamin C to the food.

Saffron is a spice material derived from the dried anthers (pollen-bearing part of the stamen) of a crocus plant (*Crocus savitus*). The natural pigment is crosin, a water-soluble carotenoid. Saffron is highly valued for its subtle flavoring and bright yellow coloring, but its extremely high cost limits its use.

Annatto and annatto extracts are colorings derived from the seed coat of a tropical tree (*Bixa orellana*). Its primary carotenoid is bixin. In concentration, the color is red, but depending on the degree of dilution, the hues range from peach to butter yellow.

Annatto is one of the oldest plant coloring materials, and

has been used widely in dairy products (butter, margarine, cheese, and ice cream). Also, it is used in batters, confections, nondairy coffee whiteners, and whipped toppings. At low levels of use, annatto does not contribute any flavor to the food.

If a solvent/dispersant or dry carrier is used with annatto, this information must appear on the ingredient listing of the food label.

- *Chlorophylls.* Chlorophylls, green pigments in plants, are available in very large quantities, yet have been underutilized as food colorants. They are very unstable and break down to pheophytins, which are olive-green in color. They have been used to a limited extent with food products, such as in dehydrated spinach and green pasta. They are used in nonfood items such as soaps and other toiletries. At one time, chlorophylls were promoted for their purported deodorant quality. This claim has not been proven.

Xanthophyll (*lutein dipalmitate*), extracted from alfalfa, has a hue that ranges from light to very dark yellow. This pigment is found in the egg yolk, marigold petal, and alfalfa. Dried alfalfa meal is permitted in chicken feed to "enhance" the yellow color of poultry skin and egg yolks. Also, tagetes meal (from Aztec marigold petals) and yellow corn endosperm oil are permitted for similar purposes in animal feed. Also, partially defatted, cooked, and toasted cottonseed flour is permitted to be added to feed as a colorant.

- *Other Plant Colors.* Among other noncertified plant-based colors are riboflavin, turmeric, and caramel coloring. Both riboflavin (vitamin B_2) and caramel coloring can be synthesized.

Riboflavin, an intensely yellow color, occurs naturally as a nutrient, and is found in small amounts in all plant and animal cells. It is especially rich in yeast, and found, too, in leafy vegetables, milk, egg, organ meats, and malted barley. Riboflavin is not only used as a food colorant, but as a vitamin to fortify food and feed, and as a component in nutritional supplements.

Riboflavin is light-sensitive. For this reason, fluid milk suffers riboflavin loss if the container is clear and it is stored in a lighted case in a grocery store. Under similar circumstances, riboflavin as a colorant deteriorates if the food or beverage product is exposed to light.

Turmeric, a bright yellow pigment, is extracted from the rhizome of an herb (*Curcuma longa*). The pigments responsible for the color are curcuminoids, with curcumin as the major one. The main applications for turmeric are in curry mixes, with seafood, egg-based products, in chicken dishes, and for pickles and pickle relishes. At the typical level used for coloring, turmeric does not contribute any significant flavor or aroma; at high rates, for spicing, turmeric contributes both taste and aroma to the finished food.

Some individuals report unfavorable reactions after eating foods containing turmeric. For such individuals, label sleuthing may be necessary. Turmeric may be a hidden ingredient in mixes such as curry powders and pickling mixtures.

Caramel is used both as a color and a flavoring agent. Caramel coloring consists of heated food-grade sugars such as fructose, dextrose (glucose), invert sugar, sucrose (table sugar), and/or starch hydrolysates. Depending on which acids, alkalis, and/or salts are used in processing, caramel can be caustic caramel, sulfite caramel, ammonia caramel, or sulfite ammonia caramel. Different processes yield caramel coloring that ranges from golden brown to dark brown. Caramel coloring has an odor of burnt sugar, and is somewhat bitter in taste.

When sulfite is used in caramel manufacture, it can be detected, chemically, in the finished food. The FDA requires sulfite to be listed on labels if it is present in the food or beverage above 10 parts per million (ppm). This listing is important for individuals who need to avoid sulfiting agents.

A European study found that some individuals who are marginally deficient in pyridoxine (B_6) may be sensitive to caramel coloring. This coloring is difficult to avoid in processed foods and beverages. It appears, commonly, in baked goods, commercial soups, gravies, gravy bases, steak sauces, powdered flavors, table syrups, vinegars, textured vegetable protein, seasonings, mixes, soy sauce, colas and other types of soft drinks, liquor, canned meats, ice cream, ices, candy, preserves, and pet food.

Caramel coloring was classified by the Joint FAO/WHO (Food and Agriculture Organization of the World Health Organization) Expert Committee on Food Additives as "D," signifying that virtually no toxicological data are available for this colorant. Because there are many different methods of manufacture, it is nearly impossible to characterize caramel coloring for regulatory purposes.

Colors from Animals. Cochineal is the main pigment obtained from the dried female insect (*Dactylopius coccus*). Sometimes, it is erroneously termed a beetle; in reality, it is a scale insect. It feeds on red berries of the cochineal cactus, and the pigment in the berries is carminic acid. The female insect encloses young larvae with carminic acid from the cactus berries. The red pigment is present in the yolks of the insect's eggs and also in the fatty parts of the female insect. After producing the eggs, the female dies. The eggs are covered over by her dead scalelike body. The whole dead bloated female insect, which contains hatched larvae and some eggs, are brushed off from the cactus, collected, boiled, dried, and used as colorant.

Cochineal extract or carminic acid ranges in hue from orange to pink to red to purple. The color has been used for centuries in various parts of the world, especially for ceremonial purposes. Now, it is used widely with foods, drugs, and cosmetics. Being both heat- and light-stable, cochineal has been used to substitute for synthetic red colors, many of which have been delisted. Cochineal extract and carminic acid are used in candy, ice cream, juice drinks, drink mixes, soda, yogurt, wine, frozen popsicles, fruit fillings for baked goods, port wine cheese, artificial lobster and crab (surimi), and pudding. Also, they are used in cosmetics such as lipstick, mascara, blush, eye shadow, and other make-up, for dietary supplement coatings, and as a medical diagnostic dye.

HISTORY OF NONCERTIFIED COLORS

In 1960, the U.S. Congress, passed legislation that covered color additives and created a unique legal classification for coloring substances that have become identified as "noncertified" colors (also known as "uncertified color additives" or "colors exempt from certification"). These substances have permanent status of acceptability for coloring uses in foods for humans. Some are solely for use in feed for animals.

Since 1960 there have been few additions to the list. For example, the list now includes synthesized carotenoids termed "nature identical," as well as pigment material of inorganic origin (titanium dioxide), and an extractive of insect origin (carmine from cochineal). Most of the noncertified food colors are allowed at levels consistent with good manufacturing practice to achieve the intended effect. This means that the food or beverage processor determines the level. A few are restricted, either to a specific level or only for specific products.

Although few restrictions are placed on the amount of a

Case histories have been reported in medical journals of reactions to cochineal and carmine. Occupational allergy has been noted in workers who inhale carmine powder in factories where color additives are manufactured. Consumers have experienced allergic reactions, especially after consuming numerous food and beverage products that contain cochineal or carmine coloring, along with additional exposures from toiletries and medications containing this coloring.

These potential allergens are hidden within a phrase such as "color added," "artificial color," or "artificial color added." The FDA is reviewing data to determine if a warn-

noncertified food color that can be used, technical difficulties may limit their applications. These colors may not be as uniform in intensity, not have the stability of their counterparts. Some may fade, due to light, long storage, heat, or other factors. However, some (such as caramel color and titanium dioxide) are quite heat-stable and resist changes. Also, modern technical advances have improved the stability of many noncertified food colors. Formerly, they were more expensive than their synthetic counterparts. This feature, too, has changed, making the noncertified colors more attractive to food processors.*

*In the past, food and beverage processors favored synthetic food colors for additional reasons. Supplies of synthetics were dependable; natural ones were not. Many plant-derived colorants were imported. Crop failures, shipping irregularities, and even political turmoil in other countries could result in erratic deliveries. Furthermore, the composition of a synthesized color could be identified more accurately, and monitored more easily by food technologists than the complex combinations that occur with noncertified colors. With advances in technology, many of these problems have been overcome.

ing is warranted on labels of foods and beverages that are colored with cochineal or carmine. Instead of a warning statement, the FDA has another option: a declaration on the label of the specific coloring agent, cochineal or carmine. The agency established a precedent for this by making it mandatory to specify FD&C Yellow No. 5 (tartrazine) on labels of foods, drugs, and cosmetics, if present, because many people react unfavorably to this color.

Either the warning or declaration of the specific color, cochineal or carmine, would be welcomed by those individuals who need to avoid these substances. Also, it would serve the interests of others. This color, derived from an animal, is unacceptable in kosher food products, as well as in food products used by vegetarians.

The health problems created for some individuals by this colorant illustrate an important point. "Natural" cannot be equated with "safe." Regarding cochineal and carmine, H.I. Silverman, D.Sc. from the Massachusetts College of Pharmacy, noted: "The so-called 'dangers' in the use of synthetic, highly purified chemicals may be only in that we know them too well. Alas, we do not know the dangers of material of natural origin."

Colors from Minerals. Titanium dioxide is a mineral compound that provides whiteness or opacity to food products. It is the same pigment, in a less purified grade, which is used in white house paint and for other industrial applications. For purposes of food coloring, titanium dioxide is produced synthetically, and regulated to limit undesirable substances that may be present, such as lead, arsenic, antimony, and mercury, to official tolerance levels.

As a food coloring, the principal uses of titanium dioxide are for sub-coating confections, and with icings. Also, it is used to sub-coat tablets of pharmaceuticals.

Ferrous gluconate, an iron compound, has a limited use.

It is permitted as a coloring for black olives, and its presence is declared on the food label.

Ultramarine blue, a naturally occurring blue pigment, is used to color salt intended for animal feed. The use of the color is limited to 0.5 percent by weight of the salt. This is the same blue pigment that has been used as bluing in laundry, and in fabric dyes and other industrial uses that largely have been replaced by synthetic blue dyes.

Why Are Food Colors Used? Colors in foods and beverages are important to consumers. Colors are associated with ripeness in produce or "richness" in gravy. Food products that appear to lack the expected color value may be regarded as inferior. Fruit that is pink, rather than red, may imply a lack of maturity. Very light brown bakery goods may be considered to be baked insufficiently. Or, if the food has an unnatural color, it may be assumed that the food is spoiled.

Colors in foods and beverages are important to consumers. Colors are associated with ripeness in produce or 'richness' in gravy. Food products that appear to lack the expected color value may be regarded as inferior.

Certain colors are traditional. Butter, egg noodles, and lemon-flavored cakes are expected to be yellow; mint-flavored jelly, green; and orangeade, orange colored.

Food colors affect our perceptions of odor, taste, and texture. Experiments have shown that if a food does not have the color we associate with it, we hesitate to accept it. Blue-colored strawberries or yellow-colored blueberries would be rejected. Despite this conventional wisdom, by the late 1990s, child focus groups shattered this concept. Children clamored for green and purple ketchup, blue margarine, and other nontraditional colors for food products.

In processing food and beverage products, due to heat,

pressure, light, or long storage, much of the original color from the food or beverage may degrade. In turn, consumers reject such products as unacceptable. The addition of color is an attempt to recompense for this loss. (The addition of flavoring agents to processed foods and beverages is a similar attempt to recompense for flavor loss, due to the same factors.)

In recent years, research in creating noncertified food colors has developed to such an extent that these substances now possess qualities that make some food and beverage manufacturers prefer them to the certified colors. The noncertified colors provide a "clean label" that is perceived as consumer friendly. Some of the noncertified food colors can yield hues unobtainable with synthetic ones. This quality is especially apparent with a golden yellow. Annatto actually excels in producing a hue that consumers recognize as acceptable for cheeses. The synthetic, certified versions tend to give a hue that is too bright for cheese such as cheddar.
In addition, some physical properties of noncertified food colors cannot be achieved with synthetic ones. Many noncertified colors are oil-soluble, whereas none of their synthesized counterparts are truly oil-soluble. This is an important feature for oil-based foods such as salad dressings and popcorn oils.

Some of the noncertified colors offer benefits beyond their coloring ability. Many of them are effective antioxidants. Paprika is a source of vitamin C, riboflavin, and carotenoids with phytochemical activity.

The Downside of Added Food Colors. Use of colors (and flavors) to compensate for losses mask the decline in food quality. Federal laws prohibit any attempt to make a food product appear better than it is in reality. This practice is regarded as adulteration and economic fraud. Yet federal officials have rarely taken actions to correct this aspect of added colors (and flavors). For example, white potatoes have been dyed red because new red potatoes could be sold at a higher price. Or, seasonal and regional oranges have been dyed orange for sales appeal, even though the greenness in the skin did not indicate a stage of unripeness.

Use of colors (and flavors) to compensate for losses mask the decline in food quality.

Such practices still persist widely in food manufacture. Caramel coloring, used in bakery products such as bread, makes the product made with white flour appear to be made from wholegrain flours.*

Farmed fish, such as salmon, lack the vivid pinkness of salmon in the wild. To compensate, colorants are permitted to be added to the fish feed in order to approximate the hue of wild salmon. (The lack of flavor and decreased level of omega-3 fatty acids due to the unnatural feed given to the reared fish are also important, but unaddressed issues.)

Consumers prefer yellow-skinned poultry and rich-yellow egg yolks, traditionally achieved in free-range birds. Now, yellow-pigmented colorants may be added to the feed of intensively reared birds, to approximate the yellow skin and yellow egg yolks that shoppers want. The colorants may give more eye appeal, but do not offer the nutrients present in feed that produces the color.

Even when noncertified colors seem benign, does the

---

*Packaging practices may add to the deception. A golden brown-colored bread wrapper makes the loaf appear darker. Or, an orange-striped bag makes carrots appear deeper in color than they actually are. A black stripe at the bottom of a bag of parsnips hides any deterioration of the tips of this vegetable. Lighting practices in food stores also may add to the deception. Green-colored lights at the produce section make green vegetables look greener; pink-colored lights at the meat section make meats look redder.

consumer really expect to find beet juice in yogurt, or red cabbage juice in processed meat? For the rare individual who reacts unfavorably to beet or cabbage, introduction of such colorants in unexpected places presents an unanticipated problem.

The addition of many colors to foods and food products may become superfluous in the future. With the growing interest in functional foods, traditional breeders of agricultural commodities as well as bioengineering scientists have the means to produce foods with increased coloration from phytochemicals that are beneficial and are good colorants, too. More lycopene can be bred into tomatoes; more carotenoids into carrots; and more betacyanins in grapes. Food scientists may develop innovative techniques to improve retention of colors, as well as flavors and nutrients in cooked foods.

Cooks have come to recognize that it is unnecessary to add baking soda to retain the color in cooked green peas, simply by steaming them briefly. The bright green of other vegetables can be retained by careful cooking. Cooks know that the conversion to drab gray-green in cooked broccoli, string beans, or asparagus is a sign of overcooking.

Consumers can avoid many of the colors added to foods, both certified and noncertified, by selecting foods that have not undergone extensive heat and/or pressure, and long storage. This means limiting the use of highly processed foods, and expanded dependence on basic whole foods.

"CONSUMER-FRIENDLY" FOOD ADDITIVES

Increasingly, consumers are reading the ingredients on food labels. In a survey of consumer attitudes, 31 percent of the consumers polled claimed that they sought "natural ingredients" and 16 percent were concerned about "chemicals or preservatives."

In response to these concerns, food scientists and technologists are attempting to produce "consumer-friendly" food additives that are safe and effective alternatives to those regarded suspiciously. Many alternatives now appear on food labels.

Sulfiting agents are a group of preservatives widely used to prevent browning in cut fruits and vegetables that can induce life-threatening allergic reactions in some individuals. (See the article "Sulfites: Preserving Foods at a Price" on page 279.) In response, food technologists developed non-sulfiting antioxidants for use by food processors. The substitute compounds consist of various combinations of citric and ascorbic acids, sodium erythorbate, calcium chloride, and sodium acid pyrophosphate. These compounds are advertised as being equally as effective as the sulfiting agents.

Some suppliers of dehydrated produce, including potatoes and apples, as well as frozen, concentrated, purees, or fibers of fruit, now offer "sulfite-free" commodities to food processors.

Alternatives to Toxic Preservatives. Spices such as cinnamon and clove, herbs such as rosemary, and onions and garlic have antimicrobial activity that helps retard food spoilage from yeast growth.

Some microbes, too, show antimicrobial activity; they can suppress the growth of competing microorganisms.

Some substances have long been recognized as natural preservatives with antimold and antibacterial activity. Vinegar is used as a mold retarder in bread. Propionic acid, a substance that occurs naturally in the ripening process of Swiss cheese, is the basis for sodium or calcium propionate. These compounds are synthesized and used as mold retarders for baked goods. Lactobacillus fermentation in yogurt produces lactic acid, an antibacterial agent that inhibits the growth of the pathogen *Staphylococcus aureus.*

A natural, cultured skim milk-based preservative, now

available commercially, can extend the shelf life of acidic foods if it is introduced at the beginning of processing. This preservative acts as an antibacterial agent against molds, yeasts, and other food spoilage organisms, yet it does not interfere with the growth of beneficial dairy culture organisms. This preservative is used with cottage cheese, yogurt, sour cream, salad dressings, and sauces.

Alternatives to Synthetic Antioxidants. One group of preservatives, the synthetic antioxidants used to retard fat rancidity (BHT, BHA, octyl and propyl gallate, and TBHQ), has had a long controversial history. At present, safe, and effective alternatives are being offered to food processors.

"Choose What Works Naturally" is the headline of one food trade journal ad, urging food processors to use natural, mixed tocopherols (vitamin E) as antioxidants to extend product shelf life and to "deliver an all natural labeling appeal." The ad notes that the mixed tocopherols, derived from vegetable oils, are 100 percent safe, natural, and effective. They extend shelf life just as well as synthetic antioxidants. "And given today's concerns about synthetic substances," the advertisement notes, "going to the natural source makes even more sense."

Ideally, food should be freshly prepared and consumed promptly. However, in our urbanized, developed world, many of us are far removed from this ideal arrangement.

Other "all-natural antioxidant systems" offered for use in processed poultry products combine natural tocopherols and rosemary extract that "have proven to retard oxidation to keep your products just as fresh, just as long, as the synthetics. So you can label your poultry products 'all natural.' Consumers will be happier . . ."

Alternatives to Synthetic Emulsifiers. Emulsifiers are a group of food additives that serve various purposes to improve volume, uniformity, and texture. In keeping with the consumer-friendly trend, one manufacturer advises food processors that its emulsifier products can totally replace the controversial synthetic emulsifiers. "Only one statement is required on the label of ingredients: polyglycerol esters of fatty acids. Naturally, this goes a long way toward making those ingredients sound more like food instead of reading like a chemical formula."

Alternatives to Synthetic Flavors and Colors. Synthetic food flavors and colors have long been regarded as questionable. Many food processors now use alternative yellow colorants from annatto or turmeric. Similarly, red colorants, derived from strong red pigment in foods, are used as alternatives to the controversial synthetic red colorants. (See the article "U.S. Certified Food Colors: A Guarantee of Safety?" on page 261.)

Ideally, food should be freshly prepared and consumed promptly. However, in our urbanized, developed world, many of us are far removed from this ideal arrangement.

Long shipments, long storage, and demand for ease of preparation are some major factors that contribute to various attempts to preserve food, retard its spoilage, and restore lost flavors and colors. The growing use of consumer-friendly additives demonstrates that safer substances can be found or developed that are effective alternatives to those with a poor record of safety.

Chapter 9

Avoiding Foodborne Illnesses

INCREASING THREATS OF FOODBORNE ILLNESS

Changes in farm practices, the environment, and lifestyle, as well as in food processing, distribution, and consumption, are all related to increased food-poisoning outbreaks.

One major change has been the increase in available food products. In the 1950s, a typical grocery stocked about 300 items; currently, supermarkets stock some 30,000. To keep all of these foods fresh and wholesome strains the system.

Several decades ago, the classic foodborne outbreak might have been from *Salmonella*-contaminated potato salad, locally prepared, served at a church picnic, and affecting dozens of people. Today, *Salmonella* may be present in very low numbers, but in a mass-produced food item distributed to tens of thousands of people far from the processing source. Mass production and international distribution, as well as worldwide travel, create the potential for global foodborne outbreaks.

Of the billions of dollars that Americans spend yearly on food, increasingly more dollars are spent on foods prepared outside the home. To meet consumer demand, the types of foods served in eating establishments have changed. Formerly, many cooked foods such as soups and stews were offered on a limited menu. Currently, many offerings are cold foods, including raw vegetables and fruits, which require extensive handling by preparers, with greater possibilities for transmission of contaminants.

In recent years, news-making outbreaks of foodborne illness have brought more attention to the federal food-safety inspection system. Not all the efforts to improve safety inspection may be helpful. Also, technologies that could prove helpful, such as food irradiation, may serve to lull the

How Large Is the Risk of Foodborne Illness?

Official statements have been issued that since 1985, the reported number of cases of foodborne diseases in the United States has declined. However, many public health officials dispute this statement, and report that actually, the number is increasing. What accounts for this contradiction?

The U.S. Centers for Disease Control and Prevention (CDC) had not taken a count of foodborne illnesses and deaths since 1983. Due to this lack of information, public health officials were unable to affirm whether foodborne diseases actually were increasing or decreasing. Many believe that they were increasing due to numerous factors, some of which are described in this article. Many cases are unreported or wrongly ascribed to other conditions. The problem is that tracking of disease outbreaks nationwide, and even within the states, is extremely uneven. Certain foodborne illnesses have been added to the public health surveillance lists only in recent years. An extremely conservative estimate of 6.5 million to 12.6 million cases of food-poisoning annually is the range cited frequently. However, many epidemiologists and public health officials believe that a more accurate figure goes as high as 81.4 million cases yearly. Estimates of deaths from these illnesses range from 525 to 7,000 annually, which may also be higher.

public into a false sense of security—a condition that may already be at work under the current system—because these technologies cannot kill all food pathogens, and recontamination is usually possible.

Since 1975, more than twenty new microbes have been identified that can cause foodborne illnesses. Existing ones may develop into more virulent strains, as with *Escherichia coli* 0157:H7. Additional new microbes continue to emerge in a never-ending procession. It is important to recognize that various pathways of foodborne illness exist.

Some Environmental Conditions. Humans may be experiencing more microbiologically induced infections because of the existence of fewer lactic acid-producing bacteria, once prevalent in the natural environment.

These beneficial organisms in the food chain, formerly abundant in soils, plants, and in raw milk, have declined dramatically. According to Dr. Clem Honer, a dairy technologist, the severe loss of these beneficial bacteria in the soil results from modern agricultural practices dependent on pesticides, weed killers, and the types of fertilizers used.

In milk processing, near aseptic handling and rapid cooling of raw milk make it difficult for lactic acid-producing bacteria to survive and multiply. To compensate, these organisms may need to be added to raw milk before pasteurization. This practice is permitted with Grade B milk. In processing milk, an important goal is to reduce the total bacterial count in the raw milk to produce a better quality product. Bacterial counts are lower, flavor freshness is maintained, and the milk is safer. But, at the same time, the lactic acid-producing bacteria are reduced or eliminated.

Ironically, this processing improves the chance of survival for psychrotrophs (undesirable bacteria that can flourish even in cold temperatures) and other pathogens that may be present in raw milk. Without the presence of lactic acid-producing bacteria, the undesirable pathogens have less competition, and can take over. The result is that pathogens such as *Listeria monocytogenes*, numerous strains of *Salmonella*, and *Yersinia entericolitica* have emerged as problems in many dairies. These pathogens are not new. They have always existed in raw milk, but were held in check by competition with the vigilant lactic acid-producing bacteria.

Another factor in foodborne illness is the contamination of the food supply by polluted water. Imported produce may be irrigated with water containing raw sewage. Crops may be fertilized with raw manure. A 1991 outbreak of *E. coli* 0157:H7 illness in Massachusetts was traced to apple cider from trees fertilized with contaminated raw manure. Such food, if not thoroughly washed and/or cooked, can result in food poisoning.

The expansion of aquaculture is another factor. Sulfur drugs and antibiotics are used to treat bacterial outbreaks in ranched fish that are penned and for a portion of their lives released into the ocean. The drug residues from the fish wastes may promote the growth of antibiotic-resistant bacteria. Some biologists are concerned that bacterial plasmids (units of DNA that replicate within a cell independent of the chromosomal DNA) carrying the genes for antibiotic resistance could be transferred to human pathogens in the same water. In the United States, antibiotic-resistant bacteria were found in fish and fish culture systems by Food and Drug Administration (FDA) researchers, who concluded that antibiotic resistance "indeed may be spread and maintained by bacterial plasmids in aquaculture systems."

Some Farm Practices Are Risky. Farming has undergone radical changes, and many current practices increase foodborne illness risks. One of the best recognized and most criticized practices involves the use of subtherapeutic doses of antibiotics with farm animals. As a result, many *Salmonel-*

la strains responsible for food poisoning have become resistant to antibiotics. As early as the 1950s, it was recognized that the same strains of *Salmonella* found in poultry feed and in processed poultry also are found in people who have eaten such contaminated poultry and have been made ill.

Approximately 90 percent of all foodborne illnesses can be transmitted from animals to humans, according to John Schmitz, head of the Department of Veterinary Sciences at the University of Nebraska at Lincoln. In most cases, a few animals harbor the pathogens and become the sources of contamination that reach other animals. With current practices of intensive rearing, as many as 100,000 head of cattle may share one feedlot, or tens of thousands of chickens may be crowded into one hen house. Under such conditions, a few animals can contaminate the entire herd or flock.

Another current practice with poultry compounds the *Salmonella* problem. By manipulating light patterns to increase egg laying, *Salmonella* colonization is increased. Also, more than a billion pounds of dead chickens and turkeys are recycled every year into poultry feed. The contamination rate of rendered birds can range from zero to 100 percent, depending on the specific product and producer. In a recent year, the industry-wide incidence rate was approximately half.

Another problem has been created by supplementing animal feed with the nutrient selenium. Even a few *Salmonella* organisms thrive in the presence of selenium. Within an incubation period as brief as twenty-four hours, the organisms can multiply a millionfold in this medium.

Risky Processing, Shipping, and Storing. Food contamination may occur in slaughtering, processing, shipping, and storing foods. Some risks have increased because of certain changes from traditional to novel practices. Much public attention has been directed to the inadequacies of current meat, poultry, and fish inspection. Other factors have not been well publicized.

Defeathering machines pound any contamination present into the carcasses of chickens while pressing feces out of their bodies. Microbial spray may land on nearby carcasses as well as on workers and on processing areas, thus spreading the contamination further.

After evisceration, poultry carcasses may be contaminated with fecal matter containing *Aeromonas hydrophila*. Then, the carcasses may be dipped in chill water, an important source of cross contamination. The chill water has been dubbed a "fecal bath."

A. hydrophila has become resistant to several types of antibiotics.

In slaughtering larger food animals, feed may be withheld prior to slaughter. This practice may enable *E. coli* to colonize more readily.

Food may become contaminated during processing from bacterial attachments to the equipment, which has become a widespread problem known as "biofouling." Microorganisms, to maintain their viability, seek solid surfaces conditioned with nutrients sufficient for growth. Food processing equipment is ideal for such attachments. The microorganisms grow and multiply, and the newly formed cells attach to each other, as well as to the machinery, forming a confluently growing colony. When the mass of cells becomes sufficiently large so that it can entrap food particles, nutrients, and other microorganisms, a microbial biofilm is established.

Biofilms have become a pervasive machine contaminant, especially with *Staphylococcus aureus* in poultry processing, *Listeria monocytogenes* in meat and dairy operations, and *Bacillus cereus* on dairy equipment.

Numerous outbreaks of *Salmonella enteritidis* (SE) with

raw eggs were well publicized in the early 1990s. One of the less publicized aspects is the continued use of centrifuge egg-breaking machines, favored by many bakeries and food service establishments to separate the liquid from the shell. Unfortunately, this convenient practice increases risks of contamination. Minute shell fragments, which may harbor bacteria, are expelled along with the egg liquid. Although the practice continues, in the past decade, the egg industry, along with state and federal health agencies, has sought to have such machines banned from use.

Consumer Eating Patterns. Changing eating patterns play a role in foodborne risks. Red-meat consumption has fallen by nearly 50 percent and whole-milk consumption by 14 percent in recent decades, accompanied by increased consumption of low-fat milk, cheese, poultry, fish, and produce.

Ironically, the enormous expansion of new low-fat foods, formulated purportedly to increase health benefits, may increase risks of food poisoning. Low-fat products have a greater potential for contamination than their traditional counterparts. For example, low-fat butter replacers may have higher water content than butter, making such products more susceptible to microbial growth. Similarly, the fat in whole milk inhibits bacterial growth more readily than skim milk lacking in fat.

Consumer interest in low-calorie and low cholesterol foods has led to the development of numerous newly formulated products, and some of them pose new safety problems. For example, federal regulations require commercially manufactured products made with unpasteurized eggs, such as mayonnaise, to have a specific level of pH and acidity, and a holding period of seventy-two hours before the product is shipped. The new type of mayonnaise cannot meet these requirements, especially the acidic level, for it has only half the acid level of traditional mayonnaise, in order to make it palatable. Processed low-acid foods are more hospitable to pathogens such as *Salmonella* and *Listeria*.

Commercially available freshly pre-cut packaged produce, convenient for salad preparation for the busy shopper, has become popular. Surveys were conducted to determine the effect of factory conditions on the microflora of such produce. Field contamination was reduced by removing outer leaves and peels. Sprays and water baths reduced microbial counts to some extent. However, shredders and some slicers were found to be sites for serious microbial build-up.

Ground meats are popular for their versatility and lower costs than whole cuts of chops, steaks, and roasts. However, ground meat, in handling, becomes more susceptible to contamination. Most bacteria find it easier to spread across the meat's surface instead of burrowing deep inside. When meat is ground, its surface area is spread across each long strand that comes out of the grinder. Bacteria present on the original surface of the meat become mixed throughout the ground batch. Later, in forming patties, the original surface area is spread further, throughout the patties. Unless the patties are well-cooked throughout, live bacteria can survive.

A relatively recent practice involves shipping large boxes of coarsely ground beef from packinghouses to supermarkets where the meat is reground more finely and repackaged in smaller quantities for sale. This practice increases the likelihood of higher microbial levels in the meat, due to extensive handling.

Richard Lechowitz of the National Center for Food Safety and Technology at the Illinois Institute of Technology, is critical of the systems in transportation and storage of refrigerated foods in the United States. He charges that, frequently, insufficiently low temperatures exist throughout the entire food-distribution chain, from trucks to supermarkets, and contribute to microbial growth and proliferation.

Although the FDA requires refrigerated foods to be stored no higher than 45°F, according to Lechowitz, ideally, it should be between 32°F and 34°F.

Consumers desire attractive foods as fresh and unprocessed as possible, which has led to the development of perishable refrigerated "fresh" foods. Packaging techniques have been devised to keep foods "fresh" and extend their shelf life. Among these techniques are vacuum packaging, sous vide (a system in which food is cooked in its own juices, chilled, and reheated, all within the packaging), and both modified and controlled atmosphere packagings. These techniques may extend shelf life, but increase risks of foodborne illnesses.

According to the U.S. Department of Agriculture (USDA), vacuum packaging may inhibit the growth of spoilage bacteria, yet encourage pathogens, notably *Clostridium botulinum,* which thrives in low- or no-oxygen conditions. The agency warns that vacuum-packaged steaks should be regarded as perishable—as risky as raw chicken.

The potential for botulism increases, too, with newer types of nonprocessed foods. Researchers at the University of Wisconsin report that, under certain conditions, novel packaging of mushrooms creates a potential source for spore development and toxin formation if *C. botulinum* is present.

Jeffrey M. Farber of the Canadian Bureau of Microbial Hazards reported that modified atmosphere packaging may allow pathogens such as *Listeria, Yersinia,* and *Aeromonas* to grow at low temperatures. If quality control is poor, sous vide packaging may favor the development of *Listeria* and *C. botulinum.*

Preservatives are added to foods to extend their shelf life and prevent food spoilage. In recent years, nearly half of several hundred large food companies announced plans to increase reformulation of many food products so that

MAJOR FOODBORNE PATHOGENS

• *Campylobacter jejuni.* Symptoms from *C. jejuni* infections range from a mild illness with diarrhea lasting a day, to severe abdominal pain, severe diarrhea (sometimes bloody), sometimes accompanied by fever, occasionally lasting for several weeks. The incubation period for most cases is two to five days and the illness usually lasts from two to ten days, depending on its severity. Although the illness is generally regarded as a relatively mild disease, death can occur in some cases, especially for the very young, very old, or the immunocompromised. *C. jejuni* frequently contaminates raw poultry, but also contaminates other foods.

• *Clostridium perfringens.* Illness from *C. perfringen* intoxications typically occurs six to twenty-four hours after ingestion of food bearing large counts of this bacterium. The illness in humans is frequently a mild gastrointestinal distress, lasting only about a day. Deaths are uncommon. *C. perfringens* contaminates raw meat and poultry, and other foods, too.

• *Escherichia coli* 0157:H7. Usually a mild gastrointestinal illness that occurs three to five days after eating contaminated food. However, *E. coli* 0157:H7 disease can result in illness requiring hospitalization such as hemorrhagic colitis and hemolytic uremic syndrome (HUS). Hemorrhagic colitis is distinguished by the sudden onset of severe abdominal cramps, little or no fever, and diarrhea that may become grossly bloody. Although less than 5 percent of *E. coli* 0157:H7 disease cases develop HUS, it is a severe, life-threatening illness. HUS is a disease characterized by red blood cell destruction, kidney failure, and neurological complications, such as seizures and strokes. Most of these HUS cases are children under five years old, although the feeble elderly may also be at risk. *E. coli* 0157:H7 usually contaminates raw ground meat, but also contaminates other foods.

• *Listeria monocytogenes.* Illness caused by this bacterium may be either mild or severe. Milder cases are characterized by a sudden onset of fever, severe headache, vomiting, and other influenza-type symptoms. Severe cases can result in chronic illness and death. Listeriosis may appear mild in healthy adults and more severe in fetuses, the elderly, and the immunocompromised. Outbreak data show that the incubation period ranges from three to seventy days. *L. monocytogenes* contaminates many types of foods, including deli meats, a Mexican-type cheese (quesa blanca), raw vegetables, unpasteurized fruit juices, etc.

• *Salmonella.* Illness from this bacterium usually appears six to seventy-four hours after eating contaminated food and lasts for a day or two. Common symptoms are nausea, diarrhea, stomach pain, and sometimes vomiting. In rare cases *Salmonella,* like many other bacterial and parasitic infections, can cause chronic disease syndromes such as arthritis and meningitis. Although the illness is generally regarded as a relatively mild disease, death can occur in some cases—especially for the very young, very old, or immunocompromised. Numerous strains of *Salmonella* contaminate foods. *S. enteritidis* contaminate raw eggs; *S. typhimurium,* raw sprouts and raw-milk cheeses, etc.

• *Staphylococcus aureus.* Intoxications occur usually within one to six hours following consumption of the toxin produced by the bacteria. In fact, onset of symptoms may occur within thirty minutes of consumption. Illness caused by *S. aureus* enterotoxin (the toxin from *S. aureus,* produced in the intestine) is characterized by severe nausea, vomiting, cramps, and diarrhea. Although the illness generally does not last longer than one to two days, the severity of the illness may indicate the need for hospitalization and possibly for surgical exploration.

- *Toxoplasma gondii.* This parasite can cause acute or chronic human illness when people eat raw or undercooked pork, mutton, and some other meats. The acute illness has mild flu-like symptoms. People can also be exposed to *T. gondii* through contact with cats or cat excrement. Most people infected with the parasite do not have any symptoms, and some people are at higher risk of getting sick from this parasite. A woman infected with *T. gondii* during pregnancy may transmit the infection to her fetus, possibly leading to still birth or a baby born with birth defects ranging from hearing or visual impairments to mental retardation. People with suppressed immune systems, such as AIDS and cancer patients, are also at higher risk than others from this parasite. One outbreak associated with undercooked meat indicates that the incubation period ranges from ten to twenty-three days.

labels read "all natural/no additives." Supermarkets are ill-equipped to implement safety controls required by such products. The reformulated products may increase food-borne illnesses.

Certain supermarket practices, developed for convenience, pose risks. Prestuffed turkeys may be contaminated. Pop-up indicators for doneness of fowl may be inaccurate and untrustworthy for safety. At times, produce such as melons are precut. One incident involved cutting of unwashed cantaloupe into smaller portions for sale. Apparently, the knife picked up pathogens present on the melon rinds and transferred them to the edible portions. People who ate the melons were made ill from salmonellosis.

In supermarkets, hydration systems maintain moisture in certain fresh produce. They help maintain freshness and reduce shrinkage, but contribute to foodborne illnesses.

Eating Away from Home May Be Risky. Restaurants account for many foodborne illness outbreaks. Although incidents with undercooked hamburger have well publicized, other risky restaurant practices are less well known. Restaurant workers may be poorly trained in food safety. Some may be infected and contaminate foods that they handle. In commenting on nouvelle cuisine, Julia Child remarked, "it is so beautifully arranged on the plate; you know someone's fingers have been all over it." A recent study showed that *L. monocytogenes* was present on 11 percent of all restaurant dishcloths examined. Doubtless, contamination is prevalent on other commonly used kitchen aids, including can openers.

Some risks result from certain restaurant practices. For example, *B. cereus* contamination of fried rice may result from the way the grain is prepared, especially in some Asian restaurants, where cooked rice is left at room temperature.

The popularity of salad bars in restaurants has generated greater use of cold entree salads based on meat, poultry, pasta, potatoes, and soy-based protein products. With this development, there is a new risk posed by the enterotoxic (toxic in the intestine) *Staphylococcus aureus*. In studies, after twenty-four hours, the toxin was found in all salad dressings examined from salad bars.

People tend to associate botulism with food improperly canned at home. In the past, certainly this was true. However, due to changing patterns and a decline in home canning, botulism outbreaks in recent years have occurred in restaurant settings. In one case, potato salad had been prepared from leftover baked potatoes, improperly stored. In another instance, onions used in patty-melt sandwiches resulted in twenty-eight restaurant patrons being hospitalized with neurological signs and symptoms of botulism. The sautéed onions had been covered with a thick layer of melted margarine and set aside for use during the day. The onions were not reheated before being used in the sandwiches.

"Takeout Continues to Skyrocket!" was the title of an article about the growing popularity of take-out food. Unfortunately, this burgeoning industry offers a new possibility for food poisoning. Take-out and delivered food service increase the chances of infection if recipients fail to reheat the food to a sufficiently high temperature or length of time to kill off bacteria that might be picked up en route to delivery.

In a study of take-out foods, low-level contamination by *Listeria* was detected in about 15 percent of cooked poultry, 8 percent of ready-to-eat meats, 5 percent of vegetables, and 2 percent of milk and dairy products tested. In another study, 22 percent of all take-out foods purchased in supermarkets was found to be microbially contaminated.

In commenting on nouvelle cuisine, Julia Child remarked, "It is so beautifully arranged on the plate; you know someone's fingers have been all over it."

Preparing Food at Home May Be Risky. It is estimated that about 21 percent of all foodborne illnesses result from faulty home-kitchen practices, compared to 79 percent from dining out. Many of these illnesses are preventable. Much emphasis has been placed on kitchen and personal cleanliness, avoidance of cross contamination, and the need for thorough cooking, prompt storage, and adequate reheating. However, additional factors, less well appreciated, also contribute to food poisoning.

With lifestyle changes, many children and young adults grow up without having learned any basic principles of safe food preparation. Emphasis on convenience may focus attention away from safe methods of food preparation, cooking, and storing. One lifestyle change that is a risk factor is the prevalent use of microwave ovens in home kitchens. This appliance may be a major new factor in the incidence of salmonellosis and other food infections. Microwave ovens cook foods unevenly.

Commonly, people freeze meat, poultry, or fish in the same packaging in which it was wrapped when purchased. According to Martha Patnoad of the Cooperative Extension Service of the University of Rhode Island, such flesh foods should be washed thoroughly and repackaged before they are frozen. Patnoad claims that any bacterial contamination from processing may remain in the packaging material and proliferate. The practice of defrosting and refreezing flesh foods increases the risk of food poisoning by allowing any contaminants present to continue growing and multiplying.

Your Health May Be a Risk Factor. The health status of an individual determines the health of the intestinal tract and the efficiency of the immune system. Both factors are important to resist or minimize the effects from infections caused by foodborne pathogens.

Use of prescription drugs and over-the-counter medications may lower resistance by impairing the body's normal defense mechanisms that help ward off infections. Anyone using a prescribed antibiotic for a medical purpose is at risk. So are ulcer patients who take antacids that reduce the stomach acid, which normally kills invading bacteria. The elderly, especially, may be affected. About 20 percent of sixty year olds, and about 40 percent of people older than eighty, have atrophic gastritis—an inability to secrete sufficient stomach acid to kill bacteria. Use of cortisone encourages microbes to proliferate. Normally innocuous bacteria may be transformed into noxious ones, including *Streptococcus*, *Staphy-*

lococcus, Pneumoniae, Brucella, and *Typhoid,* as well as spirochetes and viruses responsible for influenza, coxsakie, and poliomyelitis.

One's individual nutrition status may be crucial in determining the mildness or severity of viral infections. In mice, deficiencies of antioxidant nutrients such as selenium and vitamin E turned a normally benign virus (coxsakie B_3) into a disease-causing strain. Similar transformations may occur with other viruses, and may influence the severity of such infections as influenza, hepatitis, and human immunodeficiency virus (HIV).

Adequate intake of dietary fiber may play a beneficial role in minimizing the risks of foodborne illnesses by lessening the effects of pathogenic agents. Fiber can change the quantity and composition of mucin (a secretion from intestinal cells). Mucin is known to constitute the major defense mechanism against pathogenic agents. In animal tests, rats were fed various types of fibers in their diet for four weeks. Fibers increased mucin secretions. However, the amount of fat in the diet was important. A high-fat level lessened mucin production, whereas a low-fat level enhanced its production.

SHORT-TERM ILLNESS, LONG-TERM HEALTH DISORDERS

"I've had the bug," is a common statement. Foodborne illness is thought to affect every American yearly with at least one bout of enteric (diarrheal) disease. While most food poisoning is an unpleasant experience of short duration, some common bacterial and parasitic diseases of foodborne origin can cause or predispose us to numerous chronic illnesses such as joint diseases, central nervous system disorders, heart complications, intestinal inflammation, or kidney disease. For some time, it had been estimated that about 9,000 cases of foodborne disease result in death each year. This estimate was lowered, but many health professionals believe that the number is actually higher, due to unreported and misdiagnosed cases.

Joint Disease. Reactive arthritis, formerly called aseptic arthritis, is a joint disease that can be triggered by foodborne pathogens. At times, genetic susceptibility is a factor. It is estimated that an individual who carries a specific gene, called HLA-$B_2$7, and who suffers diarrheal infection inflicted by certain intestinal pathogens, is about eighteen times more likely to develop reactive arthritis than is a person exposed to the same pathogens but who lacks this specific gene.

Although symptoms of reactive arthritis may last for less than a year for most people, some 18 percent may continue with symptoms for longer periods. Nearly half of the latter group experience multiple arthritic episodes.

The same genetically susceptible people are much more likely to develop other joint diseases as well. They are thirty-seven times more likely to develop Reiter's syndrome (an arthritic condition in adult males, usually associated with inflammation of the eyes and urethra, and sometimes with skin lesions); and up to 126 times more likely to develop ankylosing spondylosis (a chronic, progressive form of arthritis characterized by inflammation and eventual immobility of the joints, spine, and related structures).

Certain types of foodborne illnesses from *Yersinia enterocolitica* appear to be strong initiators of arthritic conditions, which may be accompanied by debilitating symptoms that last for years.

In 1985, a large outbreak of *Salmonella typhimurium* from contaminated milk in the Chicago area resulted in reactive arthritis in 2.3 percent of the cases examined. A smaller percentage developed Reiter's syndrome. The most seriously affected individual was a person who also carried the HLA-$B_2$7 gene.

The following year, a follow-up study of the Chicago area patients showed in twenty out of twenty-nine cases that reactive arthritis symptoms still persisted. In six cases, the condition had worsened. The joint diseases tended to become chronic, and the arthritic symptoms had progressively increased.

For decades, various microorganisms have been thought to be associated with rheumatoid arthritis. To date, none has been identified specifically as a causal agent.

Autoimmune thyroid disorders, such as Graves' disease, can be initiated by one type of *Y. enterocolitica* bacterium.

Neuromuscular Disorders. Chronic neuromuscular disorders can result from certain acute gastrointestinal illnesses caused by *Campylobacter*. One type, *C. jejuni,* is thought to be the single most identifiable pathogen associated with Guillain-Barré syndrome, a disorder marked by acute weakness, autonomic dysfunction, and respiratory insufficiency. This syndrome can be life-threatening, and is reported to be the single most common neurologic cause in hospital admissions. People suffering from Guillain-Barré syndrome, and who are known to be infected with *C. jejuni,* develop a significantly graver form of the disorder.

Foodborne illnesses may be related to other neuromuscular disorders, including myasthenia gravis and lupus erythemata.

Heart Conditions. Several specific foodborne pathogens have been linked, directly or indirectly, to endocarditis and myocarditis (inflammations of heart membranes), and may result in permanent heart damage. Frequently, cardiac disorders (including aorta insufficiency and mitral valve damage) accompany ankylosing spondylitis, which had been induced by foodborne pathogens.

Foodborne gram-negative bacteria (bacteria that do not become violet in color in a stain test; gram-positive bacteria become violet in color) have been suggested as factors in the development of atherosclerosis.

Additional Disorders. Kidney diseases such as hemorrhagic colitis, caused by *Escherichia coli*, may result in acute renal failure, decreased platelets in circulating blood, and hemolytica anemia associated with small blood vessel diseases. Other renal diseases have been associated with pathogens such as *Shigella*, *Salmonella*, and *Campylobacter*.

Foodborne illness also may cause nutritional disorders. Repeated episodes of pathogen-induced diarrhea may prevent nutrient absorption, or result in large fluid losses. Both conditions can lead to malnutrition. Even short bouts of diarrhea can cause subtle nutritional changes. Diarrhea contributes to poor general health by compromising nutritional status. In turn, the immune system may become impaired. The gut may be damaged, and its permeability increased. Proteins may enter into systemic circulation where they do not belong, and where they can do harm. The ensuing serious consequences of this condition, termed "leaky gut," may include food intolerances and other health disorders.

It is thought that foodborne pathogens may play roles in some chronic diseases of unknown origin, yet be overlooked as factors. Some pathogens have not yet been studied thoroughly.

CONTRACTING TRAVELERS' DIARRHEA

An estimated 300 million people travel outside of their own countries every year. Americans comprise about half of the 16 million among them who travel from industrialized to developing countries. Of these, about one-third will develop travelers' diarrhea (TD).

TD is caused by numerous infectious agents—bacterial, viral, and parasitical—and the spectrum of clinical illness varies considerably. Travelers may experience more than one attack of TD during a single trip and also be infected by more than one agent.

The highest risk areas include most of the developing countries of Latin America, Africa, the Middle East, and Asia. Somewhat lower-risk areas include most of southern Europe, and a few Caribbean islands. There are relative risks determined by where travelers eat. Dining in private homes is the least risky. Restaurant eating is more risky, and eating foods prepared by street vendors poses the highest risk.

Typical TD results in four to five loose or watery stools daily, accompanied by symptoms that include abdominal cramps, nausea, vomiting, bloating, urgency of bowel evacuation, fever, bloody stools, and malaise. Usually, episodes begin abruptly during travel, or shortly after returning home. Fortunately, TD generally is self-limiting. The average duration of diarrhea is three to four days. However, 10 percent of cases persist longer than one week; about 2 percent, longer than one month; and less than 1 percent, longer than three months. However, TD rarely is life-threatening.

Causes of TD. Infectious agents are the main cause of TD. Enterotoxigenic *Escherichia coli* (ETEC) are the most common causative TD agents in all countries surveyed. These organisms adhere in the small intestine, where they multiply and produce an enterotoxin (a toxin produced in the intestine) that causes fluid secretion and diarrhea. Other *E. coli* differ in the degree of virulence.

Salmonella is another common infectious bacterium involved in TD. In industrialized countries, this large group of organisms commonly causes outbreaks of food-associated diarrhea. In developing countries, the proportion of TD cases caused by *Salmonella* varies, but is not high. In addition to diarrhea, *Salmonella* also can cause dysentery, characterized by small mucous-containing bloody stools.

No Ice, Please!

Many people who travel to developing countries are careful to avoid undercooked food, unpeeled fruits and vegetables, and to use safe water for drinking and brushing teeth. Yet they may accept ice in alcoholic beverages, assuming that the alcohol eliminates the risk of infection if the ice happens to be contaminated. This assumption is false.

Ice as a source of infection depends on the type and number of pathogens in the water from which ice is made, the length of time that ice is frozen, and the type of beverage in which ice melts. Over time, live pathogens progressively decrease in various frozen substances. Live bacteria decline as the freezing approaches 32°F.

Prolonged freezing of contaminated water kills many, but not all, waterborne pathogens. *Escherichia coli,* the most common cause of travelers' diarrhea, tends to cause illness only when these bacteria are ingested in large numbers. Freezing sharply reduces the population. Similarly, by freezing water, many *Salmonella* will be inactivated. But *Shigella,* bacteria that cause dysentery, are far more hardy. Live *Shigella* have been recovered in ice frozen solidly for two months. As few as 200 live *Shigella* can inflict acute human illness.

A study was designed to simulate the typical freezing of ice in commercial freezers, common thawing at room temperature, and effects on selected pathogens. Four common agents of travelers' diarrhea were used: two strains of *Shigella, Escherichia coli* and *Salmonella typhi.* Six types of drinks were tested: bottled drinking water, club soda, a cola drink, a mixture of one-part scotch to two parts soda, 80-proof scotch, and 86-proof tequila.

None of the four types of pathogens was totally inactivated

by freezing for twenty-four hours, followed by melting of the ice in any of the test drinks. There was a progressive decrease of bacterial survival in ice from water to liquor.

In drinking water, 100 percent of the live organisms were recovered on complete melting of ice. Carbonated beverages and alcoholic drinks are considered to have some mild disinfectant effect. Yet both may be incriminated in some cases of travelers' diarrhea, if added ice is contaminated.

Due to *Shigella's* hardiness, it is estimated that these bacteria account for approximately 15 percent of all travelers' diarrhea in Mexico. *Shigella* infection via ice may contribute to other sources of infection, such as that from undercooked or inadequately refrigerated foods. After heavy rainfall, common in rural and urban areas of many developing countries, ice and water can become sources of infection.

In a few countries, *Shigella* causes TD in about 5 to 15 percent of travelers. Most cases result in watery diarrhea, but a few in dysentery.

Campylobacter jejuni is responsible for a small percentage of reported TD cases, some with bloody diarrhea.

Many viruses, including adeno-, astro-, corona-, and entero-viruses are acquired commonly by travelers. Ten percent to 15 percent of travelers develop Norwalklike viruses. In several studies, up to 36 percent of diarrheal illnesses in travelers were associated with rotaviruses in the stools, although many of the people remained asymptomatic.

Parasites, too, are involved in some TD cases. In studies, up to 9 percent of people with TD were infected with *Giardia lamblia* or *Entamoeba histolytica. Cryptosporidium* has become recognized in some TD cases. Other parasites occasionally are involved in TD. Even with the best current methods to detect pathogens, from 20 to 50 percent of cases remain without recognized causes. Testers do not always search for the involved pathogen, and some are difficult to detect. For example, even the best technique may be insensitive to *E. coli* and *Shigella*. In experiments, these pathogens, although present, were not detected in 30 to 40 percent of the cases examined.

Prevention of TD. At present, no vaccines are available that are effective in preventing TD. Several nonantimicrobials (such as Lomotil) have been advocated as preventives. However, controlled studies indicate that difenoxine (the active metabolite of Lomotil's diphenoxylate) actually *increased the incidence* of TD in addition to producing other undesirable side effects. No antiperistaltic agent (such as Lomotil and Imodium) are effective in TD prevention. No data support the effectiveness of activated charcoal as a TD preventive.

TD is best prevented by paying meticulous attention to food and beverage choices. Uncooked foods are risky. High-risk ones include raw vegetables and raw or undercooked meats and seafood. Other risky items include ice made from tap water, unpasteurized milk and other dairy products, and unpeeled fruits. Even cooked foods are risky if they are not thoroughly heated, handled improperly, or contaminated by handlers.

Drinks considered safe include bottled carbonated beverages, bottled water, beer, wine, hot coffee and tea, or water that has been boiled sufficiently or treated appropriately with iodine or chlorine. Wipe the cap of the bottle before removing it. In addition to paying meticulous attention to food and beverage choices, travelers must practice good personal hygiene, especially frequent hand washing.

MULTIDRUG RESISTANCE TO A VIRULENT PATHOGEN

"The 'superbug' has arrived with *Salmonella typhimurium* DT104 (definitive type) which is multiply-resistant to five antibiotics used in human therapy, being widely distributed in animal populations throughout the United States," reports Michael Doyle, head of the University of Georgia's Center for Food Safety and Quality Enhancement. *S. typhimurium* has become resistant to five important antibiotic groups: ampicillin, chloramphenicol, streptomycin, sulfonamides, and tetracycline. Also, some strains of the pathogen have acquired resistance to fluoroquinolones, which represents the last line of defense for treating serious *Salmonellae* infections.

Antimicrobial resistance from some strains of *Salmonella* has become a worldwide health problem. In 1984, *S. typhimurium* was reported as an emerging pathogen in the United Kingdom. Subsequently, it has become a major cause of illness in humans and animals in Europe, especially in the United Kingdom, and also has emerged in the United States and Canada as a widespread pathogen with multidrug resistance.

According to the Centers for Disease Control and Prevention (CDC), the annual number of *S. typhimurium* cases in the United States has not increased significantly in the past fifteen years, but the percentage of isolates (pure strains) that are drug-resistant has risen sharply. From 1979 to 1980, less than 1 percent was multidrug-resistant. However, by 1994–1995, multidrug-resistance had risen to 34 percent. The greatest resistance was displayed to chloramphenicol.

Although many *Salmonella* strains are mild and killed readily with adequate heat, a few strains, including *S. typhimurium* and *S. enteritidis,* are far more virulent, and can be fatal. An estimated two million to four million cases of salmonellosis occur each year in the United States, with 40,000 culture-confirmed cases, and 500 deaths. Of the culture-confirmed cases, one-fourth are identified as *S. typhimurium.*

Causes for Resistance. Researchers believe that the thera-

S. typhimurium Outbreaks in United States

- In November 1993, seven culture-confirmed cases of *S. typhimurium* were reported among residents of Gideon, Missouri, a small town with an unchlorinated water supply. The water was found to contain fecal coliforms. Radio announcements advised residents to boil drinking water, but no reason was given, nor was the possiblity of illness even mentioned. The radio message was quite ineffective. Eventually, nearly half of the entire population became ill (650 people out of a population of 1,100). Fifteen required hospitalization, and seven nursing home residents died of the infection. *S. typhimurium* was confirmed as the cause of the waterborne outbreak. The contamination probably resulted from birds entering a 100,000-gallon water-storage tower through an uncovered hatch. Flushing—the most extensive that had been done in three years—of the unchlorinated distribution system, just before the outbreak, had emptied water from this tower into the general water supply.

- In 1994, an outbreak of *S. typhimurium* infection occurred during the winter holiday season. Physicians in Dodge County, Wisconsin reported that they had treated seventeen patients. At least fourteen had eaten raw ground beef, either plain or seasoned with onion and an herb mix, during the seventy-two-hour period before the onset of illness. Stool samples showed *S. typhimurium* in seven specimens. Before the outbreak ended, 107 cases were identified and confirmed, of which fifty-one required hospitalization.

- In October 1996, elementary school children in a Nebraska farm community were served cold chocolate milk from cartons during school lunch and subsequently became ill. Culture of the stool samples of the children showed *S. typhimurium.* Many of the milk cartons showed expired "sell by" dates. In addition, some children had handled a turtle, as well as a reportedly ill kitten, both brought to school for "show and tell." Neither animal was available for testing.

peutic and nontherapeutic uses of antibiotics in food animals is an important factor in the trend of growing antibiotic-resistance that has developed for many bacterial strains, including *S. typhimurium.*

More than 40 percent of the 50 million pounds of antibiotics produced yearly in the United States is used with animals. More than 80 percent of this amount by weight is used for growth promotion; the remainder, to treat diseases. Scientists agree that antibiotic use for growth promotion should end, and antibiotic use be reserved to treat diseases.

Similarly, antibiotics are misused with humans. Doctors may prescribe antibiotics for children with colds, upper respiratory tract infections, and bronchitis. But these conditions do not benefit from antibiotics, which are ineffective with viral infections. Each year, this misuse represents a substantial proportion of all antibiotic prescriptions for children in the United States.

In 1997, experts from the World Health Organization (WHO) repeated the same two recommendations made on numerous earlier occasions: (1) to minimize further resistance to antimicrobial agents, drugs used as human medicines should not be used as growth promoters in food animals; (2) the use of antimicrobial agents, whether for humans or animals, must be used judiciously and sparingly, and used solely for therapeutic purpose. The CDC concurred.

Sources of Human Infections. Humans are at risk from

S. typhimurium infections through direct or indirect contact with infected livestock and other creatures, and from contaminated food and potable water. Vehicles of infection include human-to-human transmission, as well as from farm animals such as cattle, pigs, poultry, sheep, goats, and horses; pet dogs, cats, and birds; and rodents, foxes, badgers, sea gulls, and exotic psittacines (such as parrots, macaws, and parakeets). Also, infections have been traced to the consumption of unpasteurized dairy products, chicken, pork sausage, meat paste, and municipal drinking water.

Efforts to reduce *S. typhimurium* on farms are difficult because the pathogen can infect such a wide range of animals. To date, little is known about its epidemiology, and what kinds of controls may be effective. There are gaps in fundamental information about this especially virulent strain of *Salmonella*. This pathogen is ranked fifth in the present list of priority pathogens associated with beef at slaughter. The top four are *E. coli* 0157:H7, *Salmonella enteriditis*, *Listeria monocytogenes*, and *Campylobacter*. Significantly, all five of these major food pathogens have emerged or have become virulent only in recent years.

Efforts to reduce *S. typhimurium* transmissions through the food chain offer challenges. Contamination can occur on the farm with animals and animal feed; at slaughterhouses; in food processing, storing, and distributing; at retail outlets; and in kitchens of institutions and homes, where raw foods are handled and prepared.

One factor that may play an important role in *S. typhimurium* infection is the large population of pet cats. These animals can shed *S. typhimurium* DT104 in their feces for twelve weeks or longer after they recover from acute infections.

In the state of Washington, this pathogen was suspected for possible association between ill animals and human infections. In Washington, a high proportion of persons with

S. typhimurium live in counties with large numbers of dairy cattle.

Antimicrobials Become Ineffective. Resistance to two classes of antibacterials—trimethoprim and ciprofloxacin (a fluoroquinolone)—were confirmed in the United Kingdom in 1993. It is thought likely that this resulted from the veterinary use of these two antimicrobials. In 1994, enrofloxacin (another fluoroquinolone) was licensed for veterinary use in the United Kingdom. Subsequently, humans infected with *S. typhimurium* in the British Isles have not responded fully to fluoroquinolones.

In 1995, the Food and Drug Administration (FDA) approved use of sarafloxacin (another fluoroquinolone) to treat *E. coli* in poultry flocks in the United States.

Reducing Infection

Experimentally, pulsed electricity has been used to destroy *S. typhimurium* on chicken carcasses, followed by water rinses. In 1995, researchers reported that this technique reduced the pathogen, and none was detected in the treatment water. However, changes in chicken skin color occurred, which might make the unappealing birds unsaleable.

An oral vaccine against *S. typhimurium* UK-1, the most common strain of *typhimurium* in chickens, has been developed by Roy Curtiss, a biologist at Washington University in St. Louis, Missouri. Curtiss genetically engineered the bacteria, and then weakened them by deleting the two key genes. This allowed the vaccine to develop an immune response in chickens, without triggering their illness. The lifetime immunity bestowed by the vaccine on breeder birds and laying hens was transferred to their eggs and offspring.

To date, *S. typhimurium* infection in the United States has not shown resistance to these two fluoroquinolones. However, there is no assurance that with continued use, resistance will not develop.

Frederick Angulo, a CDC medical epidemiologist, warned veterinarians not to misuse fluoroquinolones in animals, because the practice would result in more *Salmonella*-related deaths to humans exposed to *S. typhimurium*. Angulo reported that people exposed to fluoroquinolones as residues in meat and chicken develop permanent resistance to this group of drugs. Angulo warned that, "should fluoroquinolones be widely used in food animals in the United States, we would fully expect fluoroquinolone resistance to . . . emerge (extensively) in humans."

Food safety scientists are especially concerned with *S. typhimurium* in the presence of a multiresistance pattern to the main classes of antimicrobials. Molecular studies show that resistant genes are encoded chromosomally. Thus, even if use of these important antibiotics is reduced, resistance to them is not expected to be reversed.

Many infected people report that they have been given antibiotics, especially penicillin-type, prior to infection. Studies show that antibiotic use with humans and animals is a predisposing factor for *S. typhimurium* infections.

Official Actions. As *S. typhimurium* emerged as a public health issue, the U.S. Department of Agriculture (USDA) launched a group effort, by its Office of Public Health and Science, a branch of the Food Safety and Inspection Service, along with its Animal and Plant Inspection Service. The group was joined by the FDA's Center for Veterinary Medicine and CDC. Cooperatively, the group studied this newly emerging *Salmonella* strain, with a goal of recommending a course of action for its control.

In 1998, the group released its report. Depending on

which statistical model is used to calculate the cost of *S. typhimurium* nationwide, the financial burden of its infection is estimated to be from $67 million to $900 million annually in the United States.

The group recommended that researchers test *Salmonella* isolates in animals and humans for their multiresistance to the main antimicrobials, and to test carcasses and food products. On the farm, researchers need to study risk factors for ill animals, such as animal movement, antibiotic use, and environmental contamination. During processing, researchers need to evaluate the effectiveness of HACCP systems (Hazard Analysis and Critical Control Points) to reduce carcass contamination, and treatment techniques to reduce infection. The group urged that the role of antibiotics be addressed. Although "pathogen reduction in the production segment of the farm-to-table continuum will be difficult with *S. typhimurium* DT104," the group admitted, "proper handling and thorough cooking of meat animal products will decrease exposure risks."

GERM-PROOFED PRODUCTS?

Foodborne diseases from bacteria, viruses, and parasites have become major health problems as significant as cardiovascular diseases and cancers, according to the Centers for Disease Control and Prevention (CDC). Among numerous strategies being developed to prevent food contamination, numerous household products and objects are being treated with antimicrobials. Are they essential? Are they effective?

Although sanitation is important, some products are turning concerns about germs into phobias. Promotional advertisements suggest that bugs are everywhere, and that consumers need to wage warfare, whether on the kitchen counter or in the toilet bowl. Many products exploit this phobia.

Since the 1990s, hundreds of antibacterial agents have

been incorporated into a wide array of consumer products. They range from soaps, toothbrushes, facial tissues, diapers, cotton swabs, baby wipes, to kitchen cleaners, window cleaners, and even to ball-point pens. Plastic cutting boards, trays, bread and bagel slicers, and kitchen sponges, pretreated with antimicrobials, have been introduced to inactivate or inhibit the growth of pathogens. Pretreated furniture and fixtures are sold, not only for home use, but also for meat-cutting establishments, breweries, restaurants, and supermarkets.

To produce such treated products, antimicrobial pellets are bonded permanently to plastic or fiber. The pellets do not wash off or wear out. The chemical components are reported to be extremely stable during the products' lifetime.

Antimicrobials are incorporated into some food-contacted papers and paperboards. Also, they are impregnated in products such as children's toys and plastic trays attached to children's high chairs. They are used in hospital mattresses, pillow covers and surgical drapes, as well as in carpeting and athletic shoes. Such treatment reportedly inhibits the growth of many pathogens, including *Escherichia coli, Proteus vulgaris, Salmonella pullorum, Salmonella dysenteriae,* and *Staphylococcus aureus.*

False Sense of Safety. Health professionals, governmental officials, and even some industry executives regard some of the germ-fighting claims for these antimicrobial products as exaggerated or misleading. There is "no proven infection-prevention benefit in the use of these products," warns the Association of Professionals in Infectious Controls, an organization of physicians, nurses, and other healthcare workers involved with infection control in medical settings.

The effectiveness of these products has been questioned by Mitchell Cohen, director of the CDC's division of bacterial and mycotic diseases. These products will kill pathogens in laboratory settings, but, asks Cohen, will they kill pathogens "when they are routinely used in the kitchen? Will they result in a decrease in foodborne disease?" Studies are lacking to confirm their benefits beyond the old-fashioned control of hand washing with ordinary soap and water.

The Environmental Protection Agency (EPA) shares responsibility with the Food and Drug Administration (FDA) for surveillance of different types of antimicrobial products used to manufacture packaging materials and substances used in food processing. Under certain conditions, the EPA can transfer its regulatory authority to the FDA. The two agencies have agreed to split jurisdiction over antimicrobial treated products. Actions may be initiated by either agency.

The EPA ordered a company to stop selling unregistered kitchen sponges with pesticide-type claims that the product kills harmful germs. The agency ordered another company to stop advertising claims that its treated kitchen cutting boards "kill infectious bacteria." There was no proof that the products killed organisms such as *Salmonella* or *E. coli.* The EPA reported that the use of the treated cutting boards was acceptable, but consumers should not depend on the treatment for safety. Instead, users should follow the customary practice of washing the boards in hot soapy water after each use.

In another action, the EPA fined a toy company and ordered it to retract a claim that its antimicrobially treated toys would not develop mold, mildew, fungi, or bacteria. Although the antimicrobial used by the company had been registered by the EPA to inhibit bacterial growth in plastic, the chemical had not been approved for public health-oriented claims.

Potential Resistance Problem. The problem of resistance has been raised with the widespread use of the antibacterial agent, triclosan, in treated soaps and detergents. Stuart

B. Levy, M.D., director of the Center for Adaptation Genetics and Drug Resistance at the Tufts School of Medicine, demonstrated that triclosan can trigger genetic changes in bacteria, and might create a more troublesome breed.

Consumers should not be lulled into reliance on antimicrobially treated products as a magic bullet that eliminates the risks of contaminated objects as sources of infectious foodborne illnesses. Such an illusion may end up lowering reliable safeguards.

Levy says, "if you continue to use this antibacterial agent in your home, you'll recruit two kinds of bacteria: one formerly susceptible to the agent but now resistant, and other bacteria that never had a chance to come out in significant numbers before because they were crowded out by the normal bacteria."

Formerly, triclosan was used mainly in hospitals, where infection control is vital. Now, its use has proliferated into total household use. This overconcern with infection control is worrisome, according to Levy. Antibacterial soaps and detergents may be self-defeating by causing resistant strains to develop. (See the article "How Important Is Hand Washing?" on page 345.)

In addition to the potential resistance problem germ-proofed consumer products present, their use may give a false sense of safety. Consumers should not be lulled into reliance on antimicrobially treated products as a magic bullet that eliminates the risks of contaminated objects as sources of infectious foodborne illnesses. Such an illusion may end up lowering reliable safeguards. The prudent approach for all food handlers remains to constantly practice good sanitation in the food preparation area, and practice good personal hygiene.

HOW IMPORTANT IS HAND WASHING?

The Food and Drug Administration (FDA) is convinced that significant numbers of foodborne illnesses are transmitted by food preparers, and that vigorous and rigorous interventions are needed. To achieve this goal, the agency added regulations to its Food Code that assists local, state, and federal government to ensure that foods provided by retail establishments are not vehicles of communicable diseases.

The additions prohibit ill and/or infected food employees from preparing food, and prohibit preparers' bare-handed contact with ready-to-eat food.

Because the latter prohibition is controversial, the FDA requested a review by the National Advisory Committee on Microbiological Criteria for Foods, as well as input from various groups and individuals. Admittedly, scientific data and information are incomplete.

Some Questions that Need Answers. The FDA seeks information about several aspects of the issue. What is the amount of hand contact that can result in pathogen transfer? Does the placement of a garnish, such as a parsley sprig on a plate or a lemon wedge on a glass, transfer pathogens? Can pathogens be transferred to raw produce by bare-handed workers who wash the produce? Can pathogens be transferred by bare-handed workers to dry foods such as toast or rolls? The FDA also seeks information about what constitutes a properly performed hand wash.

Are Gloved Hands the Answer? Despite lack of agreement, the FDA has imposed a "glove rule" or "no-bare hands" contact with ready-to-eat foods (such as sandwiches and salads). The National Advisory Committee on Microbiological Criteria for Foods finds that sufficient data are lacking. Representatives from affected groups also voiced uncertainties. They argue that a ban on bare-handed food contacts is unnecessary if proper hand washing and basic sanitation measures are followed.

The National Restaurant Association (NRA) reports that in the few states with mandated glove use, there is no evidence demonstrating that the glove practice reduces foodborne illness. Instead, California, Florida, and Texas have opted for increased hand washing compliance.

Steve Grover, representing the NRA, reports that there are some types of food handling that make glove use impractical. He demonstrated by donning a pair of foodworker gloves and showed how difficult it was to peel shrimp without tearing the gloves. Grover concluded that mandatory glove use, though tempting, is not the solution.

A program that mandates food handlers to wear gloves may backfire. The use of gloves actually may discourage food preparers from practicing good hand washing. "Gloves are not effective for preventing cross-contamination of food, unless proper personal hygiene practices are followed by the foodservice personnel," notes the Food Marketing Institute (FMI). "Gloving is not and should not be considered to be an effective substitute for proper hygienic practices."

The FMI reports that "if individuals do not wash their hands thoroughly before donning gloves, the food-contact surface of the gloves may become contaminated with the very microorganisms from which the gloves are intended to form a barrier."

Within the warm, moist glove environment, high bacterial levels multiply on the skin. Therefore, if gloves are used, immediately after they are removed it is vital that the hands be washed thoroughly. Otherwise, any surfaces or foods contacted after glove removal may become contaminated.

Bacteria on gloved hands can double every forty minutes when the hands are dry, according to the International Association of Milk, Food, and Environmental Sanitarians.

In some cases, gloves also worsen the problem, because the food preparer does not realize that the gloves are dirty.

The structure of the gloves also may contribute to the transmission of pathogens. Oils adhere to gloves and can promote adherence of microorganisms to the gloves.

Some 80 percent of food-grade vinyl gloves have preexisting punctures or tears. Studies on the use of vinyl gloves "strongly suggest that the increased safety margin thought to be derived from wearing gloves to prevent the transmission of disease from contaminated hands may be grossly overestimated," according to the Compliance Control Center, an industry group.

Are Antibacterial Soaps the Answer? The widespread use of antibacterial soaps may cause problems worse than the ones they are intended to prevent. Stuart B. Levy, M.D. and his associates at the Center for Adaptation Genetics and Drug Resistance, Tufts University School of Medicine, investigated triclosan, a common antibacterial ingredient in soaps and detergents. They demonstrated that triclosan behaves a lot like an antibiotic, and could encourage bacteria to mutate in ways that make them resistant to antibacterials, including antibiotics. (See the article "Germ-proofed Products?" on page 341.)

Are Hand Sanitizers the Answer? Although regular use of soap and water hand washing procedures is the gold standard, other solutions may be important when hand washing is hampered by lack of ready access to sinks. The use of alcoholic or peroxide solutions to clean hands is judged to be safe and effective for those who process and handle foods. These liquids work by dissolving the membrane walls of bacteria. They are nonspecific. Unlike triclosan, they do not promote resistance

Waterless hand sanitizers, consisting of about two-thirds ethyl alcohol, are reported to be capable of killing 99.95 percent of pathogens within fifteen seconds. These sanitizers, intended for bare-handed use, are compatible with rubber glove use, too.

Some alcohol-free hand sanitizers also are reported to kill 99.9 percent of most disease-causing pathogens. Unlike the antibacterial soaps that lose their effectiveness over time, these sanitizers reportedly have sustained antimicrobial activity.

Iodine-coated wipes are available to sanitize either wet or dry hands of food preparers. Also, wipes coated with a quaternary sanitizing compound can reduce microbial levels on food-contact surfaces.

Hand sanitizers, however, have limitations. Applying sanitizers without hand washing first is a futile exercise. "You cannot sanitize a dirty surface," warns Dennis Bogart, an industry sanitation expert. Debra De Vlieger, from the FDA, adds that sanitizers cannot penetrate organic materials to get to the bacteria.

Sanitarians tested instant hand sanitizers, and found that their use could significantly increase bacteria on hands. Researchers report in Dairy, Food, and Environmental Sanitation that the use of instant hand sanitizers in foodservice establishments could be ineffective.

Are Antibacterial Hand Lotions the Answer? Some restaurants have opted to provide food preparers with antibacterial lotions in lieu of rubber gloves. These lotions reportedly eliminate pathogens and other organisms from the hands. The antibacterials (registered with the FDA) form an invisible polymer coating, that bonds electrochemically to the outermost layer of skin. The active disinfectant, at 0.3 percent in the lotion, is reported to kill *E. coli, Salmonella, Staphylococcus, Listeria,* and *Streptococcus* on contact, and to minimize chapping that results from frequent hand washing. These lotions are reported to last up to four hours after application, and to remain on the hands despite repeated hand washings. There is no mention about the possibility that these lotions might transfer from the treated hands to the foods being prepared.

Are Automated Devices the Answer? To help reduce pathogen transmission in foods, mandatory use of hands-free water taps in food processing facilities has been suggested. Automated faucets already exist in many settings, including restaurant bathrooms and public facilities in airports, bus terminals, and railway stations.

The Centers for Disease Control and Prevention considers proper and frequent hand washing to be one of the most important interventions in preventing the spread of infectious diseases.

Studies show that restaurants with "no touch" automated hand-washing stations, whether for bare-handed or gloved food preparers, can reduce levels of pathogens significantly over manual faucet operations. Also, the automation eliminates the time variability in manual washing.

Along with automated faucets, additional automated devices have been introduced that present a new technique for compliance. One system simplifies hand washing to its most basic level for foodservice food preparers. A "no touch" hand washing system makes use of two cylinders into which employees are required to plunge their hands. This action initiates spinning of the cylinders, triggered by electric eye sensors. A high-pressure, low-volume warm water spray containing an antimicrobial solution is ejected through a nozzle with twenty jets, for twenty seconds.

This automation is carried to a new dimension with electronically controlled hand wash monitoring and verification systems. The first one was introduced in 1997, and displayed at the National Restaurant Show. The system monitors the employee, who is required to wear a badge that begins to blink when the employee enters the bathroom. A badge continues to blink if a person does not use the soap dispenser, or fails to spend adequate time in front of the sink. Employers can obtain daily printouts about the hand-washing practices of individual employees. This paternalistic approach may backfire. Just as some smokers find ways to bypass smoke detectors, employees may seek ways to thwart automated hand washing systems.

Automated systems fail to instill in employees the habit of hand washing. One study of more than a million employee hours evaluated hand-washing compliance. Findings were dismal. Employees averaged less than one hand wash per day. After electronic hand-washing control and verification systems were installed at test locations, and employees were given individual badges to activate water flow, the number of hand washings increased dramatically. However, after the systems were removed, hand-washing performance returned to the same lax level of less than one hand washing per day per employee.

Is Proper and Frequent Hand Washing the Answer? The Centers for Disease Control and Prevention (CDC) considers proper and frequent hand washing to be one of the most important interventions in preventing the spread of infectious diseases.

The CDC's annual update (1999) of pathogens transmitted through food-handling includes: Norwalk and Norwalk-like viruses, hepatitis A virus, *Salmonella typhi*, *Shigella* species, *Staphylococcus aureus*, and *Streptococcus pyogenes*. Pathogens occasionally transmitted include: *Campylobacter jejuni*, *Cryptosporidium parvum*, *Entamoeba histolyitica*, enterohemorrhagic (causing to hemorrhage in the intestine) and enterotoxigenic (causing to be toxic in the intestine) *Escherichia coli*, *Giardia lamblia*, nontyphoidal *Salmonella*, Rotavirus, Taenia *solium* (tapeworm), *Vibrio cholerae* 01, and *Yersinia enterocolitica*.

Hand Contacts in Nonfood Settings

At the beginning of life, hospital-acquired infections with respiratory syncytial virus (RSV) are a major problem, spread primarily by infectious nasal secretions. By separating infected infants, and encouraging hospital staff and parents to wash their hands before contacting the infants, the incidence of RSV infection is reduced significantly.

A study showed that generic liquid dishwasher detergent was up to 100 times more effective against RSV transmission than antibacterial soaps commonly used in hospitals.

Daycare centers need to adopt strict hand washing policies and become far more vigilant in disinfecting surfaces to prevent the spread of bacteria that cause diarrhea in young children. In a study, licensed day care centers were found to have high levels of coliform contamination, especially in kitchen areas and on the hands of daycare workers. Researchers took cultures from the hands of staff workers and children, as well as from faucets, toilets, walls, floors, diaper-changing areas, furniture, tabletops, toys, and countertops. The highest rates of contamination were found in the kitchen areas where 19 percent of the surfaces sampled were contaminated. Sixteen percent of staff workers had fecal coliform on their hands—nearly three times the contamination rate of the children. Centers with hand-washing rules had significantly lower contamination rates than centers that were lax.

Residents in long-term care establishments are at risk of acquiring facility-associated infections. Laxity in hand-washing practices and lack of glove use have been found to be important factors.

More Americans die yearly from hospital infections than from car wrecks and homicides combined. Many of these infections can be avoided if hospital personnel practice hand washing.

According to Duncan W. Clark, M.D., "hand washing is the most simple and effective method for preventing hospital-acquired infection." Dr. Clark wrote a resolution for the American Medical Association, adopted unanimously. The resolution, "Ten Dirty Digits," brought to the attention of health professionals the failure to practice routine hand washing. Studies show that only 14 to 59 percent of physicians, 25 to 45 percent of nurses, and 23 to 73 percent of other health workers routinely wash their hands between patient examinations. Dr. Clark noted that 1997 marked the 150th anniversary of the pioneering efforts of the Austrian physician, Ignaz Semmelweiss to stress the importance of hand washing in order to reduce infection transmission. His message still needs to be heeded.

Infected food handlers can transmit pathogens to others through bodily fluids from diarrhea, vomit, open skin sores, boils, fever, urine, or jaundice. The objective is to break the chain of infection, either by eliminating the causative agent (through good personal hygiene and good sanitation practices) or breaking transmission by means of proper hand washing.

In the food industry, improper hand washing is perhaps the main factor in cross-contamination. Some estimate that as many as one in four cases of foodborne illnesses is due to poor hygiene practices. At times, poor hand washing practices result because of the inaccessibility of water and soap sources. Sometimes, pathogens resist insufficiently hot water, or insufficient scrubbing. Frequently, hand washing is not practiced.

Hand contact by food preparers at foodservice establishments is a global concern. Numerous surveys indicate poor practices in numerous settings where food is prepared. These are some findings:

- One third of all cases of foodborne illnesses result from contaminated food preparers. In the CDC's surveillance data of nearly 3,000 outbreaks, poor personal hygiene was a contributing factor.
- According to the U.S. Department of Agriculture (USDA), people think that they wash their hands, whereas in reality they are only rinsing them.
- According to the Texas Department of Health, nobody is monitoring certain risky practices, such as a restaurant employee who fails to wash hands after handling raw meat, and then picks up a platter of food for serving.
- In a 1998 FDA/USDA Consumer Food Safety Survey, 24 percent of consumers admitted they do not wash their hands with soap after handling food such as raw meat; and 21 percent do not wash their cutting boards after cutting these foods. In addition, 32 percent admitted to not washing their hands before cooking the main meal.
- A study of more than 300 Detroit school children found that youngsters who washed their hands four times a day had 24 percent fewer sick days due to respiratory illness, and 51 percent fewer days lost because of stomach upset than children who had poor hand-washing practice.
- In a home-safety survey of 121 households in eighty-two cities in the United States and Canada, registered dietitians observed food preparation practices for one meal. The observers applied the same standards of food safety and sanitation required for restaurants. Hand washing deficiencies were found in 20 percent of all households,

> with a 57 percent frequency of critical violations. The poor practices were failures to wash hands before handling foods; after using telephones; after touching one's face, hair, body, or other people; after handling garbage, soiled dishes, or using the bathroom.

Household sponges and dishcloths tend to harbor bacteria. If used, they should be changed frequently. Use of disposable paper towels is more sanitary than cloth towels. If cloth towels are used, they should be washed frequently.

CUTTING BOARDS: WOOD OR PLASTIC?

For many years it was assumed that hard plastic cutting boards were impervious, could be cleaned thoroughly, and were more hygienic than porous wooden ones. This untested assumption led the U.S. Department of Agriculture (USDA) to urge use of plastic cutting boards in home kitchens, and for sanitarians to endorse them for commercial use.

Pathogens Thrive on Plastic. In 1993, this assumption was challenged by unexpected findings of microbiologists at the Food Research Institute of the University of Wisconsin at Madison. With concerns about the increasing problems of foodborne illnesses, Dean O. Cliver and Nese O. Ak were attempting to find ways to decontaminate wooden cutting boards and make them as safe as plastic ones for home use. To their surprise, they discovered that pathogens disappeared on wood, but thrived on plastic.

Experimentally, Cliver and Ak contaminated five-centimeter blocks from both plastic and wooden cutting boards with two nonpathogenic strains of *Escherichia coli;* the virulently pathogenic strain, *E. coli* 0157:H7; *Listeria innocus; L. monocytogenes;* or *Salmonella typhimurium.* Cliver and Ak reported that "bacteria inoculated onto plastic blocks were readily recovered for minutes to hours and would multiply if held overnight. However, "recoveries from wooden blocks were generally less than those from plastic blocks, regardless of new or used status; differences increased with holding time." Clean wood blocks usually absorbed the inoculum completely within three to ten minutes. If the fluids contained the amount of bacteria likely to come from raw meat or poultry, the bacteria generally could not be recovered after entering the wood. At much higher levels, they might be recovered after twelve hours at room temperature and with high humidity, but their numbers were reduced by at least 98 percent, and more often by more than 99.9 percent. The small remainder was readily removed with hot water and detergent. Cliver and Ak concluded that "cross contamination seems unlikely if the bacteria cannot be recovered by the procedures used in these experiments."

Surprised by their results, the researchers repeated the experiments several times. Each time, after exposure of only three minutes, in each type of wood tested, more than 99.9 percent of the bacteria disappeared. Yet, all bacteria on plastic surfaces survived. Old knife-scarred wood performed as well as new wood in its antibacterial effect. Yet similarly scarred plastic seemed to encourage growth. The bacteria on plastic survived soap and hot water scrubbing.

Despite these findings, the USDA's Meat and Poultry Hotline, in response to numerous consumer calls, continued to recommend nonporous materials such as plastic. Susan Conley, the Hotline director, urged the use of unmarred surfaces of nonporous materials, and mentioned plastic, marble, or glass. (Yet all three do become knife-scarred.) The USDA's Agricultural Research Service (ARS) found bacteria more difficult to remove from some wooden boards, and suggested that plastic cutting boards are preferable for safe food preparation. The ARS reported that "results of the majority of past studies also seem to support the traditional viewpoint that nonporous surfaces such as plastic are more easily cleaned and sanitized than wood."

Follow-up Studies of Cutting Boards. In 1994, Cliver and Ak, joined by C.W. Kaspar, did additional studies with four blocks of polymers (plastics), hard rubber, and nine hardwoods. Bacteria were applied in a nutrient broth or chicken juice, and recovered by pressing the blocks onto nutrient agar. Bacteria inoculated onto plastic blocks readily recovered after minutes to hours. They multiplied when held overnight. Recovery of bacteria from the wooden blocks generally was less than those from the others.

Although new plastic cutting surfaces were relatively easy to clean and were microbiologically clear, plastic boards with extensive knife scars were difficult to clean manually, especially if they had chicken fat deposits on them. Cleaning of the wooden boards with hot water and detergent generally removed remaining bacteria, regardless of bacterial species, wood species, and whether the wood was new or used.

Additional follow-up tests were made by microbiologists at the University of Michigan. By scanning with an electron microscope, viable bacteria were detected on wooden cutting boards. But the researchers concluded that as long as surfaces were maintained in a hygienic fashion and sanitized frequently, there would be no danger of cross contamination either from a wooden butcher's block or a plastic block.

An ideal cutting board for commercial operations would be stainless steel, according to Dr. Mansell Griffiths, a microbiologist at the University of Guelph in Canada. But, he added that it would be "prohibitively expensive and impractical."

During early 1997, Cliver, joined by P.K. Park, updated the findings from the University of Michigan. They, too, used an electron microscope to study three types of plastic cutting boards. The scanning revealed new surprises. Plastic cutting boards had holes, grooves, punctures, and cavities that can shelter bacteria from manual cleaning. Polyethylene and foamed polypropylene were found to contain holes and perforations, even when the plastics were new. During normal use, these surfaces acquired large numbers of deep knife mark grooves, punctures, and cavities. Although acrylic cutting boards acquired fewer knife marks, with use they became much more splintered and fractured. All three surfaces were inoculated with a nutrient broth containing *L. monocytogenes, Staphylococcus aureus,* and *E. coli.* Vigorous washing with detergent and hot water did not remove the bacteria from cavities in the board. Dried bacteria deposits formed a biofilmlike attachment to the surface of the acrylic board. These results may help to explain the findings in recent studies: used plastic surfaces are more difficult to clean manually than old wooden surfaces.

Cleaning Advice. What are consumers to make of all this confusing information? The last pronouncements probably have not been made. Meanwhile, whatever type of cutting board you use, keep it clean. Wash it with hot soapy water, especially after handling raw flesh foods. Allow the board to air dry, or use clean paper towels. Sanitize it frequently by using a solution of two teaspoons of chlorine bleach in each quart of water. Rinse well in clear water. If possible, invest in two cutting boards. Reserve one for cutting raw flesh foods, and the other for cutting all other foods. Play it safe.

BENEFICIAL BACTERIA COMBAT PATHOGENS

Bifidobacteria were identified as early as 1899 at the Pasteur Institute in Paris. Since then, research continues to add to our knowledge of these beneficial bacteria.

The intestine of the human fetus is sterile, but after birth many bacteria begin to colonize. Bifidobacteria are among the first to establish themselves in the infant's intestinal tract, and in the healthy infant, they predominate. They continue to be found in the mature intestinal tract, albeit at lower levels than those in the infant.

Bifidobacteria thrive in human milk. They grow better in human milk than in cows' milk due to differences in protein content and abilities to buffer against invading pathogens. Breast-fed infants have more bifidobacteria than do formula-fed infants. Also, breast-fed infants have lower amounts of harmful bacteria such as *Streptococci* than do formula-fed infants. As growing infants are given solid foods, the beneficial bifidobacteria remain, but decline in numbers.

Bifidobacteria, by predominating as the major intestinal flora, lower the pH (acid-alkaline balance) of the intestinal contents. The increased acidic level discourages growth of acid-sensitive pathogens such as *Clostridium perfringens.*

Diarrhea and Other Intestinal Problems. Bifidobacteria help control diarrhea and other intestinal problems and help reestablish or maintain healthy microfloral balance in the gut. Foods supplemented with bifidobacteria may offer additional benefits, by helping good digestion, strengthening the immune system, reducing serum cholesterol, preventing tumor formation, improving lactose tolerance, synthesizing fractions of the B vitamins, and helping to improve overall health.

In one study, children with chronic diarrhea were given traditional drug therapy, antibiotics, and special diets, but the diarrhea persisted as long as ten weeks. When given bifidobacteria preparations, the chronic diarrhea lessened in all children within three to seven days.

In another study, volunteer adults with diarrhea were given bifidus-supplemented yogurt three times daily, in addition to a common antibiotic treatment. After three days, the patients had less abdominal discomfort and fewer bowel movements.

For many elderly people, intestinal movements are weak. Constipation is common, and lack of exercise can make the problem worse. In a study of bedridden elderly people, stool frequency was noted before and after bifidus-supplemented yogurt was eaten. Before, the stool frequency was poor; after supplementation, it improved. After the bifidus-supplemented yogurt was withdrawn, the stool frequency became poor once again, as before the test. The findings demonstrated the benefit of long-term, continuous supplementation.

Infections. In recent years, there have been many investigations of bifidobacteria's ability to prevent infections from pathogens that invade the intestinal tract. In the last two decades, both animal studies and test-tube experiments have shown bifidobacteria's capacity to reduce infections from strains of *Shigella, Escherichia coli,* and other pathogens.

Among the studies were bifidobacteria's antitumor activities. Whole cells, or cell-wall preparation of bifidobacteria, were able to inhibit tumor cells in test mice.

Vitamin B Fractions. Bifidobacteria's ability to produce some fractions of vitamin B was demonstrated. Some strains were found to produce high levels of riboflavin (vitamin B_2) and pyridoxine (vitamin B_6). One strain produced biotin. These findings suggest that when bifidobacteria-supplemented food is eaten, some vitamin B fractions may be produced in the intestine.

Development of Bifidus-supplemented Foods. In Japan, where bifidobacteria have been studied since 1950, bifido-supplemented yogurt is manufactured by a process similar to the one used to process traditional yogurt, except for a different inoculating culture. Strains of bifidobacteria are selected that grow well in milk. The lactic acid starter must be compatible, to ensure lower acid production which affects cell viability. Because bifidobacteria are anaerobic, oxygen must be excluded when the product is manufactured, packaged, and stored. The packaging must have low oxygen permeability. For this purpose, glass bottles or aluminum-laminated packages are used for most types of products. Some plastics are satisfactory, if they are good oxygen barriers.

In the United States, some dairies have begun the practice of adding bifidus, as well as acidophilus, another beneficial bacterium, to yogurts, in addition to the starter bacteria used to convert milk to yogurt. As more information is generated regarding the values of these beneficial bacteria, they may be introduced into more products. Label information is helpful for knowing the ingredients in fermented milk products, including any added bacteria.

In the future, no doubt, there will be greater interest in the development of bifidus-supplemented foods, as their benefits are more widely acknowledged.

Chapter 10

CONTAMINANTS IN OUR FOOD

MONITORING PESTICIDES IN OUR FOOD

How safe is our food? And who is monitoring food safety? As federal regulatory agencies devote resources and energy to monitoring the food supply, it is important for consumers to know what programs exist to cope with reported problems. The following discussion is limited to the existing programs and their effectiveness in one area of food safety: the monitoring of pesticide residues in food.

The Food and Drug Administration (FDA) has the greatest responsibility for monitoring pesticides in foods. However, it shares some responsibility with the Environmental Protection Agency (EPA), and the U. S. Department of Agriculture (USDA).

The EPA's Role. The EPA is responsible for registering pesticides and establishing tolerances for any pesticides that may leave residues in food. The tolerance level is the maximum amount of residue that is presumed not to present an unacceptable health risk.

Over the years, the concept of what constitutes an unacceptable risk has widened. Safety tests of pesticides now are required to determine, among other effects, a pesticide's potential to cause chronic illness in humans, including reproductive disorders, birth defects, and cancer, as well as environmental damage. In 1972, Congress required the EPA to reregister older pesticides in accordance with current requirements.

Pesticide producers who seek approval by the EPA for use of a new pesticide must submit results from toxicological studies, data on the pesticide's environmental fate, and results of actual field testing. Before registering a compound, the EPA evaluates these data—balancing risks against benefits—the safety of the residue level, the necessity of an adequate and economical food supply, and other ways in which consumers might be affected by the specific chemical as well as other chemicals related to it.

In 1978, in an attempt to improve pesticide regulations, Congress mandated the EPA to begin reassessing the safety of some 35,000 registered pesticide products. The program was reviewed by the General Accounting Office (GAO) in 1980. The GAO reported that the EPA had restricted or canceled uses of some pesticides, but many remained unevaluated. The GAO concluded that the EPA's limited actions left the public largely unprotected, and faulted the EPA for being hopelessly behind schedule, with many unresolved and procedural issues that jeopardized its success.

In 1986, again the GAO reviewed the EPA's reassessment program. By then, the EPA's responsibility for registered pesticides had risen to some 50,000 products. The GAO found that most of the older registered products had not yet been fully tested and evaluated in accordance with current requirements. The EPA's efforts at reassessments and reregistrations had progressed so slowly that completion would require several decades. The GAO recommended that the EPA reregister older pesticides "in the most expeditious manner practicable" and cancel registration of those products whose labels were not in compliance with registration standard requirements.

The USDA's Role. The USDA is responsible for pesticide surveillance solely with meat and poultry. The agency has authority over food animal inspection. Its division of Food

Safety and Quality Service (FSQS) samples and tests for various pesticides and other chemicals.

The USDA shares some responsibility with the FDA, the agency that has authority over food animals before slaughter and after the USDA's inspection is completed. The USDA shares responsibility with the FDA, too, in monitoring eggs and egg products.

The two agencies work jointly under the Food Safety and Inspection Service (FSIS). This group notifies the FDA whenever an inspection reveals a tissue with an illegal level of a pesticide (or other chemicals, including animal drugs) in meat and poultry. The FDA conducts a follow-up inspection of those involved in the production and marketing of the meat or poultry in question, and is empowered to take regulatory action when warranted.

In order to increase communication between the two agencies, the Residue Violation Information System (RVIS) was initiated. This nationwide interagency database contains information about tissue residues found in all domestically slaughtered livestock and poultry. The RVIS offers access to information nearly round-the-clock, seven days a week. The data enable both agencies to identify and track repeated violators, especially across regional boundaries. Formerly, it was difficult to track repeat violators because they would ship to multiple slaughter facilities using different identities. Now the system provides additional information about violators, such as "also known as . . . " and "doing business as . . ."

The FDA's Role. The major responsibility for pesticide monitoring rests with the FDA. The agency monitors all foods shipped interstate, including domestically raised and imported foods. The agency has developed a number of programs over the years to cope with an ever-mounting volume and complexity of problems.

In the 1960s, the FDA established a program to monitor the nation's food supply for pesticide residues. According to the FDA, data gathered over the years demonstrated that, in general, pesticide chemicals are used according to label directions, and violative residue levels are the exceptions. Above-tolerance residues can result from misuse of pesticides, poor agricultural practices, or at times, from unusual weather conditions.

More commonly, according to the FDA, violations involve pesticides for which no tolerance has been established for use with certain crops. Aldicarb, for example, was used on watermelons in 1985 by some growers, although it had not been registered for use with this crop. The illegal use resulted in acute food poisonings before the watermelons could be located and destroyed. This incident, and others, caused the GAO to criticize the FDA for not preventing the marketing of most of the food found to contain illegal pesticide residues. The GAO criticized the FDA, too, for not penalizing growers who market food with illegal pesticide when the FDA is unable to remove it from the market.

The FDA may take legal action to remove foods from the market if they have violative pesticide residue levels. With domestic foods, the FDA can seize the foods or order injunctions; with imported foods, it can detain shipments at ports of entry.

The FDA may establish a regulatory limit for long-lasting pesticides that had been in use but subsequently were banned. An example is DDT, a pesticide banned in the late 1970s, but which persistently continues to contaminate foods.

- *The FDA's Testing Program:* The FDA collects domestic food samples as close as possible to the point of production in the food distribution chain. This procedure offers the best opportunity to identify shipments of fresh produce and other foods that may contain illegal pesticide residues, and if necessary, to take prompt regulatory action. The FDA selects samples of crops based on how often the food is used in the diet, or if there is a history of residue problems with the food.

The FDA analyzes samples of both domestically raised and imported foods for pesticide residues. Generally, the techniques used for these tests are capable of determining residues at levels below the established tolerance, but not as low as more sensitive techniques can test.

The GAO reported that the FDA did not test foods regularly for a large number of pesticides that might be used or present on foods, including many that—by the FDA's own admission—required continuous or periodic monitoring because they were known to be potential health hazards. Since the GAO's charges, the FDA has attempted to lessen this problem by conducting selective surveys. The agency determines the occurrence of a particular pesticide or a group of chemically related pesticides in a number of different crops. Or, the agency may concentrate efforts on sampling one crop for one or more different pesticides. These surveys may examine food-pesticide combinations that may not normally be covered as part of ongoing monitoring.

The FDA recognizes that for some pesticides, several residues, including various forms, breakdown products, or alteration products, need to be considered in order to evaluate the total amount of residue for a specific pesticide. For example, an analysis of the total residue for DDT must include its numerous breakdown products. At times, the breakdown product is more toxic than the parent compound.

- *Market Basket Study*. The Market Basket Study, also known as the Total Diet Study, is another tool for the FDA's pesticide monitoring. This ongoing study attempts to estimate how much total pesticide is consumed by males and females, in eight different age groups ranging from infants to the elderly.

In conducting this study, the FDA staffers purchase foods from common retail outlets throughout the country. Seasonal purchases are made four times yearly. The samples are chosen from three cities in a specific region, and each year the chosen cities are different. The sampling contains several hundred individual food items, with selections based on nationwide dietary surveys. The foods are prepared as they would be if consumed, and then analyzed for pesticide residues (and other substances).

The results, along with data on the amounts of the foods likely to be consumed, allow for calculations of the probable dietary intake of pesticide residues. The amounts provide estimates of the actual amounts consumed in foods as they are eaten, because pesticide levels may be changed in washing, peeling, and cooking. Usually, such preparations succeed in lowering residue levels.

In the Market Basket Study, as well as in regulatory monitoring, the FDA analyzes foods for some several hundred pesticides for possible residues. This number includes a wide variety of commonly used pesticides, but does not represent the larger total of all that are in use.

FDA officials believe that the residue levels and corresponding intake of the pesticides not tested in the samples probably are similar to those that are tested.

Data from the Market Basket Study are used to develop dietary intake information on pesticide residues and to compare these intakes with "acceptable daily intakes" (ADIs). These amounts are defined as the daily intake of a chemical that, if ingested over a lifetime, appear to be without appreciable risk. The ADIs are established by the United Nations' Food and Agriculture Organization (FAO) and the World Health Organization (WHO).

Effective Enough? Well-publicized incidents have led to increased awareness and actions that have strengthened

How Effective Are Controls on Imported Food?

Imported foods account for an ever-increasing proportion of the American food supply. A GAO review of the FDA's pesticide surveillance of imported foods recommended that better sampling and enforcement were needed with imported foods. The GAO noted that the FDA was sampling only a very small percentage of imported food shipments (less than 1 percent of about one million shipments of imported foods), and that the selections of samplings were left to individual judgments of the FDA inspectors, who tended to sample foods imported in large quantities, leaving many other types unsampled. The GAO noted that the FDA laboratories relied on tests capable of detecting less than half of all of the pesticides potentially available in world markets. The FDA was limited in targeting tests due to a lack of knowledge about which pesticides are used in foreign countries.

The FDA, acting on some of the GAO's recommendations, improved its ability to monitor imported foods, especially fresh produce. The agency purchased the Battelle World Agrochemical Data Bank. This computerized data base contains information on worldwide pesticide use, and helps the FDA target its monitoring of individual imported foods for specific countries.

Imported foods now comprise more than half of all samples analyzed, due to our increased use of imported foods. The rate of violative levels of pesticide residues in samples of imported crops is far more than the rate on domestic crops. If the FDA discovers violative import samples for a specific commodity, the agency may invoke a certification requirement. In effect, this is an automatic detention.

Certification may be required from all shippers from a country where widespread use of illegal residues commonly is tolerated. The certification requirement has clout by making the regulated industry responsible for correcting pesticide residue problems. The automatic detention was further strengthened by the FDA adoption of a procedure to invoke automatic detention if a single shipment contained a violative level of pesticide residue.

Certification requires the importer to be responsible for having each shipment in question analyzed and certified by a private laboratory that the food is free of violative levels of the residue(s) in question. A certificate of analysis must accompany the import documents for each shipment subjected to certification, which is reviewed by the FDA.

monitoring. The system is incredibly complex. Despite its shortcomings, our system compares favorably, and functions better than most pesticide-monitoring programs elsewhere in the world. Our system is not foolproof. It can be improved by using state-of-the-art testing, careful monitoring, systematic re-evaluations, and vigorous enforcement of regulations. Although 100 percent safety cannot be guaranteed, the food supply can be made as safe as possible by means of the entire body of monitoring programs and enforcement regulations.

ASBESTOS CONTAMINATION OF FOODS AND BEVERAGES

Although the hazards of human inhalation of asbestos fibers are well established, the hazards of human *ingestion* of these fibers are largely unknown. Several incidents and investigations would seem to indicate that asbestos contamination of beverages, foods, and drinking water may add another and very important dimension to the environmental problem of asbestos pollution.

The high incidence of both abdominal neoplasms and gastrointestinal cancer among asbestos workers, and the knowledge that asbestos fibers may penetrate the mucosa of the stomach and the intestinal wall of animals prompted the Health Protection Branch of the Canadian Department of National Health and Welfare to investigate the presence and distribution of asbestos fibers in beverages and foods. In 1968, asbestos fibers had already been found and reported in beer. In the United States, state health officials making inspections in 1972, found asbestos fibers in products from a brewery and a distillery. The brewery switched to cellulose filters, and the distillery attempted to find a suitable substitute filter medium for clarifying its products. Canadian authorities suggested that such material might find its way through filtering systems into city drinking water supplies, as well as filtered beverages, both alcoholic and nonalcoholic.

Tested samples of beer, wine, sherry, port, vermouth, and soft drinks from Canada, the United States, Europe, and South Africa. All of the samples contained asbestos fibers.

The physicochemical properties of asbestos make it highly suitable for purposes of filtration. In beverage and food processing, as well as in preparation of drugs, filtration is widely used in various stages of manufacturing processes, from the preparation of raw materials, through intermediate steps, to final filtration of products. In order to minimize or prevent the growth of bacteria and their toxins, the speed of final filtration may be critical. Chrysotile, a variety of asbestos, allows for such rapid filtration, and is widely used in food and beverage processing, with products such as sugar, lard, edible oils, fruit juices, soft drinks, beer, wine, liquor, and drinking water.

Tests for Contamination. Dr. H.M. Cunningham, head of the Canadian Department on Food Additives and Contaminants, and Dr. R. Pontefract, research scientist in the department's biochemistry division, tested samples of beer, wine, sherry, port, vermouth, and soft drinks from Canada, the United States, Europe, and South Africa. All of the samples contained asbestos fibers. Many of the fibers were hidden in clumps of debris such as mineral matter in water, and in diatomaceous earth (an extremely fine, inert dust composed of the shells of diatoms—microscopic algae), which, in some cases, was used as a filtering aid. Asbestos contamination in the filtered beverages may not necessarily be the result of filtration, but may have been present in the water used to produce the beverage.

Drs. Cunningham and Pontefract analyzed tap water from three Canadian cities that have modern filtration systems. All of the samples of the water contained asbestos fibers. Samples of unfiltered water, taken from an asbestos mining town, had a far higher count of asbestos fibers. In some tests of water samples from 82,000 to 296,000 fibers per liter were found. The use of water pipes made of a mixture of asbestos and cement further complicates the problem of asbestos-contaminated water. In the United States, some 800,000 miles of water pipes contain some asbestos.

On the basis of these findings, the two researchers conducted experiments to learn what happens when asbestos is present in the stomach. When asbestos was injected into the stomach of rats, the fibers passed through the walls of the digestive tract, traveled through the blood, and ultimately became deposited in vital organs such as the brain, spleen, lungs, liver, and kidneys. The researchers suggested the need for further studies, to determine the extent to which asbestos fibers may penetrate the walls of the human digestive tract, the degree to which they may be transported to organs of the body, and the biological significance of their presence in various tissues.

The water of Lake Superior had long been regarded as the most uncontaminated of all the Great Lakes. That was true until the Environmental Protection Agency (EPA) disclosed that high concentrations of potentially dangerous asbestos fibers had been found in Lake Superior, which supplies the drinking water for Duluth and several other Minnesota communities, as well as to Wisconsin and Michigan. The source of the contamination, the agency announced, was probably a taconite (iron ore) processing plant, located seventy miles from Duluth, which had been discharging many thousands of tons of taconite waste daily over a period of years. Because the health effects from drinking asbestos-contaminated water are unknown, communities using Lake Superior water were advised to find alternate sources of drinking water for very young children. As a result, school systems and parents switched to well water and bottled drinking water.

Asbestos in Food and Food Packaging. Asbestos fibers may be introduced into the human digestive tract from other sources. Asbestos and talc are both silicate compounds, and frequently they are found intermixed in the same ore deposits. They differ in physical structure rather than in chemical composition. Asbestos is fibrous, while talc is flaky or granular. Medical warnings were issued as early as 1972 regarding the use of asbestos-contaminated talcum powder with infants. Studies had shown that some talcum powders contained from 5 to 25 percent of asbestos, which could be inhaled by infants and caregivers.

Talc is officially approved as a food additive for certain purposes. Thus, ingested talc, which happens to contain asbestos fibers, is a distinct health hazard. Talc was first approved as a flavor-fixative coating on polished rice, under the Food and Drug Act of 1906. Additional uses for talc as a food additive were sanctioned later: in paper, paperboard, cotton and cotton fabrics used for dry food packaging; on confections and chewing gums, as release and dusting agents; and in table salt, vanilla and vanilla-vanillin powders, garlic and onion powders, dry soup mixes, baking powder, as an ingredient of dried egg yolk, icing sugar, and certain dietary supplements, with labels showing silicate compounds, and as anticaking agents to render such dry substances free flowing.

For the Japanese market, polished rice is first treated with glucose, and then with talc. Microscopic examination of such treated rice, produced and sold in California, showed asbestos form fibers. The rice contained both pathogenic amphibole asbestos and chrysotile, the most popular commercial form of asbestos fiber. Such treated rice, cooked in Japan and sent to the United States for analysis, showed similiar contamination.

Epidemiologic data support a cause-and-effect relationship between the talc additive and stomach cancer. Stomach cancer is most prevalent in those areas in Japan where the main staple is rice, and less prevalent where rice is supplemented by other cereal grains and fermented soybean products. The incidence of gastric neoplasms (abnormal morbid new growths or tumors in the stomach) is highest among Japanese who eat rice with every meal, but the incidence declines as preference increases for vegetables and milk. Reuben R. Merliss, M.D., an investigator in this field, suggested that talc, not rice, is the cancer-causing agent, because "in other oriental countries where talc-coated rice is not popular the incidence of stomach cancer is not unduly high."

Stronger Protection for the Consumer. Tests conducted by the Food and Drug Administration (FDA) confirmed the presence of asbestos fibers on talc-coated polished rice. In August 1972, the agency proposed that talc used in food and food packaging must be free from asbestos fibers. The agency admitted that the detection of asbestos by analytical methods is complex and generally inadequate for purposes of surveillance of food and beverage products. The agency announced that it intended to monitor and eliminate asbestos impurities from drugs and cosmetics, because these consumer products also may be contaminated with asbestos.

The multiple threats of asbestos contamination in air, foods, and beverages should serve as a convincing illustration of the complexities of environmental pollutants. The combined exposures from this accidental, as well as intentional, additive, have increased the total body burden of a substance that is an acknowledged carcinogen. Talc had been considered to be innocuous in foods, and was a "prior sanctioned substance" in use before the 1958 amendment to the Federal Food, Drug and Cosmetic Act. It has enjoyed the privilege of being exempt from the legal definition of "food additive" and was therefore not subject to regulations that govern food additives due to the fact that it had "Generally Recognized as Safe" (GRAS) status. By June 30, 1973, FDA proposed to require that the words "free of asbestos form particles" be added to labels. Such a requirement, vigorously enforced, results in stronger protection for the consuming public.

PLASTICS IN CONTACT WITH FOOD

Plastic food wraps and plastic food containers have become commonplace in kitchens and in food stores. How safe are these plastics when they come in contact with food?

Many plastics contain plasticizers, which are used to increase flexibility. Some plasticizers have been found to migrate from the plastic. One, for example, is di-(ethylhexyl) adipate (DEHA), a suspected carcinogen. DEHA is used commonly with polyvinyl chloride (PVC) film wrap, popular for covering stored food and for food that is to be cooked in a microwave oven.

Migration Levels in Film Wrap. In a study of home use of PVC film wrap, the migration level of DEHA was found to increase in proportion to the time that the food was in contact with the PVC wrap, and with the rise in cooking temperature. The highest migration levels were found when the plastic film was in direct contact with food that had a high surface fat content. The highest migration levels were found with microwave oven-cooked meats (pork spareribs and roast chicken); and bakery products (cakes, scones, and biscuits made with peanuts). Somewhat lower levels were detected in microwave oven-cooked potatoes and carrots; the lowest levels in fruits and vegetables (except avocado, due to its high fat content). Migration levels were low when there was little or no direct contact between the food and the wrap, including microwaved food.

Examination of the use of PVC film with foods in retail stores showed similar results. The amount of DEHA that migrated into the food depended on how long the film was in contact with the food's fatty portions. The highest amounts were found in cheeses, baked goods, and sandwiches; lower amounts in cooked meat and poultry; and the lowest amounts in fruits and vegetables.

Food Freezer Bags and Wraps. Polyethylene, a popular plastic film commonly used for food freezer bags and wraps, does not contain plasticizers, and is considered to be generally safe for microwave oven use. However, if any printing has been applied to the surface, polyethylene

SOME OTHER UNANTICIPATED INTERACTIONS

- *Styrofoam.* An ordinary styrofoam cup was found capable of disintegrating when it held hot tea and lemon. Discoveries of such unanticipated interactions still occur from time to time.

- *Benzene.* Benzene from multilayer, oxygen-barrier, laminated bags has been found to migrate into meat, poultry, cheeses, and other packaged foods. This problem surfaced when an off-odor was noted in a roast beef shipment. Investigation showed that the meat contained benzene from the packaging, ranging from less than 5 parts per billion (ppb) to 17.8 ppb in raw meat. The benzene volatilized when the meat was heated.

- *A Dye to Stamp Meat.* For many years, a purple dye (FD&C Violet No. 1) had been used to stamp inspected meat. The dye was suspected as a carcinogen. There was no assurance that the portion of the meat with the dye would be cut away before being consumed. In 1973, the FDA banned the dye as a meat marker.

- *Nitrosamines.* Nitrosamines (carcinogenic compounds) were discovered in rubber nipples used to cap baby bottles. The rubber was reformulated to eliminate nitrosame formation. More recently, nitrosamines were discovered in hams that had rubber netting to encase them after boning and curing. The rubber was reformulated to eliminate this problem.

should not be used for microwave oven cooking. The primer applied to the plastic prior to printing, as well as the applied inks, when heated, may subject the plastic to conditions quite different from those for which they had been approved. Similarly, formed plastic containers used for carry-out fast foods should not be reused to heat foods in microwave ovens. Such containers, when heated, may be subjected to conditions unlike those for which they had been judged safe.

Increasingly, plastic food wraps and containers have become popular for microwave use. This practice creates a potential hazard. High heat can release components from the plastics, including base monomers, plasticizers, colorants, and stabilizers.

"Active Packaging." Of growing concern to the FDA is "active packaging" which involves the placement of metallic heat "susceptors," about the size of a Band-Aid, into plastic food packaging intended for microwave cooking. The susceptors focus microwave radiation to produce extremely hot surfaces (400°F to 500°F) within the package. The high heat permits the food to be browned or crisped—features usually lacking in microwave cooking. At such high heat, however, substances such as polymers and their breakdown products, adhesives and their components, and other additives in the plastic, can migrate into food.

The plastic packaging materials approved by the FDA now used for cooking food in microwave ovens have never been given clearance for use at such high temperatures. The most severe conditions for such packaging recognized by the FDA's protocol are only from 212°F to 275°F, conditions that formerly prevailed. In recognition of the change that has occurred, FDA scientists are working with members of the packaging industry to study new testing procedures, and to learn if packaging materials could be modified in order to assure safety at high heat.

The term "microwaveable" printed on some plastic wrap products may create a false impression. The term does not denote that the FDA has granted approval for that use. The plastics industry is self-regulated, and conducts its own research to determine the safety of its products. FDA spokesmen have cautioned that existent migration data are not directly applicable to freezing or microwave cooking of foods in packages labeled "microwaveable."

Minimizing Unnecessary Exposure. At present, it is not known if any long-range adverse health effects result from repeated daily consumption of low levels of plastic components. To minimize unnecessary exposure to plastic component migration into foods, do not place foods in direct contact with plastic wraps before cooking in a microwave oven. If you use plastic wrap, limit its use to serve as covers for food containers, without coming into direct contact with the food. Use plastic containers only for their original purposes. If containers were intended for storing food, do not reuse them for heating food in the microwave.

REDUCING UNWANTED RESIDUES ON FOOD

Various types of unwanted residues may be present on foods, including pesticides, heavy metals, industrial compounds, animal drugs, mycotoxins (molds that are highly toxic and probably cancer-causing) that can develop on plant crops, and harmful bacteria. Fortunately, many of these residues are reduced significantly in food processing as well as by practices in the home kitchen.

Of course, we live in an imperfect world. We must realize that the food supply—safe and healthful—nevertheless does contain some unwanted residues, from farming, processing, and the environment. Even if concern with residues makes us decide to purchase only certified organic foods, this still does not provide a safeguard against all potential contaminants. Thus, it is useful to understand the nature of residues, and the ways to reduce them, insofar as possible.

Minimizing undesirable residues on food is a shared responsibility of surveillance officials, growers, distributors, processors, and consumers. The following examines the nature and extent of various types of unwanted residues, and what we can do to minimize them.

Pesticides. In a U.S. Department of Agriculture's (USDA) report under the Pesticide Data Program, researchers noted that pesticide residues generally are well below the level of established tolerances and that this finding is to be expected because of "the dissipation of residues between the farm and the marketplace and the standard food preparation techniques applied prior to testing. (See the article "Monitoring Pesticides in Our Food" on page 361.)

During processing, as produce is washed, sorted, peeled, blanched, and canned, any pesticide residue is reduced dramatically. For example, according to Henry Chin of the National Food Processors Association, about 85 percent of the tomato crop is processed for sauce and salsa, up to 45 percent of apples, for juice and sauce; and up to 79 percent of oranges, for juice. According to Chin, the residues on fresh vegetables and fruits often are those from post-harvest pesticide application used to keep the produce pest-free while in transit to markets. However, there is no need for post-harvest treatment of produce intended for processing, because the time between harvesting and processing perishable produce is very brief. In one study, for instance, residues from pesticides such as methyl parathion and chlorpyrifos were found on ten samples of raw unwashed apples. After being processed into apple juice and apple sauce, no residues were detected in any of the finished products.*

---

*In general, pesticide residues are reduced in cooking, but exceptions have been discovered. Processing actually may increase the level of some undesirable residues. For example, EBDC (ethylenebisdithiocarbamate) is a fungicide that is officially restricted for use with crops, due to the hazards discovered with its breakdown product, ETU (ethylene thiourea). ETU, fed to laboratory animals, was shown to cause

Many pesticides penetrate the peel. Others are absorbed through the roots. Nonetheless, according to researchers, washing and peeling produce can remove about one-fourth of pesticide residue.

What is the extent of pesticide residues in the food supply? California supplies more than half of our nation's fruits and vegetables, so findings from pesticide residue monitoring in California are of interest to everyone. The 1995 annual report of California's Department of Pesticide Regulations noted that more than 98 percent of the produce sampled by the state had "either no detectable residues or residues within legal limits." Based on 5,502 samples of 132 different commodities taken from seaports, packing sites, and both wholesale and retail outlets, 33.7 percent had residues within the U.S. Environmental Protection Agency's (EPA) acceptable tolerances. About 1.6 percent of the samples contained illegal residues. The remainder had no detectable residues. These findings approximate those from the annual reports of the Food and Drug Administration's (FDA) Residue Monitoring Program, conducted in various locations, nationwide.

Official Canadian findings are similar. According to a review by the National Cancer Institute of Canada, published in 1997, an expert panel reported that most foods did not contain detectable pesticide residues, and those that did were well below permitted levels.

Pesticide residue levels may decline further as Integrated Pest Management (IPM) is practiced more widely. IPM combines minimal amounts of pesticides with biological and

---

liver and throat cancer, as well as fetal abnormalities. When raw EBDC-treated tomatoes were cooked, the ETU level increased ten to ninety times as much in the cooked tomatoes. Depending on the amount of EBDC residue on the harvested produce, the amounts of ETU residues were generally about forty to fifty times higher in cooked than in raw vegetables.

cultural practices to control agricultural pests effectively. In addition, the increasing growth of organic farming may contribute to a further decline in total pesticide residues.

Future applications of new technology might further reduce the need for pesticides in post-harvest applications. Pulsed ultraviolet lasers might replace or lessen pesticide applications.

Reducing pesticides in the kitchen. Use some of the same techniques used by food processors. Wash produce thoroughly in running water to rid it of surface pesticides that are water-soluble, as well as soil remnants and insects. Wash lettuce leaf by leaf, says Ross Davidson, a clinical microbiologist at Mt. Sinai Hospital in Toronto. After an outbreak of foodborne illness traced to *Escherichia coli* on lettuce, Davidson experimented by purposely contaminating lettuce with bacteria. He found that rinsing or dipping a cored intact lettuce head—a common practice of food preparers—was insufficient for removing the bacteria. Washing the leaves individually was more effective.

According to a consumer food-marketing specialist at the University of California at Davis, about 90 percent of pesticide residues can be removed by washing the produce thoroughly under running water.

You can wash grapes more efficiently if you remove them from the stems, and place them in a colander for rinsing. Soak produce briefly in a container with water and some vinegar, and then rinse thoroughly. Avoid a long soak to prevent water-soluble nutrients from leaching out. Do

---

* Some groups have recommended washing produce in a weak solution of dishwasher detergent. Scientists at the EPA and the FDA discourage this practice. Chemicals used in dishwashing detergents could be absorbed into porous foods and be ingested. These two agencies reported that detergents, soaps, and special commercial products designed to wash produce are unnecessary.

not use detergents in the water.* Peel and discard the outer leaves of lettuce. If you peel and discard fruit skins from fruit such as apple or pear, remember that there is a trade-off: you may reduce pesticide residue somewhat, but lose dietary fiber.

Heavy Metals. Heavy metals can contaminate foods from soils, packaging materials, or processing techniques. Jeffrey Morgan, at the EPA's National Exposure Research Laboratory in Cincinnati, reported how toxic metals can contaminate foods. For example, grapefruit juice, stored in opened tin-coated steel cans for two weeks, showed increased heavy metal contamination. Morgan found that coffee, prepared in a lead-containing glazed ceramic mug, leached considerable lead during the first half hour, and lower levels for up to twenty-four hours. Also, old dinnerware with lead-containing glazes can leach high lead levels into foods if the dinnerware is used in microwave ovens.

Morgan tested the effects of different cooking techniques on mercury-contaminated walleye fillets. The mercury level was not reduced either by pan-frying or by smoking the fish.

Low levels of arsenic, commonly used as a growth promoter in feed used with laying hens, can accumulate both in the egg yolks and whites. As with mercury, Morgan found that cooking did not lower arsenic residue levels. In some cases, this metal actually increased in the cooked eggs.

Reducing heavy metals in the kitchen. Transfer any remaining food from opened cans to inert storage containers such as glass. Avoid undesirable interactions of foods with metals that can leach lead, cadmium, or other toxic metals. For example, do not store acidic foods in galvanized vessels, or make lemon sherbet in a metallic ice-cube tray. Use microwave-safe containers in this appliance. Limit your consumption of lake fish from any area known or suspected of being contaminated with heavy metals. Some fish, such as swordfish, are natural mercury accumulators. Restrict your consumption of such fish.

Industrial Contaminants. Although U.S. manufacture of polychlorinated biphenyls (PCBs) was discontinued in 1977, PCBs deposited in the sediment of rivers and lakes have led to continued PCB residues in fish and other aquatic organisms. Dredging, shipping, storms, and marine organisms disturb the sediment and cause the reintroduction of PCBs into water, and result in fish contamination.

Reducing industrial contamimants in the kitchen. Processing and cooking can reduce PCB residues, as well as PBBs (polybrominated biphenyls) and TCDD (2,3,7,8-dibenzo-p-dioxin) in fish and fish oils, according to Mary Zabik, at Michigan State University's College of Human Ecology. These residues are fat-soluble; so any process that reduces fat effectively reduces their levels. Zabik found that by trimming visible fat from fish, PCB levels could be reduced up to 95 percent.

Others found that, by removing the bellyflap and the fat-containing lateral line in raw fish, PCBs could be reduced in chinook salmon by 40 percent; in carp and blue fish, from 19 percent to 33 percent; and in walleye, by 20 percent.

By baking, broiling, or pan-frying, from 20 to 35 percent of the PCBs could be removed from Great Lakes fish. Although char-broiling and smoking of foods are undesirable practices because they produce mutagens, it was found that PCB residue could be eliminated completely by smoking Lake Michigan carp. Char-broiling reduced the contaminant by about 45 percent. Baking and pan-frying also reduced PCBs by about 45 percent.

In other studies, residue reduction of PCBs by cooking fish was less effective, and depended on the species. Residues were reduced only slightly in striped bass, and minimally in chinook and coho salmon. However, broiling of siscowets (lake trout) reduced PCBs by 53 percent; and roasting or microwaving, from 26 to 34 percent.

In PCB-contaminated blue crabs, the hepatopancreas contains the highest concentration of residue. By removing this organ before blue crabs are boiled or steamed, PCBs could be reduced in the claws by 25 percent; and in the body muscles, by 33 percent.

In experiments, residues of Aroclor, a PCB compound, were found to remain during various stages of processing edible oils, until the step of deodorization. At that point, the residues were eliminated. In other experiments, residues were eliminated or reduced by other treatments. Shrimp sun-dried for thirty-six hours lost all Aroclor. Shrimp treated with sodium nitrate lost all Aroclor after thirty hours. Freeze-drying reduced Aroclor residues in shrimp by about 40 percent; and in eggs, by about 25 percent.

Processing and cooking of meat, poultry, and fish can reduce PCB levels significantly, mainly by rendering out the fat, which goes into the broth. It was found that PCB reduction from the raw to the cooked state in chicken was 56.1 percent in the drumstick, 69.7 percent in the breast pieces, 55.9 percent in the thigh meat; 60.8 percent in the thigh skin; and 91.2 percent in the fat-containing flesh (the adipose tissue).

Because PCB residues are higher in fatty tissues of fish, reduce the residues by trimming all visible fat before cooking the fish. Avoid eating the internal organs of crab and lobster. Discard the broth in which flesh foods have been cooked, if they are suspected of having PCB residues. Select ocean fish rather than fresh water fish.

Animal Drugs. Monitoring drug residues in the food supply from food-producing animals is a responsibility shared by the USDA's Food Safety and Inspection Service (FSIS) and the FDA's Center for Veterinarian Medicine (CVM).*

The CVM Tissue Residue Reduction Program has both a preventive and regulatory approach, to ensure that consumer exposure to drug residues in edible tissue of food animals is minimized. A database collects, stores, and recovers information gathered during the FDA and state on-site follow-ups of reported violative tissue residues. In tracking these cases, the data, identified from FSIS's monitoring and surveillance programs, can identify specific slaughterhouses and animals. Data are collected from the Tissue Residue Information Management System (TRIMS), a database of information generated by the FDA follow-up investigations and from FSIS's violative residues information with domestic meat and poultry. The number of cases fluctuates, but several thousand violative residue cases occur yearly. The drugs most frequently identified as causing residues are antibiotics that include penicillin, streptomycin, oxytetracycline, sulfamethazine, tetracycline, gentamicin, and neomycin.

Reducing animal drug residues in the kitchen. Studies of drug residues in meats showed that reduction of these medications varies widely, depending on the type of compound

---

*Both agencies have several branches devoted to this program. FSIS operates a Hazardous Analysis and Critical Control Points Program (HACCP) for surveillance and testing, to ensure that the nation's meat and poultry supply does not contain unlawful drug residue levels. The FDA's Center for Veterinarian Medicine (CVM) is responsible for ensuring that edible products intended for human consumption such as meat, milk, and eggs obtained from animals, treated with new animal drugs, do not contain unsafe drug residue levels. Also, CVM enables the marketing of animal drugs, food additives, feed additives, feed ingredients, and animal devices that are judged to be safe to animals, humans, and the environment.

and the cooking method used. According to William Moats, of the USDA's Meat Science Research Laboratory at Beltsville, Maryland, some antibiotic residues are reduced "in ordinary cooking of meat by procedures such as frying, grilling, or roasting, even to 'well done' temperatures in the center." Moats found that these cooking procedures decreased residues of some drugs (oxytetracycline, chlorotetracycline, and penicillin G) depending on the duration and temperature of the cooking. However, even after the meat was well cooked, residues of some drugs remained, including clenbuterol and sulfamethazine.

Heating meat only to "rare," in addition to posing a risk of foodborne illness, results in very little reduction of drug residues. More significant reduction occurs when the meat is cooked to a "well-done" stage. However, results vary from drug to drug.

Unless you have access to organic meats, the sole means of reducing drug residues that may be present in flesh foods is to cook them thoroughly in liquid, and then discard the liquid. Consumers need to rely on the safety network developed jointly by the USDA and the FDA, with various monitoring programs devised by these agencies, and seizures of foods that are found to have violative levels of drug residues.

Mycotoxins. Another worrisome group of residues are mycotoxins, produced by molds that may contaminate crops. Some 400 mycotoxins have been identified. Some can cause acute or chronic toxicity; others are regarded as carcinogenic. Many grain crops and soybeans can be contaminated, and indirectly affect other foods such as milk, cheese, and meat if the animals are fed mycotoxin-contaminated feed. The important grain mycotoxins include aflatoxins, fumonisins, zearalenone, and deoxynivalenol.

Considerable differences exist in the effectiveness of various processings intended to destroy mycotoxins, reported

L.B. Bullerman, of the University of Nebraska's Department of Food Science. Methods used to reduce mycotoxin residues include programs of breeding, control of storage conditions, and decontamination of grains by physical, chemical, and biological means. Heating or roasting of aflatoxin-contaminated grains produced only small reductions of the toxins. Hand sorting reduced the contamination level somewhat. The most effective method was the use of ammonia. However, this method is not approved by the FDA for grain that is intended for human consumption.

Reducing mycotoxins in the kitchen. Store grains, flour, and peanuts in tightly closed containers in a dry place. Discard any that smell or appear moldy, without sniffing or tasting.

Bacteria. Many types of harmful bacteria can contaminate foods. Thermal heating of food, such as cooking or pasteurization, has been used traditionally to kill harmful bacteria. Several new techniques have been developed that do not depend on heat.

One approach uses brief pulses of high-intensity white light to kill microorganisms on the surfaces of perishable foods. Laboratory tests demonstrated that the technique could reduce *Salmonella* up to 95 percent on meats. The same process can be used with water, food packaging, and medical and pharmaceutical products. Other approaches include oscillating magnetic fields, high hydrostatic pressure, and bacterial destruction by low-voltage, low-current electrical treatment in various salt solutions used as electrolytes. All of these techniques bypass irradiation, a system that has official approval but has not been embraced enthusiastically by most food producers or consumers. For milk, the process known as microfiltration removes nearly all bacteria prior to its minimal heat treatment of pasteurization.

In the future, ozone may be used as a safer substitute for chemical disinfectants and sanitizers in food processing. It is more powerful than chlorine in deactivating a very large number of virulent organisms. Although ozone use has not yet been approved in the United States for food use, it is approved as "Generally Recognized as Safe" (GRAS) to treat bottled water, and in bottle water plants. It has long been used in Europe by the food industry.

Ozone does not remain in water for any length of time. Thus, its use may be considered as a process rather than as a food additive. There would be no safety concern about consumption of residual ozone in food products. Any byproducts produced by ozone in treating foods are similar to normal oxidation products. They do not contain chlorine, and therefore are thought to be less likely to have any deleterious health effects than the byproducts of chlorine treatment.

Reducing bacteria in the kitchen. The oft-given advice deserves repetition. Kitchen cleanliness and personal hygiene are important. Thorough cooking, prompt refrigeration, thorough reheating, frequent handwashing, and avoidance of cross-contamination have become mantras for food preparers. Remember that we all ingest some harmful bacteria in foods. The healthy person with a strong immune system generally can detoxify a limited amount, but a person with an impaired immune system may be at risk even with a small amount of harmful bacteria.

Chapter 11

Agricultural Practices That Affect Our Food and Health

FEEDING OUR FOOD ANIMALS: FROM GRASS TO SEWAGE SLUDGE

There was a time when our food animals grazed on summer grass and winter hay. Then, it was found that livestock gained weight more readily if fed grains or soybeans. However, by the 1970s, this practice was viewed as costly and wasteful. It was argued that, instead, such valuable food crops should be used to help feed the world's people. This turnabout stimulated a search for alternative substances—a search that still continues. It has taken us from grass and hay feeding to such nontraditional ingredients in animal feed as sewage sludge and treated manure.

The search for alternative substances in animal feed suited the new conditions that arose from agricultural changes. Formerly, agricultural wastes such as cornstalks, wheat straw, apple pomace, sugarcane bagasse, and citrus rinds were recycled on farms as mulches. Animal manures were composted and spread as fertilizers. The growth of large-scale, specialized commercial farms created problems of costly waste disposal. Also, growing concerns about water pollution and regulations instituted to curb waste disposal acted as an incentive to find solutions. "Recycle" became a buzzword of the era.

Recycled Waste for Animal Feed. This solution could turn waste into profit and, at the same time, lessen water pollution. For example, cheese producers could no longer dispose of whey, a byproduct of cheese making, by spewing it into waterways. Selling whey as an ingredient for animal feed not only prevented water pollution, but turned waste into new-found revenue sources.

With the advent of huge feedlots for cattle, and intensively reared confined poultry, tons of manure were generated in concentrated areas. Interest in manure sales had declined with the rise of commercial fertilizers. Manure, like whey, created problems of pollution. Selling manure to be used as an ingredient in animal feed could be profitable, and also prevent water pollution.

Gradually, a plethora of substances found their way into animal feed. They included agricultural wastes such as corn cobs, peanut skins, beet and potato residues, culled pistachios, almond hulls, bruised bananas, and seeds left after the edible oil is pressed from them. They included retail food wastes such as stale bakery products, candies, and potato or corn chips. Slaughterhouses and tanneries provided blood, entrails, hoofs, bristles, and feathers for use in animal feed. Some alternative substances were added to animal feed for cellulose, provided from industrial wastes such as sawdust, wood chips, twigs, and even ground-up newspapers and cardboard boxes. Others were cement dust from kilns, sludge from municipal composting plants, waste from electric generating plants that used coal, and waste water from nuclear power stations.

Much interest was devoted to recycled manure. By the 1970s, nearly two billion tons of animal wastes were generated yearly in the United States. The idea of recycling it in animal feed was estimated to save 40 million tons of grain annually. The United States Department of Agriculture (USDA) reported that the protein in cattle manure in American feedlots was equivalent to the protein in the nation's entire soybean crop.

In 1967, the Food and Drug Administration (FDA) withheld approval for the practice of using recycled manure in animal feed. Its decision was based on the recommendation of toxicologists inside and outside of the agency. Their concern was that recycled manure was risky. It could contain disease-producing organisms and parasites, residues of drugs and their breakdown products, and toxic substances other than contaminants.

Proponents argued that manure, exposed to aerobic fermentation, would be safe. The treated recycled animal manure would reduce pollution, and bring economic benefits to consumers.

Although the FDA could control the practice in interstate commerce, the agency was powerless to control intrastate commerce and state policies. By 1975, dried poultry waste (DPW) was approved for intrastate sales in Georgia, California, Colorado, Oregon, Iowa, and Mississippi; and several years later, in Alabama, Virginia, and Washington. Florida, Georgia, Iowa, and Oregon registered DPW as a feed ingredient under their existing laws.

With such widespread official approval within many states, by 1976 the FDA considered a more relaxed policy based on the recommendations of its own Bureau of Food and Veterinary Medicine. The FDA would permit the feeding of animal or poultry waste to cattle not being finished for slaughter (such as brood stock, over-wintering cattle, or calves not old enough to go to feedlots). The FDA proposed that all cattle fed animal waste and intended for human food would need to undergo a minimum withdrawal period of sixty days prior to slaughter. The agency proposed to prohibit feeding animal wastes to laying hens, breeder poultry, milk-producing dairy cows, and all poultry intended for human food.

Other Ingredients. By the mid-1970s, there was great

interest in single-cell protein for animal feed. Petroleum-derived protein was produced from yeast grown on paraffin in crude oil. Interest in this feed ingredient had a serious setback when it was discovered that the product was contaminated with a cancer-causing substance.

Industrial-grade vegetable oil byproducts were considered for inclusion in animal feed. However, the FDA would not approve them because of their high levels of pesticide residues. In 1975, the agency mandated a label statement on such products "not for food or feed use."

Another group of substances introduced into animal feed is what came to be dubbed "The Four Ds"—dead, dying, disabled, and diseased animals. In 1989, the FDA issued a Compliance Policy Guide, and considered uncooked meat derived from such animals as adulterated. Meat from such animals, shipped interstate, is required to be adequately heat-treated to make it safe.

By the late 1970s, sewage sludge from municipal sources was introduced into animal feed. To kill pathogens present, the sludge was treated with cesium 137 radioisotopes, a waste product of nuclear reactors. The treated sludge, along with other ingredients, is pelleted as a feed supplement for sheep and cattle. Also, treated sewage water serves as a liquid feed on fish farms for bivalves such as clams, oysters, mussels, and scallops, and could be extended to lobsters, crabs, and certain fish varieties.

Through the years, as additional waste products have been incorporated into animal feed, the FDA decided to approve food waste recycling into feed on a case-to-case basis. By 1991, among such food wastes were moisture-damaged or maggot-infested grains; foods contaminated by rodents, roaches, or bird excreta. The FDA expressed concern about the use of airline garbage because of its possible contamination with plastic, glass, metal, and tinfoil.

Dr. Daniel G. McChesney, leader of the Feed Safety Team of the FDA's Center for Veterinary Medicine (CVM), reported in 1996 that the "variety of waste products, byproducts, and co-products that are being considered for use in animal feed is growing rapidly, and the FDA anticipates even more rapid growth in the future. Government, whether it be federal or state, cannot develop regulations rapidly enough to address each product and the nuances associated with it."

. . . additional waste products have been incorporated into animal feed . . . By 1991, among such food wastes were moisture-damaged or maggot-infested grains; foods contaminated by rodents, roaches, or bird excreta.

Current Concerns. McChesney reported that CVM's principal concerns with the use of garbage, waste products, byproducts, and co-products are related to the "poorly defined nature of the product; the numerous sources that can range from restaurants, to laundries, to industrial manufacturers; the collection vehicles/receptacles which can vary from designated trucks and receptacles to collection by the same trucks used to pump septic systems; the variety of contaminants possible; and the level of control (or lack of control) encompassed by local and state laws/regulations." McChesney continued: "The processing of potentially recyclable material can vary from minimal—with no testing for contaminants—to commercial processing such as rendering with pesticide and chemical screens. . . . Regulating the materials [other than on a] case-by-case basis at the federal level is currently not feasible."

One of the current issues, according to McChesney, concerns the use of sewer grease. "The FDA is opposed to the use of sewer grease or any product which has come in contact with or passed through the same drain as sanitary sewer water or solid matter as a component of human or animal food. . . . The FDA is opposed to the use of grease trap waste from floor drains, pot wash drains, dishwasher drains, sink drains, etc.; in animal feed unless the contaminants were known (or not present) and did not result in unsafe tissue residues in milk, meat, and eggs or present a health hazard to animals. The Agency has not opposed the use in animal feed of 'restaurant grease' or 'sludge' when it consists entirely of edible byproducts used in, or obtained from, the preparation of human food." (Note that there is no mention made of the quality of the restaurant grease. By the time it is discarded, it has been rendered toxic by peroxidation.)

Another current concern, according to McChesney, is the use of dehydrated cafeteria garbage in animal feed. This product is defined as "artificially dried animal and vegetable waste collected sufficiently often that harmful decomposition has not set in, and from which have been separated crockery, glass, metal, string, and similar materials. . . . It must be processed at a temperature sufficient to destroy all organisms capable of producing animal diseases." If part of the grease and fat is removed, the substance is designated as "degreased, dehydrated garbage."

. . . the FDA's Center for Veterinary Medicine reported in 1996 that the "variety of waste products, byproducts, and co-products that are being considered for use in animal feed is growing rapidly, and the FDA anticipates even more rapid growth in the future. Government, whether it be federal or state, cannot develop regulations rapidly enough to address each product and the nuances associated with it."

The FDA does not object to a product meeting this definition from being used in animal feed, provided it is not adulterated with anything that would result in animal health problems, or produce residues such as pesticides, industrial chemicals, pathogenic microorganisms, or drug residues in meat, milk, or eggs.

An issue that has not been addressed, according to McChesney, is whether it is appropriate to include biodegradable packaging and utensils in dehydrated cafeteria garbage. The agency has not reviewed the safety of this practice.

One objection that the FDA has raised is the use of newsprint, both as a feed ingredient and as a bedding material for food animals. Often, bedding is consumed by animals. The basis for this objection is the same for both uses. Initially, the FDA objected to the use of newsprint because of concerns that the process used in bleaching wood pulp could lead to dioxin residues in the paper, and that the ink might contain chemicals that could present an animal safety problem, or a residue problem in products intended for human consumption. However, in the past few years, the process of bleaching wood pulp has been changed, and the FDA now considers the dioxin contamination problem to be minimal. However, the ink problem remains as a concern. Some newspapers have switched to vegetable-based inks and approved color dyes, but the practice is not industry-wide. Thus, the FDA continues to object to the general use of newsprint as a feed ingredient and bedding material.

Distillers dried grains, a byproduct of breweries used as an ingredient in animal feed, is of special concern to CVM as a risk, for both animal health and human safety. In April 1994, over 4,600 cattle from seven Kansas feedlots became ill. More than 700 of the cattle died. Investigation showed that animals in all of the feedlots had been fed distillers dried grains from milo (a sorghum grain used in animal feed), along with a substance from a local ethanol production facility and an antibiotic. The FDA's investigation further showed that the added substance was contaminated with several antibiotic analogues (substances similar to the antibiotics in structure and form). The ethanol production facility had processed and distilled some waste ethanol that contained antibiotics and several antibiotic analogues just before the outbreak of the cattle deaths. A laboratory feeding trial duplicated the circumstances, and affirmed what CVM inspectors had suspected during their on-feedlot investigations. The same clinical signs and lesions were produced. In this incident, not only were feedlot cattle killed, but the contaminant posed a potential risk for unsafe residues in the meat of surviving animals. The same contaminant had been sold to dairies in several states, with a potential to cause unsafe residues in milk.

McChesney cautioned, "As recycling becomes more common and nontraditional sources of ingredients enter the animal feed market, the FDA wants to stress to this segment of industry that they . . . have an obligation to produce a safe and wholesome product. . . . Only ingredients of the highest specifications and with a past history of safe use should be used. Industry should . . . avoid the use of ingredients or processes that might result in poisonous or deleterious substances entering animal feed."

Feed and "Mad Cow" Disease. McChesney's cautionary advice should be heeded. With the emergence of bovine spongiform encephalopathy (BSE), popularly dubbed "mad cow's disease," the subject of recycled animal manure, as well as the "Four Ds" as components of animal feed deserve careful reevaluation. BSE was first recognized in 1986 as a newly emerging disease. There are indications that the first clinical case was observed a year earlier.

Among the risk factors for BSE, the USDA has identified the changes in rendering processes and the feeding of large amounts of meat and bone to young dairy calves. The only common factor in the cattle with BSE is that feed containing meat and bone meal was fed to the affected animals. Further epidemiological studies, including computer simulation of the British epidemic, suggest that feed contaminated by a transmissible spongiform encephalopathy (TSE) agent caused the disease.

In Britain, dead sheep—many having died of scrapie, a sheep disease that bears some resemblance to BSE in cattle—as well as dead cattle with BSE, were picked up by "knackers" (a British term for individuals who carry away dead animals from farms and render them into animal feed). The product, only partially rendered, contained large quantities of the scrapie/BSE agents, and was fed in large amounts to dairy calves. The spread of BSE appears to have been aided by the feeding of rendered BSE-infected cattle back to calves. The BSE agent was recycled from cows to calves, until a 1989 ban of ruminant-to-ruminant feeding.

Also, in the late 1970s and early 1980s, many British rendering plants switched from an effective solvent-extraction rendering process using live steam, to a different heat-extraction method. Apparently, the new method was less effective and allowed BSE present in the cattle, to survive the treatment.

BSE outbreaks in Britain have been well publicized. However, other European countries also experienced incidents, although fewer cattle were affected. Various rendering processes used in the European Union were tested for their ability to deactivate the BSE agent. Four out of fifteen processes in use were shown to produce meat and bone meal with detectable BSE infectivity. One process showed absolutely no reduction whatsoever over the original raw materials. As a result of these alarming findings, the processes were banned from use in the European Union.

As a result of the outbreaks in Britain and other European countries, the feeding of ruminant-derived protein supplements to other ruminants was banned. The feeding of specified offal (organ meats) or their products to farm animals and to all pets was banned. The slaughter and incineration of suspect cattle was made compulsory. British officials banned from human food and all animal feed the use of specified bovine organs (brain, spinal cord, thymus, tonsils, spleen, intestines, and products derived from them) from cattle over six months of age.

As a result of the European outbreaks of BSE, certain precautionary measures have been taken in the United States. In 1989, the USDA's Animal and Plant Health Inspection Service (APHIS) prohibited the importation of live cattle and zoo ruminants from Britain. In the same year, the National Renderers Association, as well as the Animal Protein Producers industry recommended to their members that they refrain from rendering sheep offal for inclusion in cattle feed. However, the voluntary effort was judged not to be adequately effective when the FDA conducted a 1992 survey of current rendering practices in the United States. Some rendered adult sheep protein was found in cattle feed. Fifteen plants were identified as the major processors, rendering more than 85 percent of the total amount of adult sheep rendered in the United States. The inspectors found that eleven of the plants rendered adult sheep with heads; seven rendered sheep separately from other species; and four rendered sheep that had died of causes other than slaughtering. Six of the eleven renderers who processed adult sheep with heads were selling rendered protein byproducts to cattle feed producers. The FDA concluded that the rendering industry's voluntary program was not being followed fully.

In 1993, the FDA issued letters to manufacturers of drugs, biologics, devices, dietary supplements, and animal products, urging them to use cattle products in their own production solely from non-BSE countries.

In 1994, the FDA proposed a ban on feeding tissues from ruminants to livestock, but the proposal was never implemented due to opposition from the livestock industry and lack of inspection funding. This inaction raised concerns. Paul Taylor of the National Institutes of Health reported that U.S. pigs and chickens are being fed scrapie-contaminated food. Both pigs and chickens are susceptible to BSE, and are slaughtered before the age when symptoms appear. The animals could carry BSE undetected, and transmit it to humans through the food supply. Although the FDA announced that it would expedite regulations banning ruminant protein in ruminant feed, the agency failed to prohibit ruminant feed for other livestock.

To date, no evidence has been found that BSE is zoonotic, that is, a disease that can be transmitted from livestock to humans. However, scientists are cautious and report that it cannot be ruled out that BSE may be zoonotic. Some pathogens are transmitted from animals to humans. One example is *Cryptosporidium.* In the case of BSE, the long time period between infection and its manifestation adds to the uncertainties. Meanwhile, the BSE issue provides a strong incentive for officials to reevaluate all nontraditional feed additives and the effectiveness of processes used to render animal-derived substances to make them safe for use in animal feed.

ANIMAL DRUGS AND MICROBIAL RESISTANCE: UNCERTAINTIES AND CONCERNS

In 1965, a large outbreak of severe salmonellosis in England caused widespread illness and some deaths. The outbreak was traced to a multiresistant strain of the pathogen. Researchers connected the disease in humans to the use of antibiotics in farm animals. The pattern of antibiotic resistance in the affected humans was similar to the pattern of antibiotic resistance in affected calves.

An official commission investigated the outbreak. In 1969, the commission issued its "Report of Joint Committee on the Use of Antibiotics in Animal Husbandry and Veterinary Medicine," known popularly as the Swann Report. It was the first official document to question the wisdom of using antimicrobial drugs with animals that also were used with humans.

Following the Swann Report, in 1970 the United Kingdom passed legislation strictly limiting antibiotic use. The Netherlands, all Scandinavian countries, Germany, and Canada followed. The United States considered a ban, but it was never approved.

Now, more than three decades later, the concerns are still present and have increased because of many instances of antibiotic resistance. Yet scientific understanding of the problem is incomplete, and uncertainties still exist.

The practice of using antimicrobial drugs with food animals began in the 1940s. The drugs have been used at high levels to cure or contain animal diseases. However, it was discovered that the same drugs, if used routinely at low levels, could promote animal growth. This feature still is not well understood. Systematic, low-level use enhances feed efficiency and fights infections usually not detected without clinical examination. These features translate into greater profitability in livestock management.

Unfortunately, the antimicrobial drugs used with food animals are either the same as, or related to, drugs used with humans. The low-level use with animals, especially to promote growth, has been of special concern. The practice threatens human health because drug residues can remain in the final food products and cause human illness.

The Food and Drug Administration (FDA) has established specific time periods between the last administration of the drugs and the slaughter of the animals, to limit drug residues from remaining and being consumed by humans. These rules are based on knowledge of the time needed for the breakdown of active ingredients in the drugs. Despite these regulations, the FDA conducts frequent recalls of animal-based foods because of illegal residues still present. This problem continues to pose an immediate threat to human health. However, there is another concern regarding the use of these drugs with food animals that poses an even greater long-range threat: resistance.

Scientists have found that the cautions expressed in the Swann Report were warranted. Indeed, some pathogens (especially bacteria) have become resistant to antimicrobial drugs. This finding raises concerns about the role of animal drug use in the emergence of drug-resistant bacteria in humans and the ability of health care professionals to cope with the threat to human health. Some microorganisms are naturally resistant to some antimicrobial drugs. Others become resistant, by mutation, by incorporating genetic material for resistance from other microorganisms, by ingestion, or by cellular contact.

Confounding Factors. Despite the passage of many years, scientists admit that considerable uncertainty exists about many aspects of microbial resistance. Data are limited about the public health threat. The U.S. General Accounting Office (GAO) found that differences of opinion exist among various branches of the federal government about the risk to public health posed by antimicrobial drug use in food animals, and a lack of unanimity concerning the best plan of action. The GAO recommends that various involved branches of government work together to address the critical information gaps, and then develop science-based decisions.

Scientists both at the Centers for Disease Control and Prevention (CDC) and the FDA expressed concerns that drug-resistant varieties of *Salmonella* and *Campylobacter* (two major foodborne contaminants that cause human illnesses) have been transferred from food animals to humans and caused illness. Positive traceback of drug-resistant human illness through the food chain to its source has been done on rare occasions, but not routinely. Much of the evidence is circumstantial. But sufficient evidence has accumulated to convince the CDC and the FDA officials that the problem is real.

. . . there is uncertainty about how many of the estimated 76 million annual cases of human foodborne illnesses involve organisms that are resistant to antimicrobial drugs.

Advances in medical technology, such as DNA fingerprinting, are helping to establish cause-and-effect relationships. In 1996, the FDA, the CDC, and the U.S. Department of Agriculture (USDA) established the National Antimicrobial Resistance Monitoring System: Enteric Bacteria (NARMS). Scientists in this coordinated effort examine specimens from humans and animals. They monitor changes in antimicrobial susceptibilities of intestinal pathogens that affect both humans and animals. The specimens are taken from healthy farm animals, from carcasses of food-producing animals at slaughter, and from animal-derived foods at retail sales. Laboratories of the FDA, the CDC, and the USDA examine the various types of specimens, using similar testing procedures.

Uncertainties exist about drug levels needed to cause resistance. The CDC studies found relatively high correlations between feeding low levels of antimicrobial drugs to food animals and the presence of drug-resistant bacteria in animals. However, studies elsewhere suggested that some critical thresholds of antibiotics are needed to cause microorganisms to become resistant, and these thresholds may not be reached by low-level use of the drugs.

Another unresolved issue is the extent that animal foods

are the sources of foodborne illnesses. At present, it is unknown. Only about 10 percent of people who become ill from foodborne illnesses seek medical help. Hence, there is uncertainty about how many of the estimated 76 million annual cases of human foodborne illnesses in the United States involve organisms that are resistant to antimicrobial drugs.

A confounding factor is that human resistance to antimicrobial drugs is caused, in part, by nonagricultural uses. Investigations by the Committee on Drug Use in Food Animals, the Office of Technological Assessment (OTA), and even the U.S. Congress, all found that the two greatest sources of drug-resistant pathogens in humans are misuse of antibiotics, both by doctors and patients, and the emergence of drug-resistant pathogens in hospitals.

Nearly two million Americans have hospital-acquired infections each year. Many of these infections are difficult to treat because they are caused by pathogens that have become resistant to the drugs commonly used to treat them. Often, such hospital-acquired infections occur in patients who already are medically stressed.

Short-term Cost vs. Long-term Benefit. Frequently, the recommendation to ban use of antimicrobial drugs in food animals is offered as a precautionary measure to protect these drugs' effectiveness in human health care. Would a ban of low-level use actually result in a decline of bacterial resistance in animals? Data are inconclusive. Studies that compare use versus nonuse are equivocal. Some studies find reduced resistance in pathogens in food animals when drugs are withdrawn from use. Other studies find no change or increased resistance. In Europe, where antimicrobial growth-promoter use was banned more than three decades ago, there are smaller percentages of resistant bacteria. Some European studies suggest that long-term benefits might outweigh short-term costs to farmers and consumers.

It is difficult to measure precisely the economic effects of antimicrobial resistance in animals. Changes in the costs of animal production, as well as the effects on trade, need to be examined if a ban is imposed. Estimated costs of the effect to livestock of resistant microbes range from virtually no impact on animal health to costs that exceed the value of the animal. For producers who use low levels of antimicrobial drugs, the costs of treating animal diseases could increase if pathogens are resistant and if producers have to resort to more expensive or less effective drugs to cure or contain the diseases. Currently, no data exist to suggest that this development is occurring. Producers not currently using these drugs may be able to use less expensive antimicrobial drugs to treat disease outbreaks caused by susceptible pathogens.

Other factors that require attention in economic considerations are the costs inflicted by resistant foodborne illnesses, such as productivity losses, illnesses, medical expenses, and deaths. Very little data exist on the economic costs associated with antimicrobial-resistant microorganisms. Even fewer data exist about resistant pathogens directly related to animal drug use. According to one study cited by the CDC, drug resistance to *Staphylococcus aureus*, a major pathogen associated both with food contamination and hospital exposures, imposes costs of $122 million yearly in the U.S.

In the 1970s and 1980s, studies were conducted to learn the costs of limiting or banning the use of antimicrobial drugs at low levels. The estimated annual net losses to producers and/or consumers ranged widely, from under $1 billion up to about $12 billion. The perceived benefits from curbing or banning action might not offset higher food prices. More recent studies are needed, but have not been done.

Most livestock research in the United States is focused on the benefits of these drugs for improved performance in animals, but little focus is on the pathogen characteristics, such as resistance, or the economic considerations. The FDA has proposed a framework to evaluate and ensure human safety of new antimicrobial drugs intended for food animal use. The proposed guidelines classify these drugs according to the extent of their usefulness to restore or maintain human health, their potential to develop resistance, and their effects on the pathogenic load in animal products. Also, the guidelines propose to establish predetermined thresholds, so that actions could be taken to suppress the emergence of resistant pathogens.

The USDA researchers admit that "there are voids in basic data about many aspects of antimicrobial drug use in U.S. livestock production. . . . A ban against low-level use of antimicrobial drugs in U.S. livestock production would likely raise costs to producers and consumers in the short run; long-term impacts are still unknown."

LOW-LEVEL DRUG RESIDUES IN FOOD

As discussed earlier, use of certain drugs with farm animals has long been controversial. The issue involves the potentially harmful effects on humans from repeated exposures to low levels of drug residues in foods derived from treated animals. When the same drugs are used with animals as with humans, potential problems of overdose and resistance may result. For example, an antibiotic may be ineffective when used by someone who has had chronic ingestion of residues of the antibiotic from foods.

Investigations of Drug Residues in Milk. In August 1992, the General Accounting Office (GAO), responding to congressional requests, issued the results of two separate investigations that involved drug residues in food. The first report had been prompted by two surveys, conducted by groups outside of government, concerning animal drug residues found in milk. Some 20 to 38 percent of retail milk samples tested were found to contain animal drug residues, including a suspected carcinogen, sulfamethazine , and other unapproved drugs.

After review, the GAO concluded that the "FDA could not demonstrate that the nation's milk supply was free from unsafe animal drug residues" and that the agency "did not have test methods to detect and confirm many drugs believed to be used in milk-producing dairy cows." The GAO suggested that a different strategy was needed to correct the problem.

A second related GAO report concerned the recombinant bovine growth hormone (rBGH). Regarding food safety, the GAO found "a critical consideration that was not—but should have been—part of the FDA's established research review; that is, the identification and evaluation of indirect human food safety risks that result from animal health effects caused by the use of animal drugs."

The increased milk production in rBGH-treated cows results in an increased incidence of mastitis, which would be treated with antibiotics. As a consequence, higher levels of antibiotic residues could turn up in milk and beef from treated animals. The GAO could give no assurance that at present "the nation's milk supply has not already been contaminated by antibiotics beyond acceptable levels." Use of rBGH could compound the problem.

Effect of Antibiotics in the Intestinal Tract. To understand the effect of drug residues from foods on humans, one must understand the functioning of the gastrointestinal tract. The intestinal microflora consist of those established in the tract and others briefly introduced with food.

The established microflora maintain stable relationships and occupy specific sites within the intestine. Their type and numbers vary in different sections of the tract. For example, the stomach contains mainly a low concentration of gram-positive, acid-resistant bacteria and fungi.

The microflora in the beginning of the small intestine are similar to those of the stomach. However, the population of microflora remains low in that area because peristaltic action moves the food along so rapidly that microorganisms have a difficult time remaining and multiplying there.

Further along in the small intestine, more microflora are established. However, they are less abundant and diverse than in the large intestine (colon). Because of the slow movement of food through the colon, the microorganisms have ample time to multiply. One third of the dry weight of feces consists of bacteria. About 400 different species of microorganisms are found in human feces.

Although the microflora composition in feces varies among individuals, it is fairly consistent and very stable despite continuous introduction of new organisms. Diet has a minimal effect on the intestinal microflora's composition, but the diet can have important effects on bacterial enzymes and can alter the metabolic activity of the intestinal microflora.

The microflora in the intestinal tract can be regarded as an ecosystem in which different microorganisms interact physically and metabolically with each other, as well as with the entire body.

The microflora have many physiological roles. Among their most important functions are to maintain normal wall thickness, the villi, the pH (acid-alkaline balance), and efficient functioning of the immune system. They control resistance mechanisms so that newly ingested bacteria are prevented from colonizing. They synthesize certain important vitamins, such as vitamin B_{12}. They separate estrogens, excreted in the bile, for reabsorption.

Most important, in terms of drug residues from foods, the gastrointestinal microflora metabolize ingested compounds and make them more available, or alter their activity and/or toxicity.

The total intestinal microflora ecosystem can be altered by therapeutic use of antibiotics in humans, especially if the antibiotic is poorly absorbed. In such cases, antibiotics can cause several changes in the gastrointestinal microflora. For example, any overgrowth of potentially pathogenic microorganisms can result in diarrhea, colitis, or blood poisoning, especially in individuals with impaired immune systems. Also, poorly absorbed antibiotics are ineffective in controlling bacteria and lead to an increase of antibiotic-resistant strains.

Antibiotics in the intestinal tract can alter the metabolism of the intestinal microflora, which normally change bacterial enzymes and metabolic products, and can interrupt various hormones, such as estrogens, from circulating in the intestine and liver and prevent them from being reabsorbed.

Thus, it should be appreciated that even low levels of drug residues in food can interfere with the entire ecosystem of the intestinal tract. Chronic ingestion of antibiotics and other drug residues from foods pose potential health problems.

BIOTECH ANIMALS COME TO THE FARM: CONTROVERSY MAY FOLLOW

Using techniques similar to those of gene transference that give plants new traits, scientists have turned their attention to modifying food animals by means of genetic engineering.

The scientists' efforts may give us leaner pork. The pig is among the first genetically modified farm animals that could benefit consumers directly. In addition to becoming leaner, transgenic pigs might become "enviro pigs," modified so that their waste contains less phosphorus, and thus, less harmful to the environment.

Transgenic chickens might be designed to resist illness-producing bacteria. Beef animals might be programmed to grow twice as fast and require less feed. Biotechnology advocates hope that such developments will make the marketing of genetically modified foods more acceptable to skeptical consumers.

To date, the most successful attempt at creating transgenic food animals has been with farmed salmon. By inserting genes that increase production of growth hormones, transgenic Atlantic salmon grow to market weight in about eighteen months, instead of the usual twenty-four months to thirty months for Atlantic salmon to reach the same weight in the wild. This development could benefit aquaculture farmers, who could raise fish in half the time, and with less cost for feed. Consumers might benefit from lower costs for such salmon.

Currently, transgenic Atlantic salmon are being farmed off the coast of Prince Edward Island in Canada, in a joint commercial venture of Canadians and Americans. The project has created great interest. By the year 2000, the company already had orders for 15 million fish eggs to be shipped. The company plans to supply the beneficial breeder fish to fish farms elsewhere. Approval is being sought to sell transgenic fish for consumption in Canada and the United States.

How Food Animals Are Modified. In modifying animals through traditional breeding, a type of animal is chosen that carries a desirable trait. The animal is mated in an attempt to create a new line of animals sharing the genes that express the desired trait. Traditional breeding requires time and patience to achieve the favored results. The basic principles of traditional animal modification through breeding are similar to those used with plant breeding.

In modifying animals transgenically, a scientist can isolate and manipulate a gene that carries a desirable trait. The characteristic might be for disease resistance, rapid growth, or some other favored feature. Then, the scientist inserts this single gene into the nucleus of the cell. The transplant procedure may be performed with a glass needle, viewed and guided by use of a microscope. The gene becomes integrated permanently into the chromosome, and the new gene bestows the desired trait in the mature animal.

Another technique uses disabled viruses to inject a transplant into the cell. If the surviving egg begins to grow and divide, the potential embryo is taken from the laboratory setting and implanted into a surrogate animal mother. Of the surviving offspring born, a small number will carry the new gene, integrated so that it actually will function with the desired trait.

Cloning, another technique, has been widely publicized in the production of the world-famous late sheep, Dolly. This approach makes use of a transgenic animal that already has a desired trait. Cloning creates replicas of the transgenic animal, which permits expansion of a herd of transgenic animals to form a core-breeding herd.

When any of these transgenic techniques are successful, they result in a new variety of animal, with a characteristic that previously had not existed.

Evaluating Safety of Transgenic Fish as Food. At present, no federal law specifically regulates the use or release of genetically engineered animals. Critics charge that instead, unsuitable regulations, intended for other purposes, are being applied. This emerging controversy parallels the controversy over bioengineered food crops. Critics call for stricter regulation of the "process" of genetic engineering; supporters think what is necessary is to focus on the product. Lack of consumer knowledge about the particulars of federal oversight increases the potential for public confusion.

In the case of the transgenic Atlantic salmon, the Environmental Protection Agency (EPA) and the U.S. Department of Agriculture (USDA) have bowed out, although they are responsible for certain surveillance aspects of genetically modified organisms. (These agencies play other monitoring

Potential Benefits from Transgenic Animal Research

Work with transgenic food animals might influence basic biomedical research. Laboratory animals, including rats, mice, rabbits, and monkeys, could be modified by bioengineering techniques to give them characteristics that mimic human diseases. For example, the technique might advance the understanding of oncogenes (genes that have gone awry and develop malignant tumors).

In addition, researchers are attempting to modify the organs of animals such as pigs, for possible use as donor organs for human transplantations.

Bioengineering techniques can utilize animals such as cows, sheep, and goats as vehicles for delivery of pharmaceuticals.

Inserting a single gene into an animal that is capable of manufacturing a rare protein in its milk could produce a valuable drug.

"Pharmaceutical animals" already exist. One company has created a goat that carries the gene for antithrombin 3, a blood protein that helps prevent blood clotting in humans. The company extracts the protein from a transgenic goat's milk and purifies it for drug use. Another example is alpha antitrypsin, a drug based on a milk protein, used to treat cystic fibrosis.

roles. The EPA, for example, oversees the pesticides used around aquaculture facilities and the effluent quality from these facilities.) Only the FDA is exerting any direct authority over transgenic Atlantic salmon.

The FDA has decided to treat the transgenic Atlantic salmon as a drug issue. By designating the fish's foreign genes and the growth hormone they produce as an animal drug, the agency has chosen to classify it under drug regulations. This designation subjects it to premarket requirements to determine its effectiveness and to ensure safety.

Should transgenic fish escape from fish farms, they could mate with fish in the wild and possibly even wipe out the wild populations.

Most gene-based modifications of animals for food production are regulated as new animal drugs under the FDA's Center for Veterinary Medicine (CVM). The agency has decided that the genetically modified growth hormone for the fish will be regulated by a precedent already established. The agency cites its regulation of bovine somatotropin, the genetically engineered bovine growth hormone that makes cows produce more milk. The agency reasons that transgenics merely provide another means to add growth hormone to an animal.

On the environmental front, critics charge that scientists at the FDA are less qualified and experienced than scientists at the EPA to evaluate environmental risks. Critics are concerned that transgenic Atlantic salmon may slip through numerous loopholes in federal regulations, and pose environmental threats. Should transgenic fish escape from fish farms, they could mate with fish in the wild and possibly even wipe out the wild populations. In addition, possibilities exist for unpredictable environmental disruptions. An example cited is the invasion of ecosystems by nonnative zebra mussels, a particularly aggressive species, in U.S. lakes and rivers.

The FDA reports, however, that transgenic fish farmers believe they can prevent their fish causing such environmental problems by producing transgenic fish in closed aquaculture systems (controlled, artificial environments) or by producing all female, sterile fish.

THE ORIGINS OF TRANSGENIC FISH

The science behind the transgenic Atlantic salmon was discovered by chance in the 1980s by a Canadian researcher, Choy Hew, Ph.D. Working at Memorial University in Newfoundland, he accidentally froze a tank filled with a species of flounder. When the water thawed, he was astonished to see that the flounder still lived.

Investigations showed that the species has a gene that produces an antifreeze protein. Many types of polar fish that swim in extremely cold water also have this antifreeze protein.

Researchers were able to isolate and copy the part of the flounder's DNA that triggers production of the antifreeze protein. Normally, the triggering only occurs when the fish is exposed to cold water. Hew and his colleagues attached the flounder's genetic switch to a previously isolated gene from chinook salmon that produces a growth-stimulating hormone. They inserted the new combination of the flounder's antifreeze protein and the chinook salmon's growth hormone into fertilized salmon eggs, to produce salmon with both traits. By having the growth hormone supplied continuously, the transgenic salmon could grow faster.

In the case of the farmed Atlantic salmon, a gene promoter is taken from ocean pout. This fish has a valuable trait of signaling when and where in the body to produce a natural antifreeze. The promoter is spliced to the salmon growth hormone gene, which then is re-introduced into the salmon egg. This procedure effectively changes where and when the salmon produces the growth hormone. In the wild, the dominant phase of growth hormone production is limited to summertime, when the salmon grows. In the transgenic Atlantic salmon, the growing season is virtually year round.

John Matheson, senior regulatory review scientist at CVM, defends the agency's ability to conduct environmental reviews. Matheson said that the FDA routinely investigates the environmental impact of new drugs: "We look at the environmental impacts of approving an antibiotic, how much is released into the environment, what does it do." His choice of example is unfortunate, and not reassuring. The FDA has been criticized sharply for its mishandling of antibiotic issues. Among its severest critics have been researchers from a sister agency, the Centers for Disease Control and Prevention (CDC).

Other administration officials also have voiced doubts about the FDA's ability to address environmental concerns about transgenic fish. Dr. William Brown, science advisor to the Secretary of the Department of the Interior, in which the Fish and Wildlife Service is based, comments that "we need a system that lets us check things beforehand, that shifts the burden of proof onto those that would introduce them." Brown adds: "I don't think the potential impacts on nature have been thought through as well as they should be."

Currently, the FDA is reviewing a petition to allow for the sale of transgenic Atlantic salmon as food. The agency must determine whether this fish meets the requirements for food safety as well as possible environmental effects that may result. Before coming to a final decision, the agency plans to hold public hearings on transgenic Atlantic salmon and other possible transgenic animal foods.

THE DOWNSIDE OF FISH FARMING

Increased fish consumption is developing at the very time when fish sources are dwindling, due mainly to overfishing and pollution. The growing demands for fish have given impetus to the growth of fish farming as a means of providing a dependable year-round source of certain types of fish, now available in retail stores as well as in fast-food outlets and gourmet restaurants.

To date, the most successful fish farming operations are with catfish in Mississippi and other Southern states; with rainbow trout in Idaho; and with salmon in Oregon and Washington. The newest innovation is fish farming with transgenic Atlantic salmon. (See the article "Biotech Animals Come to the Farm—Controversy May Follow" on page 407.) Aggressive promotion and marketing strategies increased the volume of domestic catfish processing elevenfold from 1976 to 1986. Most restaurant catfish are now farmed.

Rainbow trout is reared in spring water, held at a uniform 58°F temperature year-round. Nearly all rainbow trout served in restaurants is farmed fish.

Salmon is farmed in "ranches." Young salmon are reared in holding ponds of warm water, and when grown, are released into the ocean. Within one to four years, survivors return to their rearing ponds where they are caught and readied for market.

Fish farming is not new; it dates back to ancient Roman and Chinese times. What is new is that many fish farming practices are now similar to those in current land farming, including efficient operation and control of stress, disease, growth rate, flavor, nutrients and quality. These practices present challenges for fish farmers.

Fish farms encounter problems of algae growth, waterborne diseases, varying oxygen levels, and, in catfish, a perplexing "off-flavor" taste.

The pond intended for catfish rearing must be carefully sited, especially if it is to be constructed adjacent to land that has been used to cultivate row crops. The water source must be unpolluted because fish are highly sensitive to exceedingly low toxin levels.

Farmed vs. Wild Fish

Farmed fish, including transgenic ones, are lower in fat than fish in the wild. Nutritionally, this is undesirable, because the fat in fish is a beneficial unsaturated type. Also, due to the feeding practices with farmed fish, they lack the ideal ratio of omega-3 to omega-6 fatty acids present in fish in the wild. Lastly, the flavor and color of farmed fish are inferior to their counterparts. Conditions are comparable to land farming: confined versus free-range food animals.

Cultured and wild catfish are both subject to similar diseases and parasites, but the high-density rearing in fish farming can intensify problems of stress, disease, and infection.

Commonly, copper sulfate and potassium permanganate are added to the water of catfish ponds as herbicides and algicides, and to treat parasitic infections. Treating diseased fish individually is not feasible, so all the fish are given medications added to the water and/or the feed. Often, the range between an effective and a toxic dose is very narrow. At times, the treatment aggravates the problem.

Standard catfish feed consists of a fortified grain blend. Daily measured feedings are scattered mechanically to avoid excessive feeding, which would nutrify the pond, stress the fish, and promote unwanted phytoplankton bloom. At times, fish feed has been contaminated, wreaking havoc with the fish. In one incident, 48 percent of all cultivated rainbow trout developed liver cancer from aflatoxin-contaminated cottonseed meal. Aflatoxin molds are highly toxic and probably carcinogenic.

Due to the feeding practices, farmed fish may lack the coloring that is present in wild fish. Because paleness reduces their market value, farmers are searching for fish-feed pigmenters that approximate the coloring normally present in wild fish. In many countries, synthetic pigments are widely used for this purpose, but this practice is prohibited in the United States. Astaxanthin, a carotenoid pigment found in the flowers of a Romanian weed, could be a pigmenter added to the feed for reared salmon and rainbow trout. The same pigment is found in wild salmon and red snapper, as well as in crustaceans such as lobster, crab, and shrimp.

Flavor, Nutrition, Quality. How does the flavor of reared fish compare with wild fish? Just as the discriminating human palate knows the differences in flavor between domesticated and wild duck, or a pork roast from domesticated pig and wild boar, so too, there are distinct differences between the flavor of cultured and wild fish. For example, reared catfish is milder than its relative living in its traditional habitat. Fish living in warm water do not develop the same flavor as in cooler water. This is true even for marine animals in the wild. An example is the difference in flavor between lobsters from Maine and Florida.

Flavor enhancers, such as liquid smoke, are being considered as possible additions to the water in fish farms. Such additives can be picked up by catfish within fifteen minutes.

Is the nutritional content of the reared fish similar to the wild fish? While both types of fish are nutritious, different feed yields different results. For example, reared fish fed brine shrimp have very different levels of fatty acids from those fed artificial diets.

In recent times, many people have increased their fish consumption to obtain the beneficial omega-3 fatty acids present in many fish. However, these fatty acids are not obtained as readily from reared as from wild fish. When reared freshwater fin- and shell-fish were analyzed, it was found that the fats of cultured fish had higher levels of the omega-6 fatty acids and lower levels of the omega-3 fatty acids. Reared catfish, fed mainly on cornmeal, contain mostly omega-6, not omega-3 fatty acids. The omega-6 fatty acids are overabundant in the American diet, at the expense of too little of the omega-3 fatty acids.

Just as the discriminating human palate knows the differences in flavor between domesticated and wild duck, or a pork roast from domesticated pig and wild boar, so too, there are distinct differences between the flavor of cultured and wild fish.

How does the quality of cultured fish compare with its wild counterpart? A Nova Scotian salmon processor noted that what impressed him about wild salmon was its "tone." He commented that "tone is the one thing you won't find in a farm-raised salmon. . . . Farmed fish cannot move too far, and certainly do not have to catch their own food. What they do have, however, is fin-rot. In the processing of thousands of farmed salmon over the years, this was found in almost every one."

Various techniques can make farm fish grow faster and larger than normal. Fish may be manipulated hormonally—by injection or additive to feed or water—with the male sex hormone, testosterone. (See article "Biotech Animals Come to the Farm—Controversy May Follow" on page 407.) With rainbow trout, the testosterone causes immature females to develop as males.

Farm fish grow faster by being reared in warm water. In salmon ranching, the customary eighteen-month growth period of the young salmon is reduced to only six months. The salmon ranch may utilize warm water discharged from paper mills. Other considered possibilities include warm waste water used to cool machinery, or from sewage plants or nuclear power plants.

Use of strong magnetic fields is being explored as a possibility to make rainbow trout more fertile. When ova and sperm of rainbow trout were exposed to magnetic fields 10,000 times greater than the earth's magnetic fields, fertilization was enhanced.

Less Variety. "Catch-of-the-Day" may become an irrelevant term for restaurants as the supply of wild fish further declines and as fish farming ascends. The inherent characteristic of catch-of-the-day is uncertainty—uncertainty of species, sizes, and quantities. But the term also signals freshness, seasonality, and variety. The inherent characteristic of farmed fish is certainty—certainty of species, sizes, and quantities. Either fresh or frozen, farmed fish signals year-round availability, but limited choices.

"Eat a variety of food" is a time-honored slogan for good nutrition. The diversity of marine animals used as human food is far greater than land animals. As fish farming continues to develop, this rich diversity may be sharply curtailed. (See the article "Our Narrowing Food Base: A Perilous Trend" on page 18.) Retail stores and restaurants may choose to offer fewer fish choices, and restrict them mainly to the few types that are successfully farmed.

Earlier, enthusiastic accounts were given about the future developments of fish farming, with shellfish such as lobster, salt-water shrimp, crab, oyster, mussel, and abalone; red snapper; eel; and even caviar-producing sturgeon. Success with these species has been hampered for various reasons. If fish farming continues to be limited in making available only a few types of fish that can be efficiently managed and profitable, it will narrow the base of food diversity.

INNOVATIVE PEST CONTROL

The U.S. Department of Agriculture (USDA) engages in numerous cooperative research and development agreements with industrial groups that benefit the entire population. Two recent cooperative projects are notable as innovative measures of nontoxic pest control. One uses minerals; the other, sugar esters.

Mineral Particle Spray. A water spray of mineral particles may protect growing food crops such as fruits, vegetables, and tree nuts from insect pests and plant diseases. The mineral particles, microscopic in size, are specifically shaped, mixed with water, and sprayed on crops. After the liquid evaporates, it coats the crop with a white, powdery film.

The minerals used for this particle film are from kaolin (clay). The Food and Drug Administration (FDA) regards kaolin as safe, and has approved it as an indirect food additive. The spray is chemically inert, and the Environmental Protection Agency (EPA) has exempted particle film technology from pesticide tolerance regulations.

Kaolin does not harm beneficial insects. Nor does the kaolin film interfere with crop pollination or photosynthesis. The particles allow sunlight to diffuse into the leaves, with little light reduction. The reflective characteristic of the particles reduces heat stress on leaves, and lowers the temperature in the canopy of the trees or growing crops. The treated fruit develops more color, less sunburn, higher soluble solids, less deterioration, and greater weight than untreated fruit.

The particle film helps protect plants against damaging insects. The coating forms a protective physical barrier against insect pests. When they come into contact with the film coating, tiny particles adhere to their bodies. The particles agitate and repel the insects. The particles attached to nonflying insects make them unable to leave the plant. They cannot feed or lay eggs, and become confused and disoriented.

Another benefit of the spray is that it enriches the soil indirectly. Kaolin is harmless to earthworms, allows them to move freely, carry organic matter down from the soil surface, increases water infiltration, and aerates the soil. These activities improve soil structure, and in turn help plants to grow more vigorously and productively.

The mineral particle spray can be applied in fruit orchards and tree groves, and to ground crops such as peanuts, peppers, cucumbers, as well as white and sweet potatoes. The film remaining on the crop can either "weather off" or be washed off after the crop is harvested. Commonly, in conventional packinghouses, many crops are washed.

In 1997, the EPA granted an experimental use permit to field test the mineral particle spray, by fifty collaborators, including researchers from the USDA's Agricultural Research Service (ARS), university scientists, and crop growers.

The mineral particle spray has been tested in fruit orchards for several growing seasons to control a range of insect pests and diseases to which apples and pears are prone. Field tests were conducted abroad in Chile and Italy, as well as in the United States at the USDA's agricultural research laboratory research stations in West Virginia and Washington state. The treatment was found to be effective against many economically important fruit tree pests, including the leafhopper, leafminer, spirea aphid, thrip, European red mite, two-spotted spider mite, and late-season apple diseases such as sooty blotch and fly speck. Good results were achieved, too, against plum curculio and codling moth, although the sprays have not yet reached a practical economic level of control for these two difficult-to-control pests without resorting to additional measures.

To date, the most spectacular success has been the control of major problems for pear growers. The particle film completely controlled the pear psylla and pear rust.

The promising results from the field tests were confirmed with additional tests conducted in 1998 in six different fruit growing regions of the country. Fine-tuning the program increased its effectiveness and reduced the necessary number of sprayings.

Both traditional and organic growers value the effectiveness of the particle spray. Some found that it worked better than conventional controls that they had been using.

Sugar Ester Spray. Another food crop protection measure uses a form of sugar ester that is highly water-soluble, yet remains active in killing insect pests such as the whitefly, pear psylla, and other soft-bodied damaging insects. The sugar esters break down the outer coating of these insects, cause their bodies to lose water and shrivel.

In field tests, a spray consisting of a mixture of water and sugar esters, extracted from plants, killed all the pear psylla on the leaves. The spray even killed pear psylla that hatched three days later. The spray also controlled white fly, aphid, thrip, and other insect pests without harming beneficial insects.

MOVING TOWARD A BIOBASED ECONOMY

"Agriculture's role will change from food, feed, and fiber to food, feed, materials, chemicals, fuels, pharmaceuticals, animal vaccines, and many other products now derived from petroleum," noted Dr. Robert Armstrong, former executive director of the U.S. Department of Agriculture's (USDA) Alternative Agriculture Research and Commercial Corporation, a unique venture capital corporation established in 1992. New opportunities exist in the emerging biobased economy that compete with many products now derived from petroleum. According to Armstrong: "The future of the global economy is biobased, and the future of American agriculture is to be the supplier of raw materials for that biobased economy." This prediction, if realized, would be welcomed by American farmers.

The Rise, Fall and Rise of a Biobased Economy. Until the twentieth century, the economy was largely biobased.

Innovators such as George Washington Carver and Henry Ford utilized biobased materials in their pioneering efforts. Carver's research and practical developments produced hundreds of useful products from peanuts to sweet potatoes. Ford built a prototype "biological" automobile body in 1941, by making use of soybeans, field straw, cotton linters, slash pine, and bio-resin. Ford fueled the automobile with a blend of 15 percent ethanol and 85 percent gasoline. Thus, the recent interest with ethanol as a renewable energy source is not a new idea, but rather a revival.

By the twentieth century, however, powerful and efficient new technologies had allowed petroleum to be collected and refined into numerous raw materials and high-performance products. They competed with older, biologically based materials, and eventually replaced them with many products such as cosmetics, plastics, and motor oil.

"The future of the global economy is biobased, and the future of American agriculture is to be the supplier of raw materials for that biobased economy."

The shortages during World War II, and the later oil crisis, turned attention briefly to homegrown biobased materials. However, drops in oil prices and advances in oil refining, revived the oil economy. More recently, the fluctuations of supplies and prices of foreign oil, and the finiteness of its supply, has made Americans more aware of our vulnerable dependency. Once again, a biobased energy source has attracted attention.

A biobased economy is being powered across the agricultural sector by cooperative efforts among federal programs, commodity groups, private industry, and others in the private sector, along with research scientists in federal, state, and university laboratories. The researchers are investigating technologies that can convert traditional and newly introduced agricultural crops, waste residues, and animal byproducts into new products, including energy sources. These technologies, if perfected, could lower manufacturing and consumer costs, improve efficiency, and result in better performance.

Potential applications for biologically derived substances that will benefit consumers and manufacturers are numerous. They include alternative fuels, fertilizers, pesticides, detergents, paints, new fibers, paper, inks, personal care products, construction materials, insulation, nutraceuticals, packaging, pharmaceuticals, veterinary products, lubricants, coatings, absorbents, adsorbents, and adhesives.

In this shift to a biobased economy, agriculture is providing the raw materials to make consumer and industrial products. The foundations for this biobased economy are carbohydrates from plants, proteins from animal byproducts, fatty acids from oilseeds, and cellulose from trees. A biobased economy offers new opportunities to develop value-added products.

Potential applications for biologically derived substances that will benefit consumers and manufacturers are numerous. They include alternative fuels . . . insulation, nutraceuticals, packaging, pharmaceuticals . . . and adhesives

Some Success Stories to Date. The USDAs Alternative Agriculture Research and Commercialization Corporation has helped some sixty rural companies to commercialize innovative research. These efforts have led to biobased products and transfer of the technology to rural communities. Both EnvironR and Citra-Solv serve as illustrations.

EnvironR is a biocomposite that can replace hardwood and stone flooring, and also has furniture applications. The durable and attractive marblelike material looks like, but is lighter, than granite, and is harder than oak. It is made of soybeans and recycled paper.

Citra-Solv is a popular home and industrial cleaner. It is composed of natural solvents from citrus peels, rather than from petroleum-based solvents. Formerly, citrus peels were discarded as waste by Florida citrus growers, who now extract extra value at processing plants.

Research at the Ag-Based Industrial Lubricants Research Program at the University of Northern Iowa led to the successful marketing of BioSOY, SoyLINK, and SoyTRUK—a product line of soy-based industrial lubricants. The raw materials and the manufacture of the products are located in Iowa.

More than 8,700 Minnesota farm members collectively own fifteen ethanol production plants in the state. The state of Minnesota sparked its ethanol industry. Currently, 10 percent of the state's vehicles are fueled by ethanol. Each year, the ethanol production plants within Minnesota turn 78 million bushels of corn into 200 million gallons of corn-derived ethanol.

Biodiesel, a fuel derived mainly from soybean oil, has been designated as an alternative fuel by the Department of Energy. In 1998, the U.S. Congress enacted legislation that allows the use of a blend of 20 percent biodiesel and 80 percent petroleum diesel to meet the Energy Policy Act of 1992 requirements. Biodiesel is a clean-burning alternative, with similar power, fuel economy, and performance as petroleum-based diesel fuel. During 1999, more than thirty-five major fleets began using biodiesel, including 141 vehicles and equipment at one of the USDA's Agricultural Research Stations.

Research by the USDA and other scientists, plus more than $20 million in farmer checkoff funds, helped develop the U.S. biodiesel industry.

In the tradition of George Washington Carver, two students at Purdue University participated in a "New Uses for

Soybeans" competition, funded by the Indiana Soybean Board. Three years of work by a team of chemists, product developers, and marketers brought to market a new product: nontoxic soybean crayons, made with soybean oil.

Some projects are modest, as with two women farmers in Missouri who market their goat milk soaps and hand creams. All the milk used in their products is produced on their small farms. Natural moisturizing ingredients in goat's milk make it useful for skin products. The women found a niche in the natural-ingredient personal care market, and their products sell well through specialty stores in several states, and nationwide through mail orders.

New Opportunities for Agriculture. Farmers are finding new uses for raw materials from agricultural and forestry resources, some of which had previously been regarded as waste. Farmers with modest acreage can benefit from biobased products. Bioprocessing facilities are likely to be established in rural areas to crush beans for oil, or to make new fibers or materials from locally grown commodities.

Presently, four biorefineries are being built in North America. Three of them will convert cornstalks, sugarcane waste fibers, or rice straw into ethanol; and the fourth will produce ethanol from sewage sludge and organic wastes generated from municipal garbage. As alternative fuels such as ethanol are developed from farm-raised plant sources by farmer-owned cooperatives or for-profit corporations, America's dependence on foreign energy sources will lessen. Although 100 percent biodiesel for truck fuel awaits future development, currently blends of biodiesel and petroleum-based diesel are functioning. The National Biodiesel Board estimates that if only 1 percent of the agricultural diesel market were converted to biodiesel, 23 million soybean bushels would be utilized.

American farmers have new opportunities, by planting crops hitherto not raised. Plants such as vernonia, euphorbia, and lesquerella have potentials to supply materials for paints and coatings. Kenaf and hesperaloe plants have value for industrial materials such as fiber products, including paper. Guayule is being developed as a source for natural rubber and hypoallergenic latex, especially in the health care industry, to replace latex gloves for individuals who cannot tolerate them.

American farmers have greater opportunities by increasing their production of familiar plants for additional uses. Soybeans, crambe, rapeseed, and canola plants can be used to make biobased fuels and lubricants. Sunflower seed oil can produce resins used for oil-based paints. The flax plant can yield fibers for linen and paper, industrial oils for household cleaners, chemicals for paints, and varnishes used in plastics. Other vegetable oils and starches from plants can be used to make polymers. Corn, sugarcane, wheat, and milo (a sorghum grain used in animal feed) can be the stock for ethanol or ethyl alcohol production. Specialized herbs with medical benefits, in growing demand for the health care market, hold promise as high-value crops for nutraceuticals.

Partnerships Foster a Biobased Economy. A network has been created to foster a biobased economy, involving government, industry, and entrepreneurs. The USDA's Regional Agricultural Utilization Centers involve many researchers who have been engaged for over half a century in the development of biobased products. The Forest Products Laboratory, too, has played a vital role. Part of the network consists of the land-grant university system, industry scientists, and others. Federal and state university researchers can patent, but cannot commercialize, their inventions. They can license the right to commercialize the technology, developed with federal or state funds, to private companies.

State research centers carry out biobased product research to find expanded markets for commodities. Strong biobased programs exist in at least a dozen states. Center research addresses some projects that are specific to the particular state. For example, the University of Kentucky investigates new uses for tobacco, such as biochemicals, pharmaceuticals, fiber crops, and the conversion of cellulose to ethanol.

The National Academy of Sciences reported that America's abundant crop, forest, and animal resources warrant the rapid transition to alternative fuels and biodegradable biobased industrial products. The transition has begun. It will boost the agricultural economy, and at the same time improve the quality of the environment.

INDEX

Absorption, 122–133
Acceptable Daily Intakes (ADIs), 366
Acesulfame K, 173
Acids, 124
Adenosine triphosphate (ATP), 158
Agricultural Handbook No. 8, 243, 245, 246
Agriculture. *See* Farming.
Albuterol, 120
Alcohol, 76–77, 126, 140, 219, 228, 249, 332
Allergen Protection Plan, 69
Allergies, 61–73, 204, 236, 271, 274, 303–304
  peanut, 62–70
  soy, 241–242
Allyl isothiocyanate, 148
Almonds, 134–135
America's Eating Habits, 9
American Academy of Pediatrics. Committee on Nutrition, 39, 41
American Dietetic Association (ADA), 174
Amino acids, 108–109, 159, 241
  forms, 108–109, 119, 236
Anaphylaxis, 66, 68–69
Animal feed, 388–398
  See also Hen feed.
Animals, growth, 399, 410, 411
Anions, 154
Annatto, 298–299, 306, 311
Anorexia nervosa, 54–56, 60
Antacids, 126, 326
Anthocyanins, 295–296
Antibiotics, 76, 79, 383, 385, 398–404, 407
  resistance to, 335, 337, 398
Anticoagulants, 77–78, 237
Anticonvulsives, 80
Antimicrobials, 147–150, 309, 399–404
  in products, 341–344
Antioxidants, 310
Apples, 286, 287, 387
Aquaculture, 315, 408, 411
Aroclor, 383
Arsenic, 117–118, 381
Arthritis, reactive, 328–329
Artificial sweeteners, 184–187
Asbestos, 368–373
Aspartame, 173, 185–186, 194
Aspirin, 78
Association of Professionals in Infectious Controls, 342
Astaxanthin, 416
Asthma, 279, 280–281
Astragalus, 165
Atrophic gastritis, 82–83, 326
Atwater, W. O., 245
Avocados, 246

Bacteria, 386–387
  lactic-acid producing, 314–315
  resistant, 315, 343–344, 347, 400–404
Battelle World Agrochemical Data Bank, 367

Bean curd, 238–239
Beer, 140
Beets, 296, 297
Benzene, 375
Benzo(*a*)pyrene, 122
Beta-blockers, 229
Beta-carotene, 297
Betacyanins, 296–297
Beta-galactosidases. *See* Lactase.
Beverages, 369–370
  functional, 160–161
  probiotic, 159–160
  sport, 154, 158–159
Bezoar stones, 118
Bicknell, Franklin, 110–111
Bifidobacteria, 357–360
Bile, 124, 128
Binge eating, 58
Bioavailability, 98, 122–123
Biodiesel, 424
Biofilms, 317
Biofouling, 317
BioSOY, 424
Biotechnology, 407–413
Blood pressure, 257–258
  high. *See* Hypertension.
Blood sugar, 112, 170
Bone loss, 89, 90
Botulism, 324–325
Bovine somatotropin, 411
Bovine spongiform encephalopathy (BSE), 395–398
Brain, 255
Breakfast, 49–50
Breastfeeding, 31–36, 44–45
Broccoli, 113, 129, 132
Bulimia nervosa, 56–58
Buttermilk, 74

Cabbage, 140, 296
Cadmium, 218–219
Caffeine, 125, 126, 139
Calcium, 50–51, 89–90, 112–113, 124, 125, 129, 131, 154, 156, 166, 216, 220
Campylobacter jejuni, 321, 329, 333, 400
Cancer, 179–180, 205
  breast, 239
  stomach, 372
Candy plant (*Myrrhis odorata*). *See* Sweet cicely.
Canthaxanthin, 297, 298
Capsaicin, 150–154
Caramel, 300–301, 307
Carbohydrates, 111–112, 180
  complex, 170, 171
  refined, 170
Carcinogens, 121–122
Carminic acid, 301–304
Carotene, 80, 123, 128, 129–130, 280
Carotenoids, 196–197, 297
Carrageenan, 288–293
Carrots, 129–130, 246, 297
Carver, George Washington, 422
Cataracts, 87
Catfish, 414, 415
Cations, 154
Cats, 323, 338
Certified Color Industry Committee, 263–264
Chaos, 253–256
Charcoal, activated, 334
Cheese, 74
Chelation, 130–131
Cherries, maraschino, 270
Chewing gums, 168–169
Children
  eating habits, 2–3, 5, 51–52, 66–68
  nutrition, 45–52, 128, 129

obesity, 45–48, 51–52
undernutrition, 48–51
Chirality, 108–109, 118–122, 234, 235, 236
Chloride, 154, 157, 221
Chlorophyll, 299
Chocolate, 97
Cholesterol, 47–48, 99, 134, 135–136, 141–142, 176, 208, 224–232, 240
apolipoprotein components, 224
low-density lipoproteins (LDL), 224, 225, 226, 228, 242
high-density lipoproteins (HDL), 224, 225, 226, 228
tests, 224–225, 229–232
very low-density lipoproteins (VLDL), 224, 228
Cholestyramine, 79, 194
Chromium, 115, 125, 179
Chrysotile, 369, 372
Cinnamon, 148, 149–150, 309
Citra-Solve, 424
Citrus peels, 424
Clark, Duncan, 352
Cloning, 409
Clostridium perfringens, 321
Clove, 147, 148, 309
Cochineal, 301–304
Coffee. *See* Caffeine.
Colchicine, 80
Colitis, 289–293
Color Additives Amendment of 1960 (Public Law 86–618), 264
Colors
noncertified, 293–308
U.S. certified food, 261–274
Colostrum, 168
Conjugated linoleic acid (CLA), 205–207
Containers, 381
plastic, 375–376
Continuing Survey of Food Intake of Individuals (CSFII), 250–252
Contraceptives, 78–79, 229
Copper, 90, 91–92, 95, 124, 125, 178, 183–184
Cottonseed, 21–22
Creatine, 165
phosphate, 158
Curtiss, Roy, 339
Cutting boards, 353, 354–357
Cyanocobalamin. *See* Vitamin B_{12}.
Cyclamates, 185

Daycare centers, 351
DDT, 364, 365
Dehydration, 93, 137–140
Detergents. *See* Soaps and detergents.
DHA (docosahexaenoic acid), 42–41
Di-(ethylhexyl)adipate (DEHA), 374
Diabetes, 175, 177–178, 187, 229
Diarrhea, 330, 358
traveler's (TD), 330–334
Diet and Health, 251
Dietary Assessment of the U.S. Food Supply, 3–4
Dietary Supplement Health and Education Act (DSHEA), 189
Diet, 1–9, 24–28, 51–52, 318–324
away from home, 2–3, 22–23, 286, 324–325
hunter-gatherer, 24–25
macrobiotic, 48–49
portion size, 6–8
Stone-age, 25–28

Dieting, 52, 53–54
Digestion, 259
Digitalis, 80
Dishcloths, 354
Diuretics, 78, 80, 139, 222, 229
DNA, 119
Dopamine, 120
D-ribose, 158
Dried poultry waste (DPW), 390
Drugs, 326
over-the-counter, 126, 151
prescription, 120–121, 127
Dyes, 262–274

Eating disorders, 52–61
Eating habits. *See* Diet.
EBDC (ethylenebisdithiocarbamate), 378–379
Economy, biobased, 421–427
Eggs, 140–147, 318
Eicosanoids, 211
Elderly, 81–94, 129, 326, 359
Electrolytes, 154–157, 216
Emulsifiers, 310–311
Enantiomers, 120
Energy, 244
EnvironR, 423–424
Epidemiology, 255–256
Epidermal growth factor (EGF), 32
Epinephrine, 69
Equal. *See* Aspartame.
Escherichia coli, 128, 147–148, 331, 332
0157:H7, 314, 321–322
Essential fatty acids (EFAs), 110–111, 210–212
Ethanol, 422, 424, 425
ETU (ethylene thiourea), 378–379
Exercise, 8, 47, 157, 228
See also Running, compulsive.
Farming, 315–316, 388–427, 421–427
organic, 380
Fats, 110–111, 124, 125, 134, 176, 205, 206, 208–212
labeling, 208, 209, 212
monounsaturated, 134
polyunsaturated, 223
replacers. *See* Z-Trim.
saturated, 227
substitutes. *See* Olestra.
FD&C Blue No. 1 (brilliant blue FCF), 264–265
FD&C Blue No. 2 (indigotine), 265–266
FD&C Citrus Red No. 2, 266–267
FD&C Green No. 3 (fast green FCF), 268
FD&C Red No. 2 (amaranth), 271–274
FD&C Red No. 3 (erythrosine), 269
FD&C Red No. 4 (ponceau SX), 269–270
FD&C Red No. 40 (allura red AC), 270–271
FD&C Violet No. 1, 375
FD&C Yellow No. 5 (tartrazine), 271, 274, 304
FD&C Yellow No. 6 (sunset yellow FCF), 271
FDA/USDA Consumer Food Safety Survey, 353
Feces, 406
Federation of American Societies for Experimental Biology (FASEB), 252
Ferns (*Polypodium vulgare L.*), 190
Ferrous gluconate, 304–305
Fiber, 112, 125, 176, 202, 203, 327
Fish, 381–382, 383, 413–418

farmed vs. wild, 415, 416–417
fat, 382, 383
oil, 223
transgenic, 408, 409, 410–411, 412, 413, 414
Fish farming, 408, 410–411, 412, 413–418
Flavoring Extract Manufacturers Association of the United States (FEMA), 275
Fluoxetine. *See* Prozac.
Folate, 79, 83, 84–85, 100
Folic acid, 100–101, 125, 245–246
Folinic acid, 101
Food, 17, 18–24, 305–311, 418
colors and dyes, 261–274, 293–308, 311
contamination, 316–317, 323, 324–325, 360–387
convenience, 279
cooked vs. raw, 111–112, 129–130, 378–379, 382–383, 384–385
and drug interactions, 75–78
and drug residues, 326, 383–385, 398–407
flavor additives, 274–279, 416, 419
imported, 367–368
Kosher, 304
labeling, 70, 194, 208, 284, 287, 308, 309, 360
low-fat, 318–319
packaging, 307, 320, 374–377, 394
preparation, 324, 325–326, 344, 345, 350, 352–354, 382–383, 384–385, 387
preservation, 309–310
processing, 10–18, 70–71, 221, 278, 284–285, 286–287, 289–291, 305–306, 316–317, 371–372, 378
refrigeration, 319–320
residues on, 377–387
surveys, 247–253
tables, 243–247
take-out, 325
washing, 378, 379, 380–381
Food Additives Amendment of 1958, 275
Food Allergy and Anaphylaxis Network, 72
Food bars, 161–162, 165–169
energy/sports, 163–165
prebiotic, 168
Food Guide Pyramid, 5, 8, 137
Food Marketing Institute, 346
Food poisoning. *See* Illness, foodborne.
Food wrap, 374–376
Ford, Henry, 422
Formulas, infant-feeding, 36–45, 240–241
Four D's, 390, 395
Fructose, 172, 175
intolerance, 183–184
Fruits, 3, 4, 171, 379, 380–381, 420

Galactose, 181
intolerance, 181–182
Galactosemia, 181–182
Garbage, 393–394
Garlic, 147–148, 309
Genetic engineering, 407–413
Genistein, 109–110
Glycemic index, 112, 163, 165
Glycogen, 158, 170
Glycyrrhizic acid, 189
Goitrogens, 77
Grains, 385–386
distillers dried, 393–395

Grapes, 281, 282, 295–296, 380
Griseofulvin, 76
Grocery Manufacturers Association (GMA), 70–71
Guillain-Barré Syndrome, 329

Hand lotions, 348–349
Hands
  glove-wearing, 345–347
  sanitizers, 347–348
  washing, 343–354
Hazard Analysis Critical Control Points (HACCP), 69, 384
Health and Nutrition Examination Survey (HANES), 252
Heart disease, 175, 205, 242, 329
Heartbeats, 252
Heartburn, 83
Helicobacter pylori, 82
Hemagglutinins, 238
Hen feed, 143–145
Hew, Choy, 412
High fructose corn syrup (HFCS), 172, 175, 183
Homocysteine, 86
Horseradish, 148
Hospitals, 351
Human Nutrition Information Service, 251
Hydralazine, 80
Hydrangea (*Hydrangea macrophylla* var. *Thunbergii*), 190
Hydrochloric acid, 128,130
Hydrogenation, 110, 209, 241
Hypercalcemia, 107
Hypertension, 213–224, 257–258

Ice, 332–333
IgA, 31, 32
IgE (immunoglobin E), 61
Illnesses, foodborne, 312–360, 385, 402, 403
Immune defense system, 259, 387
Imodium, 334
Infants, 31–45, 128, 240–241, 250
Inglett, George E., 202, 203, 204
Insulin, 176, 177
Integrated Pest Management, 379
INTERSALT, 217–218
Intestinal tract, 405–407
Iodine, 95, 144–146
Irish moss. *See* Carrageenan.
Iron, 51, 91, 113–114, 123–124, 125, 129, 130
Irritable bowel syndrome, 183–184
Isoflavones, 109–110, 239
Isomers, 103, 106
Isoniazid, 79, 80

Joint diseases, 328–329

Kaolin, 419, 420
Katemfe (*Thaumatoccus danielli*), 187
Kefir, 159
Kessler, David A., 191, 196, 197, 198–200
Kidneys, 330

Lactaid®, 75
Lactase, 73, 74, 75, 181
Lactic acid, 309, 314
Lactoferrin, 32, 41, 114
Lactose, 124, 183
  intolerance, 73–75, 181
Lake Superior, 371
Larach, John A., 215
L-arginine, 159, 167, 257, 260
Laxatives, 126
Lead, 381
Lettuce, 380

Levodopa (Laradopa), 78
Licorice (*Glycyrrhia glabra*), 189
Limes, 141
Lipoproteins, 224
Listeria monocytogenes, 322
Livestock management, 399, 403–404
Lomotil, 334
Long-term care facilities, 351
Lycopene, 298
Lysinoalanine (LAL), 109

Macadamia nuts, 135–136
Mad cow disease. *See* Bovine spongiform encephalopathy (BSE).
Magnesium, 113, 124, 125, 154, 155–156, 221–222
Malaria, 259
Manganese, 90, 125
Mannitol, 173, 183
Manure, 389–390, 395
Marigolds, 209
Market Basket Survey, 365–366
McCarron, David A., 216, 220
Meats, 319, 385
Mercury, 381
Metabolites, 106
Metals, 116–118
  heavy, 381–382
Methyl selenol, 114, 115
Methylsulfonylmethane (MSM), 159
Microflora, 405–407
Microwave cooking, 325, 375–377
Milk, 73–74, 75, 206, 207, 219, 300, 309–310, 314–315, 404–405
  human, 31–36, 44–45, 358
Mineral oil, 79–80, 126, 195–196
Mineral particle spray, 419
Minerals, 90–91, 95–96, 112–115
Mint, 149
Miraculous berry (*Synsepalum dulcificum*), 187–188
Miso, 238
Molds, 385
Molybdenum, 125
Monoamine oxidase (MAO) inhibitors, 77
Monosodium glutamate (MSG), 78
Mountain Lake Manufacturing, 204
Muscles, 159
Mushrooms, 284
Mustard, 148
Mycotoxins, 385–386

National Advisory Committee on Microbiological Criteria for Foods, 345
National Antimicrobial Resistance Monitoring System: Enteric Bacteria (NARMS), 401
National Cancer Institute of Canada, 379
National Cholesterol Education Program, 231
National Food Consumption Survey (NFCS), 249–253
National Food Processors Association, 378
National Institute of Allergy and Infectious Diseases, 72–73
National Research Council. Food and Nutrition Board, 47
National Restaurant Association (NRA), 286, 346
Natto, 238
Necrotizing enterocolitis, 31, 39
Neomycin, 80

Neurotransmitters, 258
Newsprint, 394
Niacin, 99
Nicotinamide adenine dinucleotide (NAD), 99
Nitric oxide (NO), 257–260
Nitrosamines, 375
NSAIDs, 83
NutraSweet. *See* Aspartame.
Nutrition, 23–30, 48–51
  children, 45–51, 128, 129
  elderly, 81–94, 129
  infants, 31–45, 128
Nuts, 134–137

Oatrim, 202, 203
Obesity, 45–48, 51–53, 219, 228, 251
Olestra, 191–202
Olives, 134, 305
Omega-3 fatty acids, 142–143, 210–212, 223, 240, 415, 416–417
Omega-6 fatty acids, 210–212, 415, 416–417
Onions, 309
Orange B, 268
Oranges, 246, 378
Oregano, 148, 149
Osteoarthritis, 83
Osteomalacia, 89
Oxalates, 125
Oysters, 246
Ozone, 386–387

Pain relief, 151–153
Pantothenate, 235–236
Paprika, 298
Pasteur, Louis, 118–119
PCBs (polychlorinated biphenyls), 382–383
Peanuts, 62–70
Pears, 420
Pepper, 148
Peppers, 97, 148, 150, 246
Pesticide Data Program, 251, 378
Pesticides, 121–122, 250, 251
  monitoring, 361–368, 378, 379
  nontoxic, 419–421
Petroleum, 422
Phosphatidylserine (PS), 168
Phosphorus, 124, 125
Phytates, 125
Phytic acid, 237
Pica, 58–59
Pigments, 295–305
Pigs, 407
Pineapples, 97
Plasticizers, 374
Plutonium, 116–117
Polycyclic aromatic hydrocarbons (PAHs), 121–122
Polyethylene, 374–375
Potassium, 80, 154, 155, 216
Pregnancy, 228, 323
Prilosec, 83
Procter & Gamble (P&G), 191, 194, 201
Produce Marketing Association (PMA), 286
Produce, 319
Propionic acid, 309
Prostaglandins, 96
Proteases, 287
Protein, 92–93, 108–110, 123, 159, 163
Prozac, 121
Pyridoxine. *See* Vitamin B_6.

Recombinant bovine growth hormone (rBGH), 405
Recycling, 388–398

Report of Joint Committee on the use of antibiotics in animal husbandry and veterinary medicine. See Swann Report.
Respiratory syncytial virus (RSV), 351
Restaurants, 324–325
Retinoids, 108
Rhodiola rosea, 165
Riboflavin. *See* Vitamin B_2.
Rice, 324, 372–373
Rosemary, 149, 309, 310
Running, compulsive, 55, 56

Saccharin, 173, 184–185
Saffron, 298
Sage, 148
Salad bars, 324
Salmon, transgenic Atlantic, 408, 409, 410–411, 412, 413, 414, 417
Salmonella, 128, 312, 315–316, 322, 331, 332, 400–401
  typhimurium DT104, 334–341
Sauerkraut, 140
Schizandra, 165
Schizophrenia, 99
Scrapie, 396
Scurvy, 140, 141
Selenium, 114–115, 124, 316
Semmelweiss, Ignaz, 352
Senile purpura, 92
Serendipity berry (*Dioscoroephyllum cuminsii* Diels), 187
Sewage sludge, 391
Sewer grease, 392–393
Sexual functioning, male, 259
Sheep, 396, 409
Shigella, 332–333
Shrimp, 284, 383
Smell, 97, 255
Soaps and detergents, 351, 425
  antibacterial, 343–344, 347
Soda, 5
  diet, 184
Sodium, 14–15, 154, 156, 213–224, 305
Soil, 314, 419–420
Sorbitol, 173, 183
Soybeans, 19–21, 39, 109–110, 125, 237–242, 385, 424
  fermentation, 238
  milk, 240
  protein, 159, 164, 240
SoyLINK, 424
SoyTRUK, 424
Spices, 147–154, 309
Spirulina, 165
Sponges, 353
Staphylococcus aureus, 322–323, 403
Stearic acid, 208
Stereoisomers, 102, 103
Steroids, 229
Sterols, 107
Stevia (*Stevia rebaudiana* Bertoni), 188–189
Stress, 126
Styrofoam, 375
Substance P, 152
Sucrose. *See* Sugars.
Sugar and Sweetener: Situation and Outlook Yearbook, 4–5
Sugar Association, Inc., 174
Sugar ester spray, 421
Sugars, 3, 4–6, 111, 119, 125, 164, 170–190
  consumption, 171–181
  health risks, 175–181, 223
Sulfate, 125
Sulfites, 279–287, 295–296, 300–301, 309

Sunett. *See* Acesulfame K.
Sunlight, 89, 107, 127
Supermarkets, 323–324
Supplements, 130–133
  absorption, 130–131
Surgeon General's Report on Nutrition and Health, 251
Susceptors, 376
Swann Report, 399
Sweet cicely, 189–190
Sweet'N Low. *See* Saccharin.
Sweet One. *See* Acesulfame K.

Tagamet, 83
Tagetes, 298, 299
Talc, 371–372, 373
Taste, 97, 416
Tea, 125
  green, 159, 165
Television watching, 46–47, 52
Tempeh, 238
Tetracycline, 76
Thalidomide, 120–121
Theory of chaos. *See* Chaos.
Thiamine. *See* Vitamin B_1.
Thyroid, 229, 239
Tin, 222
Tissue Residue Information Management System (TRIMS), 384
Titanium oxide, 304
Tobacco smoking, 126
Tofu, 238–239
Tomatoes, 246, 298, 378, 379
  paste, 97
Tooth decay, 171, 172
Total Diet Study. *See* Market Basket Survey.
Towels, paper, 354
Toxoplasma gondii, 323
Trans-fatty acids, 209–210, 241
Triclosan, 343–344, 347
Triglycerides, 175, 176, 177, 224, 225, 228
Trout, rainbow, 414
Trypsin, 237
Turmeric, 300, 311
Tyramine, 77

U.S. Centers for Disease Control and Prevention (CDC), 313, 341, 350, 413
U.S. Dept. of Agriculture (USDA), 243, 246, 249, 250, 252, 253, 361, 362–363, 409
  Agricultural Research Service, 355–356
  Alternative Agriculture Research and Commercialization Corporation, 421, 423
  Animal and Plant Health Inspection Service (APHIS), 397
  Economic Research Service, 1, 3, 10–11, 173, 247, 340–341
  Meat and Poultry Hotline, 355
U.S. Environmental Protection Agency (EPA), 253, 343, 361–362, 371, 379, 409, 410, 411, 419
U.S. Food and Drug Administration (FDA), 172, 188, 189, 192, 198–200, 201–202, 208, 250, 253, 264, 276–278, 279, 284–286, 287, 303–304, 340–314, 343, 345, 354, 361, 363–367, 373, 376, 390, 392–393, 397–398, 399–400, 405, 410–411, 418, 419
  Center for Veterinarian Medicine (CVM), 384, 392, 394–395, 411, 413

Residue Monitoring Program, 379
U.S. Food Safety and Inspection Service (FSIS), 363, 383
U.S. General Accounting Office (GAO), 243–244, 250, 251, 362, 364, 365, 367, 400, 404, 405
U.S. Recommended Daily Allowances (RDAs), 29, 50, 81, 83, 84, 85, 89, 90–91
U.S. Residue Violation Information System (RVIS), 363
Ulcers, 82, 83
  gastric, 291–292
Ultramarine blue, 305

Vasodilation, 260
Vegetables, 3–4
  cooked vs. raw, 111–112, 129–130
Vegetarianism, 22–23, 48–49, 223, 237, 304
Vinegar, 309
Vitamin A, 89, 108, 123, 124, 128, 196, 235
Vitamin B complex, 235, 359
Vitamin B_1, 86–87, 124, 236, 280
Vitamin B_2, 87, 98–99, 128, 247, 299–300
Vitamin B_3. *See* Niacin.
Vitamin B_6, 78, 79, 80, 85–86, 100, 301
Vitamin B_{12}, 80, 82–84, 96, 100, 129, 133, 237, 281
Vitamin C, 79, 87, 101–102, 124, 128, 129, 131–132, 159, 233–234, 235, 236, 280
Vitamin D, 80, 89, 106–108, 124, 127, 146, 196, 235, 247
Vitamin E, 88, 102–106, 124, 125, 130, 132, 159, 196, 235, 310
Vitamin K, 77–78, 79, 80, 125, 126, 128, 196, 237
Vitamins, 233–237
  labeling, 235
Waste, recycled, 388–398
Water, 76, 93, 137–140, 156, 157, 387
  contaminated, 315, 332–333, 370–371
Weight, control and loss, 136–137, 184–187, 195–196, 219, 220, 229
Whey, 159, 164, 389
Wine, 279, 281–282

Xanthophyll, 299

Yogurt, 74, 309
  bifido-supplemented, 358, 359–360

Z-Trim, 202–204
Zantac, 83
Zinc, 51, 60, 90, 92, 125, 130, 219

About The Author

Beatrice Trum Hunter has written numerous books and articles on food and environmental issues. She has brought to public attention many subjects before general awareness with *The Natural Foods Cookbook* (Simon and Schuster, 1961), *Gardening Without Poisons* (Houghton Mifflin, 1964), and *The Mirage of Safety: Food Additives and Public Policy* (Charles Scribners' Sons, 1975). As food editor of *Consumers' Research Magazine,* Hunter continues to explore cutting-edge issues. She is an honorary member of the American Academy of Environmental Medicine, and has been the recipient of numerous awards, including the President's Award, bestowed by the National Nutritional Foods Association in 2001.

www.ingramcontent.com/pod-product-compliance
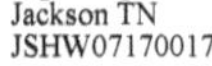
Lightning Source LLC
Jackson TN
JSHW071700170426
101040JS00022B/433